The Occupational Therapy Manager

Edited by Jeanette Bair and Madelaine Gray

The American Occupational Therapy Association, Inc.
Rockville, Maryland

Library of Congress Cataloging-in-Publication Data
Main entry under title:

The Occupational Therapy Manager.

Includes bibliographies and index.
1. Occupational therapy services – Administration.
I. Bair, Jeanette. I. Gray, Madelaine.
RM 735.6.025 1985 615.8'5152'068 85-22934
ISBN 0-910317-20-8

ISBN 0-910317-20-8

Table of Contents

Foreword

The *Manual on Administration* has for many years been a mainstay in the professional library of the occupational therapist. Its content has provided guidelines for practitioners whose vision has included moving into management positions, and it has been an up-to-date information resource with a fresh outlook for those already well established in management positions. The *Manual* has been germane to the therapist working in various settings, from the acute care hospital, to the community mental health center, to private practice.

This new text on management is an expanded version of the *Manual on Administration*. It includes all of the previous areas of interest, but necessarily goes beyond that content. Developments in technology, changes in the health care delivery system, expanding roles of therapists in traditional settings, new ventures into nontraditional settings, and the emphasis on cost containment, productivity, reduced length of stay, and accountability have added new dimensions to the ways in which occupational therapy personnel conduct their professional lives.

Although these changes have been pervasive, they have not altered occupational therapists' and occupational therapy assistants' commitment to provide the highest level of quality care in each individual intervention. Providing this level of care requires the services of highly skilled professional practitioners. It also calls for competent managers who foster a work environment in which occupational therapists and occupational therapy assistants can function effectively and creatively without unnecessary administrative encumbrances that stifle initiative and ingenuity.

This new text addresses all of the essential elements of a management system. It also recognizes the need for occupational therapy personnel to be knowledgeable about their organization, to appreciate its nuances, to be alert to trends that portend change, and to accept changes as opportunities for further growth and development.

The text provides a compendium of information critical to the effective performance of today's and tomorrow's occupational therapy manager. It succinctly describes the evolution of the health care system; the role of strategic planning in forecasting and planning for change; financial planning and budgeting; systems theory and practice; payment for services; facilities planning; ethics and professional liability; and many more core subject areas.

The chapter authors were selected because of their competence and experience in the particular subject area they address. I commend these individuals for their contribution to a text that will be state-of-the-art for years to come. I recommend this publication not only as a mainstay in a professional library, but as an effective manager's handy desk reference for everyday activities.

James J. Garibaldi
Executive Director
The American Occupational Therapy Association

Acknowledgments

Many people participated in the conceptual development, the selection of content and authors, and the review of manuscripts for this new management text. We particularly appreciate the contributions of the members of the Advisory Committee who assisted us through this complex process:

Carolyn Manville Baum, MA, OTR, FAOTA
Paul Ellsworth, MPH, OTR, FAOTA
Tina S. Olson, OTR, FAOTA
Ruth Ann Watkins, MBA, OTR, FAOTA

Other important contributors who provided publishing expertise were Anita DeVivo, the former Director of The American Occupational Therapy Association's Division of Publications, and Patricia Carpenter, former Managing Editor of *The American Journal of Occupational Therapy*. Special thanks are due Margo Johnson, who provided invaluable assistance in the day-to-day coordination of the project and in the developmental editing of the manuscripts.

Jeanette Bair, MBA, OTR, FAOTA
Madelaine S. Gray, MPA, OTR, FAOTA
Editors

Section I

Introduction

Recent data indicate that a growing percent of occupational therapists are assuming positions in management and administration. Curricula in occupational therapy, however, focus on training clinicians. The treatment of management in these curricula is usually a one-term course. *The Occupational Therapy Manager,* a completely revised version of the *Manual on Administration,* is designed to strengthen and supplement that treatment with a comprehensive introduction to management in occupational therapy. It is also intended to be a guide for new, inexperienced managers, explaining the basics of management and pointing them in directions for further study.

The Occupational Therapy Manager is organized into eight sections. The opening chapter, "The Evolution of the U.S. Health Care System," constitutes Section I and is introduced here. Separate introductions appear at the beginning of Sections II–VIII. Section I/Chapter 1 describes the broader context in which occupational therapy organizations operate. There is discussion of the part that social, economic, and political forces have played, particularly as they are represented in the federal government. The chapter also examines how the health care system has changed in recent years, from the hospital-based and physician-centered medical model to a still-developing vertical system of care that is more diversified and provided in a variety of settings. The dramatic growth in the occupational therapy profession during the 1970s is noted, and trends in the distribution of personnel are described. Finally, the chapter looks at the directions in which health care and the field of occupational therapy within it seem to be headed.

The six sections that follow focus on the six primary roles of managers: planning, organizing, directing, controlling, evaluating, and communicating. Each section is made up of one or more chapters that discuss the managerial functions encompassed in a role and relate them to the practice of occupational therapy. The chapters address both the concepts that underlie the functions and the skills that embody them. In other words, there is an attempt to balance discussion of theory and application. The concluding section covers major issues and processes that affect the practice of occupational therapy. Subjects include payment for services, regulation and accreditation of organizations, certification and licensure of practitioners, ethics, and professional liability.

The combined term *patient/client* is used throughout the book in preference to *patient* or *client* alone. In some instances, however, the context has clearly called for one of these terms alone. For example, the summary of Medicare provisions in Chapter 18 is rendered relative to *patients* because the Medicare law and regulations use that term.

Chapter 1

The Evolution of the U.S. Health Care System

Carolyn Manville Baum, MA, OTR, FAOTA

Evolution—The process of developing or working out in detail what is potentially contained in an idea or principle; the development of a design (1, p 91).

Health—The general condition of the body with respect to the efficient discharge of function (1, p 1273).

Care—To feel concern, to be concerned, to provide for (1, p 399).

System—A set or assemblage of things connected, associated or interdependent as to form a complex unity; a whole composed of parts in orderly arrangement according to some scheme or plans (1, p 3213).

It would be reasonable to assume from this terminology that the United States has designed and implemented a complex of organizations and professionals that delivers to individuals services designed to ensure that they can continue to function efficiently. This would be the stated goal of nearly all components of the health care industry: direct care, administration, research, construction, medical equipment, pharmaceuticals,

Carolyn Manville Baum currently teaches a course in occupational therapy issues and history at Washington University in St. Louis, Missouri. She has been an occupational therapy department head for 18 years and holds an advanced degree in health facilities management.

insurance, and public health care financing. The implementation of this goal is very complex.

Because of rising costs, the lack of services to meet specific needs, an imbalance of services for different populations of the society, and advances in medical technology, the health care industry has become the object of scrutiny by the government as well as the public. The public expects accessible and affordable health care and views it as a right in the same category with education, police protection, and fire protection. The latter are public services supported by a general tax base and offered by public servants. Health care monies, on the other hand, are generated by industry, third-party payers, government subsidies, private fund-raising, and individuals. Moreover, providers of care are independent, licensed practitioners.

In the past the health care system was described in terms of the extent and characteristics of health problems in the United States. The tenor of discussions has changed. Health problems today are cast in economic terms. Health care costs have risen from $41.9 billion in 1965 to over $400 billion in 1984. Currently the federal government's share of the health care bill is nearly $150 billion a year. Table 1 and Figure 1 provide details.

Occupational therapy has been a part of this system since the early 1900s. Occupational therapy personnel are affected by its vulnerabilities as well as its strengths. This chapter explores different aspects of the system now and in the future.

TABLE 1–1
National Health Expenditures, 1965–1983*

		National Health Expenditures								
		Total			Private Funds			Governmental Funds		
	Gross National Product (billions)	Amount (billions)	Per Capita	Percent of GNP	Amount (billions)	Per Capita	Percent of Total	Amount (billions)	Per Capita	Percent of Total
1983	$3,304.8	$355.4	$1,459	10.8	$206.6	$848	58.1	$148.8	$611	41.9
1982	3,069.2	322.3	1,337	10.5	186.5	774	57.9	135.8	564	42.1
1981	2,957.8	285.8	1,197	9.7	164.2	688	57.4	121.7	510	42.6
1980	2,631.7	248.0	1,049	9.4	142.2	601	57.3	105.8	448	42.7
1979	2,417.8	215.1	920	8.9	124.2	531	57.7	90.9	389	42.3
1978	2,163.9	190.0	822	8.8	110.1	476	57.9	79.9	346	42.1
1977	1,918.3	170.2	743	8.9	100.1	437	58.8	70.1	306	41.2
1976	1,718.0	150.8	665	8.8	87.9	388	58.3	62.8	277	41.7
1975	1,549.2	132.7	590	8.6	76.3	340	57.5	56.4	251	42.5
1974	1,434.2	116.3	522	8.1	68.8	309	59.1	47.6	214	40.9
1973	1,326.4	103.4	468	7.8	64.0	290	61.9	39.4	178	38.1
1972	1,185.9	93.9	429	7.9	58.5	268	62.3	35.4	162	37.7
1971	1,077.6	83.5	386	7.7	51.8	239	62.1	31.7	146	37.9
1970	992.7	75.0	350	7.6	47.2	221	63.0	27.8	130	37.0
1969	944.0	65.6	310	7.0	40.7	192	62.0	24.9	118	38.0
1968	873.4	58.2	278	6.7	36.1	172	62.0	22.1	105	38.0
1967	799.6	51.5	248	6.4	32.5	157	63.2	19.0	91	36.8
1966	756.0	46.3	225	6.1	32.7	159	70.7	13.6	66	29.3
1965	691.0	41.9	207	6.1	30.9	152	73.8	11.0	54	26.2

*Amount and per capita amount by source of funds and percent of the gross national product

Note: Per capita amounts are based on July 1 Social Security Area population estimates, which include the resident U.S. population and that of the outlying territories, plus federal military and civilian employees and their dependents overseas, plus an estimate of the census undercount.

FIGURE 1–1
The National Health Dollar, 1983: Where It Came From

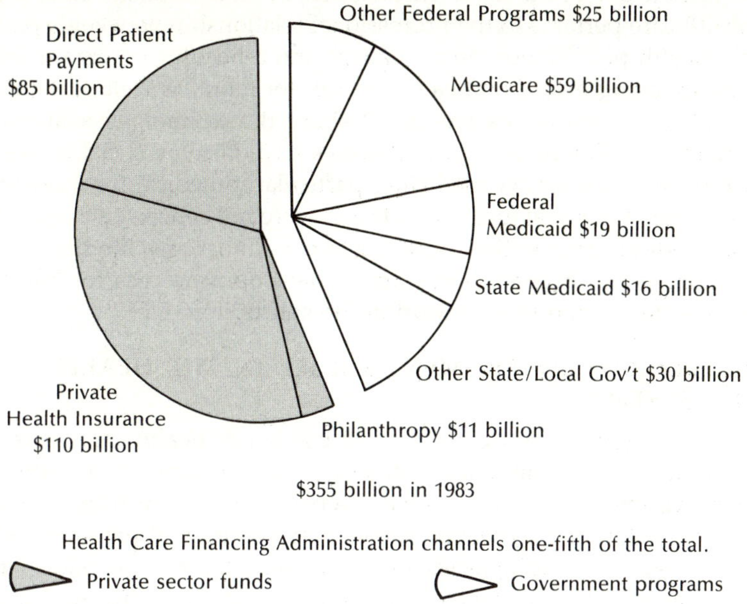

THE RIGHT-TO-HEALTH CONCEPT

The basis for much of the government's involvement in health care is the concept of the right to health. This concept was referred to in the *Congressional Record* as early as 1796. During the nineteenth and twentieth centuries it has reappeared at many points. It came to full attention in Franklin Roosevelt's Economic Bill of Rights in 1944 (2). The early meaning implied a guarantee of protection to all citizens, regardless of economic or social status, from certain health hazards. Shortly after the turn of the century the concept took on a noncomprehensive meaning. The federal government has intermittently broadened and narrowed its definition. When Roosevelt used the phrase, "The right to adequate needed care and the opportunity to achieve and enjoy good health," he was equating it with the most fundamental social and political right guaranteed to every citizen.

Very few political leaders would publicly declare that they do not support health care as a right. However, health care rights are debated daily as the system struggles to obtain a balanced budget (2). Most people would like health care to be a right. Not all people understand their responsibilities to protect that right. It is almost impossible to define the right to, as opposed to the responsibility for, a healthful status. Variation exists in government support of some known preventive measures and practices. Because of the high cost of human life and health care, state legislatures are beginning to impose stiff penalties for driving without seat belts and driving while intoxicated. Eventually, very heavy taxes may be placed on cigarettes and alcohol to support the cost of health care.

Related to the right-to-health concept is the matter of ethics, which may become one of the most critical issues in modern health care. Ethics in health care pertains to the professional relationship between a patient and a health practitioner, and a patient and a health care organization. Limits are being placed on health services for moral as well as economic reasons, as ethical issues are raised about the technology available to maintain and prolong life. Ethical issues have become social issues because of the potential of medicine, particularly medical technology, to perform functions that just a decade ago were not conceived as possible. Some medical intervention now exists for almost any life-threatening condition. It has become necessary to develop a process for handling ethical issues. Often they end up in the courts.

THE FEDERAL GOVERNMENT'S ROLE IN THE HEALTH CARE SYSTEM

The federal government pays over 40 percent of health care costs. On the grounds of economy, accountability, and consumer protection, this public investment demands a public acceptance of responsibility for health services. Historically, however, the federal government has been locked into the role of providing assistance, not control. Since the mid-1940s it has made many significant contributions to the evolving health care system. To offer a perspective on the cost and delivery of health services, major historical events are summarized in the following sections.

Construction of Health Care Facilities

Little hospital construction occurred during the depression and World War II. In 1944 the American Hospital Association and the U. S. Public Health Service organized a commission on hospital care to determine the need for hospital facilities. The work of this commission was reflected in the Hospital Survey and Construction Act of 1946, Title VI of the Public Health Service Act. Popularly known as the Hill-Burton Act, this legislation assisted the states in determining their need for hospitals and other health care facilities. Also, it provided grants to states for construction projects. Over the next two decades the Hill-Burton Act was extended and amended frequently. In the process its programs were expanded to cover diagnostic and treatment centers, chronic disease hospitals, rehabilitation facilities, and nursing homes. In 1964 and again in 1970, funds were earmarked for modernization of facilities (3).

The Hill-Burton Act was greatly modified in the National Health Planning and Resources Development Act of 1974. This legislation was especially critical in modernizing health care facilities. Many of the facilities built between 1946 and 1974 were struggling to survive, and that struggle was having a major impact on the total cost of health care. By the mid-1960s new facilities were operational, but too few health professionals were available to staff them. Also, some health facilities were obsolete, requiring nearly $20 billion a year for modernization. Construction costs of facilities increased from $470 million in 1968 to $712 million in 1971.

By the early 1970s the federal government began to recognize the need for systems to control and establish meaningful plans for future construction.

Human Resources Legislation

Since the mid-1950s the federal government has had an important role in financing human resources for health. Its first peacetime legislation to support training of health care's human resources was the Health Amendments Act of 1956, benefiting public health personnel and professional and practical nurses. In 1958, Congress established a program of formula grants to schools of public health. This was soon followed by a program of project grants for these and other schools training public health personnel (3).

The first construction grants for teaching facilities came in 1963, in the Health Professions Education Assistance Act. Schools of medicine, dentistry, pharmacy, podiatry, nursing, and public health were the eligible recipients. This act also made student loan funds available in medicine, osteopathy, and dentistry. The Nurse Training Act in 1964 provided separate funds for nursing school construction, set aside funds to expand nurse training programs, and established nursing student loan programs. Grants to improve the quality of schools of medicine, dentistry, osteopathy, optometry, and podiatry were authorized by the Health Professions Assistance Amendments of 1965. The amendments also made scholarship funds available to those schools and schools of pharmacy (3).

The first federal funds for support of occupational therapy education came in 1966, with the Allied Health Professions Personnel Training Act. This legislation authorized the award of construction and improvement grants to training centers for allied health professions. It also made advanced traineeships available to allied health professionals (3). The Health Manpower Act of 1968 extended most of the programs for health and allied health professionals, including those for occupational therapy training.

Legislation supporting training in various ways continued into the 1970s (e.g., the Health Training Improvement Act of 1970, the Comprehensive Health Manpower Training Act of 1971, and the Nurse Training Act of 1975). In 1970, however, the federal government began to limit monies for traineeships.

Health Planning

By the early 1970s the government was acutely aware of the need to control costs. Several pieces of major legislation addressed that need. A 1972 amendment to the Social Security Act created Professional Standards Review Organizations. Under this scheme, associations of physicians in a geographic area reviewed professionals' activities and institutions' services to monitor and control both cost and quality (3). The law made it possible for hospital utilization review committees to be given the responsibility of carrying out these functions. Also in 1972, Congress introduced a system of limiting the amount of reimbursements under Medicare for routine services.

Two years later came the National Health Planning and Resources Development Act, intended to ensure the development of both a national health policy and effective state and area programs of health planning and resource allocation. Under the provisions of this act each state is divided into health service areas, and health systems agencies are designated to administer them. The purposes of the agencies are as follows (3):

1. To improve the health of area residents
2. To increase the accessibility, acceptability, continuity, and quality of health services
3. To restrain costs and to prevent duplication of health services.

In 1982 came the Tax Equity and Fiscal Responsibility Act, which, among other provisions, extended the 1972 limits on reimbursements under Medicare to cover ancillary and rehabilitation services. Occupational therapy services are included under this provision.

In April 1983, President Reagan signed the Social Security Amendments (Public Law 98-21) into law, supporting a congressional mandate to alter the way in which health care was subsidized and delivered. The intent of the legislation is to impose further constraints on the level of federal spending for Medicare beneficiaries, particularly for inpatient hospital care. The law basically changes the formula for disbursing health care monies. For decades health care has been a hospital-based delivery system. On the basis of a financial formula, the payer (the federal government, an insurance company, or an individual) has reimbursed hospitals for the cost of the services that were provided. So if the services were provided, the cost of those services was paid. Under the Prospective Payment System introduced by Public Law 98-21, the Health Care Financing Administration is directed to establish a nationwide schedule defining the payment to be made for each inpatient stay by a Medicare beneficiary. The level of payment per case is determined by 470 descriptive categories called Diagnosis Related Groups (DRGs).

The introduction of the Prospective Payment System will have a profound effect on the development of the health industry. It will reduce emphasis on inpatient services and expand outpatient and community programs. It should support a greater role for rehabilitation services in the delivery of medical care. A fuller discussion of the implications of this system occurs later in this chapter.

HUMAN RESOURCES

The health care industry is labor intensive. Delivering health care requires a large number of personnel. As Table 2 indicates, there are well over two hundred occupations in health care, including many professions. New ones seem to appear continually, because of new technology and advances in procedures that require additional specialized skills.

ORGANIZATIONS PROVIDING CARE

When people think of the hospital today, they relate to a sophisticated facility providing technically advanced procedures to support life and a healthful status. Hospitals, though conceived many years ago, were not

(*continued on page 12*)

TABLE 1–2
List of Health Care Occupations

Field	Primary Title
Administration of Health Services	Assistant nursing home administrator
	Assistant hospital administrator
	Clinic manager
	Health administrative assistant
	(Health agency) administrator
	(Health agency) program representative
	Health care facility surveyor
	Health officer
	Health planner
	Health program analyst
	Health program representative
	Health systems analyst
	Hospital administrator
	Nursing home administrator
Anthropology and Sociology	Anthropologist
	Sociologist
Automatic Data Processing	Computer operator
	Computer programmer
	Systems analyst
Basic Sciences in the Health Field	Scientist
	Anatomist
	Biologist
	Botanist
	Chemist
	Ecologist
	Entomologist
	Epidemiologist
	Geneticist
	Hydrologist
	Immunologist
	Meteorologist
	Microbiologist
	Oceanographer
	Pharmacologist
	Physicist
	Physiologist
	Pathologist
	Zoologist
Biomedical Engineering	Biomedical engineer
	Biomedical engineering aide
	Biomedical engineering technician
	Biomedical engineering technologist
Chiropractic	Chiropractor
Clinical Laboratory Services	Clinical laboratory assistant
	Clinical laboratory director
	Clinical laboratory scientist
	Clinical laboratory technician
	Clinical laboratory technologist
	Specialist in blood bank technology

(continued on next page)

Dentistry and Allied Services	Dental assistant Dentist Dental hygienist Dental laboratory technician
Dietetic and Nutritional Services	Dietetic assistant Dietetic clerical worker Dietetic technician Dietitian Food service worker Nutritionist
Economic Research in the Health Field	Health Economist
Environmental Sanitation	Environmental health aide Environmental health technician Sanitarian
Food and Drug Protective Services	Food and drug chemist Food and drug microbiologist Food technician Food technologist Health inspector
Funeral Directors and Embalmers	Embalmer Funeral directors
Health and Vital Statistics	Health demographer Health statistician Statistical assistant Vital record registrar
Health Education	Health educator
Health Information and Communication	Biomedical photographer Draftsman Health information specialist Illustrator Medical illustrator Medical writer Poster and display artist Science writer Technical writer
Library Services in the Health Field	Medical librarian Medical library assistant Patients' librarian
Medical Records	Medical record administrator Medical record clerk Medical record technician
Medicine and Osteopathy	Physician
Midwifery	Lay-midwife Nurse-midwife
Nursing and Related Services	Attendant Nursing aide Orderly Home health aide Licensed practical nurse Licensed vocational nurse Registered nurse

Occupational Therapy	Occupational therapist Occupational therapy aide Occupational therapy assistant
Opticianry	Dispensing optician Ophthalmic laboratory technician
Optometry	Optometric aide Optometric assistant Optometric technician Optometrist
Orthotic and Prosthetic Technology	Orthotic-prosthetic assistant Orthotic-prosthetic technician Orthotist Prosthetist
Pharmacy	Pharmacist Pharmacy aide Pharmacy assistant Pharmacy technician
Physical Therapy	Physical therapist Physical therapist aide Physical therapist assistant
Physician Extenders	Nurse practitioner Orthop(a)edic physician('s) assistant Physician extender Physician('s) assistant Surgeon('s) assistant Urologic(al) physician's assistant
Podiatric Medicine	Podiatric assistant Podiatrist
Psychology	Psychologist
Radiologic Technology	Nuclear medicine technician Nuclear medicine technologist Radiation therapy technician Radiation therapy technologist Radiologic technician Radiologic technologist
Respiratory Therapy	Respiratory therapist Respiratory therapy aide Respiratory therapy technician
Secretarial and Office Services	Dentist's office assistant Dental receptionist Dental secretary Optometrist's office assistant Optometric receptionist Physician's office assistant Medical receptionist Medical secretary
Social Work	Social work aide Social work assistant Social work technician Social worker

(continued on next page)

Specialized Rehabilitation Services	Corrective therapist Corrective therapy aide Educational therapist Home economist in rehabilitation Manual arts therapist Manual arts therapist assistant Music therapist Therapeutic recreation aide Therapeutic recreation specialist Therapeutic recreation technician
Speech Pathology and Audiology	Audiologist Speech pathologist
Veterinary Medicine	Animal technician Veterinarian
Vocational Rehabilitation Counseling	Rehabilitation counselor aide Vocational rehabilitation counselor
Miscellaneous Health Services	Acupuncturist Cardiopulmonary technician Community health aide Electrocardiograph technician Electroencephalograph technician Electroencephalograph technologist Emergency medical systems manager Emergency medical systems planner Emergency medical technician Extracorporeal circulation specialist Medical assistant Operating room technician Ophthalmic medical assistant Orthotist

Note: From *Health Resources Statistics: Health Manpower and Health Facilities*, 1976–77 edition. U.S. Department of Health, Education and Welfare, Public Health Service, Office of Health Research, Statistics, and Technology, National Center of Health Statistics, 1979, pp. 447–458.

medically oriented until after the turn of the century. Initially they were facilities for the socially unfit, and the majority of health care was delivered at home.

From the early 1900s until the early 1970s, most health care was provided and delivered in one of two facilities—the physician's office and the hospital. Nursing homes were mostly for custodial management, and today's concept of home health care was in its early development.

Modern health care organizations are the result of scientific developments and changes in society. Hospitals have become essential to the proper care of many of the population's health problems. Other facilities are now becoming basic to providing health services to U. S. citizens (4). The system includes government, for-profit, and nonprofit facilities (see Table 3).

TABLE 1–3
Types of Health Care Organizations

Type of Organization	General Description
Federal government	Hospitals serving the armed forces Hospitals serving disabled veterans Public Health Service hospitals and clinics (includes a leprosarium) Indian Health Service
State government	Hospitals for the mentally ill State medical school hospitals and clinics Infirmaries associated with prisons and reformatories
Local government	County hospitals and public health clinics City hospitals and clinics Rehabilitation facilities
Nonprofit	Religious hospitals Charity hospitals Industrial hospitals Community hospitals Private teaching hospitals Specialty hospitals Surgical centers Home health facilities Wellness centers
For-profit	Ownership by individuals or groups for the care of their own patients/clients Investor-owned facilities (hospitals, laboratories, nursing homes, surgical centers, rehabilitation facilities, and home health facilities), including corporations and management corporations

Note: Information drawn in part from FA Wilson, D Neuhauser, *Health Services in the United States*, 2nd edition. Cambridge, MA: Ballinger Publishing Co, 1982, pp 7–18.

Multi-Institutional Systems

In a changing society and economy the freestanding hospital became vulnerable. This has led to the formation of larger health care systems in which individual facilities are linked and represent only one of several related corporate activities. The phenomenon is evident in the public sector as well as the private. In the 1970s and 1980s many types of multi-institutional systems have developed with distinct ownership and governance. They have six features in common:

1. Strong financial and organizational management.
2. A well-developed market strategy.
3. Built-in referral strategies to keep their use high.
4. A broad geographical approach.
5. An expansive service delivery model, from primary to restorative care, including home health services, ambulatory services, and skilled nursing facilities.

6. Shared services for purchasing, billing, maintenance, and marketing.

The trend toward large corporate systems taking over facilities with fewer than one hundred beds will probably continue. For-profit hospital systems will become larger through this multisystem concept. It is widely estimated that by the turn of the century 50 percent of all health care organizations will be owned by for-profit corporations and the majority of the remaining ones will be linked as multihospital systems.

Health Maintenance Organizations

Another notable development of recent years is the proliferation of health maintenance organizations (HMOs), prepaid health care plans offering comprehensive medical services to their members (Chapter 18 provides more detail). HMOs contribute significantly to lower health care costs because they provide services at little or no charge above a fixed subscription fee that members pay. Prepaid health care plans have been around since the early 1900s. They began to multiply in 1973 when the federal government, faced with spiraling health costs, passed the Health Maintenance Organization Act to foster this alternative through loans and grants. In 1971 there were thirty-nine HMOs. Today there are nearly four hundred operational ones. They serve over sixteen million people, twice the number enrolled six years ago. The Congressional Budget Office estimates that HMO enrollments will reach forty-seven million by 1990 (5).

PUBLIC HEALTH

Not all health care services are provided through the medical-industrial complex. The American Public Health Association is in its second century of service to the nation. Its activities have included and continue to be the following (6):

1. Standardization of methods (laboratory and field).
2. Control of communicable diseases.
3. Housing and health criteria.
4. Appraisal of health programs.
5. Standards for professional education.

Public health is primarily concerned with preventing disease through public programs, but increasingly it is having to provide medical care to individual patients. The prevention activities are mostly government-supported services at the federal, state, and local levels, among them, air pollution control, accident prevention, occupational medicine, occupational safety, control of sewage, solid waste disposal, clean water supplies, fluoridation of water, and neighborhood health centers.

It is in programs like the latter that the public health system has begun to administer individual care. Despite the prevalence of health insurance coverage, studies have estimated that up to twenty-three million Americans, or nearly 13 percent of the population, lack it. Among the uninsured are persons of all ages, incomes, geographic settings, races, and ethnic groups. The lack of coverage is most prevalent in certain groups—those with low income, the unemployed, those on workers' compensation disability, and racial and ethnic minorities (7). More and more, these people are going to neighborhood health centers for treatment as well as for the preventive measures such as immunizations that the centers were established to provide. For occupational therapy personnel the public health system represents a very critical link in followup with patients/clients who do not use the private health system because of their location or inability to pay.

The U. S. Public Health Service is the oldest agency of the U. S. Department of Health and Human Services, established by Congress in 1798 as the Merchant Marine Hospital Service. In 1930 the Public Health Service's Hygienic Laboratory, a research program created in 1887, was renamed the National Institute (now Institutes) of Health, and under its aegis a collection of specialty institutes has been established over the years. In 1935 the Public Health Service's budget was increased to strengthen state and local public health departments. The Public Health Service Act of 1944 brought all statutes and legislation concerning public health together. In 1946 the Communicable Disease Center, now the Centers for Disease Control, was established (3). The Office of the Surgeon General is also a part of the Public Health Service.

The Public Health Service is responsible for a number of specific programs of great interest to occupational therapy personnel. These are presented in Table 4.

THE EVOLUTION OF OCCUPATIONAL THERAPY

Only recently have historians of occupational therapy begun to document the evolution of its theories and its concepts of occupation. Historical perspectives on the profession can be studied in the works of Hopkins and Smith (8) and Reed (9). These offer an important complement to the contemporary picture of occupational therapy and should be studied in concert with this chapter.

Trends in the supply and distribution of professional personnel offer another perspective. The report of the American Occupational Therapy Association's Ad Hoc Commission on Occupational Therapy Manpower (10) provides a current and comprehensive description of the factors and forces affecting the profession's human resources. In regard to supply, the profession swelled by forty-one thousand between 1970 and 1984, "more than entered the profession in all its previous years combined" (10, p 17). During the 1970s the growth rate was 9 percent to 10 percent per year. In the mid-1980s, however, that annual rate has slowed to 5 percent. The apparent explanation for the slowdown is a stabilization of output from occupational therapy education programs.

The dramatic increase in supply, however, has not kept pace with the demand for occupational therapy personnel. Shortages of personnel are not uniformly distributed geographically or across practice settings. Geographically the greatest need for both registered occupational therapists (OTRs) and certified occupational therapy assistants (COTAs) is in the Southeast. COTAs alone are in short supply in the West. By practice setting, needs "will be particularly acute in long term care, in school systems through the early to mid 1990's, and in the newly developing alternative financing/service delivery systems [e.g., HMOs, outpatient

TABLE 1–4
Public Health Service Programs

Institute/Program	Orientation
National Institute on Alcohol Abuse and Alcoholism	Administers programs directed at the problems of alcohol abuse
National Institute on Drug Abuse	Administers programs directed at the problems of drug abuse
National Institute of Mental Health	Administers programs of research, service development, and training in mental health
Center for Health Promotion and Education	Develops health promotion and health education materials
Center for Professional Development and Training	Develops materials for professionals in the area of health promotion
National Institute for Occupational Safety and Health	Develops and maintains a safe and healthy work environment
Bureau of Medical Services	Is responsible for the safety of medical devices
Bureau of Health Professions, Division of Associated and Dental Health Professions	Designates shortages of human resources for health
	Studies distribution of human resources
	Supports education and training of human resources for health
Bureau of Health Planning	Administers programs for area health planning
National Institutes of Health	Maintain National Library of Medicine
	Carry out and support programs of basic and clinical research
National Center for Health Services Research	Conducts and supports reviews of illness, disability, and health service obligation
	Surveys patient/client use of hospitals
	Surveys nursing homes, their residents and staff
	Maintains the master facilities inventory of all U. S. inpatient facilities
National Center on Health Care Technology	Administers studies and evaluations of technological developments in health.

Note: Information quoted or paraphrased from FA Wilson, D Neuhauser, *Health Services in the United States*, 2nd edition, Cambridge, MA: Ballinger Publishing Co, 1982, pp 137–159.

work-related programs, and life skills training]. Needs will also accelerate in home health'' (10, p 6).

The growth in the number of occupational therapy personnel has been accompanied by some changes in the distribution of practitioners across practice settings. Table 5 presents data on the number and percent of

TABLE 1–5
Primary Employment Settings of OTRs and COTAs, in Percents, 1973, 1977, and 1982

OTRs

Setting	**1973**	**1977**	**1982**
College, two-year	1.4	1.2	0.8
College/university, four-year	5.6	4.9	4.1
Community health program	0.7	0.8	—
Community mental health center	4.2	4.3	2.4
Correctional institution	0.2	0.2	0.1
Daycare center	1.4	1.1	1.0
Easter Seal center	—	1.7	—
Health maintenance organization	0.3	0.2	0.2
Home health agency	0.9	2.2	3.8
Hospice	—	—	0.0
General hospital	20.5	19.8	25.3
Pediatric hospital	2.1	2.0	1.6
Psychiatric hospital	13.8	11.2	7.4
Other specialty hospital	2.3	1.2	—
Independent living center	—	—	0.2
Outpatient clinic (freestanding)	—	—	2.5
Private industry	—	—	0.7
Private practice	1.3	2.1	3.5
Public health agency	1.6	1.5	0.8
Regional medical program	0.3	0.3	—
Rehabilitation center	13.4	10.9	—
Rehabilitation hospital	—	—	8.9
Research facility	0.3	0.3	0.4
Residential care facility	—	4.4	4.0
School system (includes private school)	11.0	14.0	18.3
Sheltered workshop	0.7	0.7	0.7
Skilled nursing home/intermediate care facility	6.2	7.9	6.0
Voluntary agency (e.g., Easter Seal, United Cerebral Palsy)	—	—	1.7
Other	10.9	7.1	5.4
Total responses	99.8	100.0	99.8

COTAs

Setting	**1973**	**1977**	**1982**
College, two-year	0.8	0.9	0.6
College/univerity, four-year	0.7	0.6	0.9
Community health program	0.3	0.6	—
Community mental health center	4.0	3.5	3.1
Correctional institution	0.3	0.2	0.1
Daycare center	1.2	2.4	2.0
Easter Seal center	—	0.4	—
Health maintenance organization	0.7	0.3	0.3
Home health agency	0.2	0.4	0.8
Hospice	—	—	—
General hospital	15.1	12.7	17.8
Pediatric hospital	1.5	1.2	0.8
Psychiatric hospital	22.6	14.3	9.7

(continued on next page)

COTAs

Setting	1973	1977	1982
Other specialty hospital	1.5	1.6	—
Independent living center	—	—	0.5
Outpatient clinic (freestanding)	—	—	1.7
Private industry	—	—	1.0
Private practice	0.3	0.4	1.2
Public health agency	0.5	0.5	0.3
Regional medical program	0.4	0.4	—
Rehabilitation center	9.5	11.0	—
Rehabilitation hospital	—	—	8.4
Research facility	0.2	0.3	0.1
Residential care facility	—	8.5	7.1
School system (includes private school)	3.6	6.2	11.3
Sheltered workshop	1.4	0.9	1.9
Skilled nursing home/intermediate care facility	22.8	26.1	22.5
Voluntary agency (e.g., Easter Seal, United Cerebral Palsy)	—	—	1.2
Other	12.5	6.7	6.7
Total responses	100.1	100.1	100.0

Note: From American Occupational Therapy Association, Member Services: *Member Data Surveys*. Rockville, MD: American Occupational Therapy Association, Member Services, 1982.

OTRs and COTAs in various employment settings in 1973, 1977, and 1982. Data were not available before 1973, and no data have been collected since the initiation of the Prospective Payment System.

The data on OTRs reveal the following:

- Moderate to major increases in the percent in home health agencies, general hospitals, private practice, and school systems.
- The very beginnings of OTRs in independent living centers and private industry.
- No change in the percent in HMOs.
- Moderate decreases in the percent in community mental health programs and centers, psychiatric hospitals, and public health agencies.

In the next three to five years some dramatic changes should be evident in the percent of OTRs practicing in the community, home health, the HMO, and industry, as the vertical system of health care (see the later section of this chapter on The Changing Roles of Hospitals) is more fully operationalized.

With regard to COTAs, increases over the ten years represented in Table 5 occurred in home health agencies, general hospitals, private practice, and school systems. In 1982, COTAs were beginning to practice in independent living centers, outpatient clinics, and private industry. During the next three to five years there should be an even greater growth in the percent of COTAs in community-oriented programs. It will be important to track changes in the distribution of both COTAs and OTRs as a measure of occupational therapy's ability to relate to the changing health care system.

SUMMARY OF THE CURRENT HEALTH CARE SYSTEM

By tracing the federal government's role in the evolution of health care, the current situation can be seen in perspective:

- The government built the facilities.
- The government provided the human resources.
- The government is paying over 40 percent of the bills.
- The government supports research.
- The government has been unsuccessful in controlling costs.
- The government is responsible for providing care when individuals do not have access to health insurance.

The health care system faces these problems:

- Too many physicians.
- Too many hospital beds.
- Too many professionals competing for limited dollars.
- Too few rehabilitation professionals.
- More people with chronic conditions.
- An increase in the size of the elderly population.
- Medical technology sustaining and supporting life.

The health care system is at a crossroads. The public and private sectors must deal with these problems. The public is demanding action. The question is, Where do we go from here?

THE FUTURE

Following are some projections of the outcomes of current trends and some opinions about roles and opportunities for occupational therapy personnel relative to them. Through its Strategic Integrated Management System, the AOTA issues an Environmental Impact Statement (11) that can give the occupational therapy manager and clinician a sense of the health care environment for strategic planning purposes. The statement is updated as environmental changes dictate. At any given time the current statement can be a valuable adjunct to this chapter.

Economics

Economists are having more and more influence on the delivery of health care. They believe that the constant threat of competition and the daily struggle to protect one's program may bring out the best in the provider. The health care industry has adopted the concepts and practices basic to competition, and the government is stimulating competition to control costs. This means that successful programs will flourish and those not able to keep pace in the marketplace will fail. More mergers will occur as multi-institutional systems are established, and a much larger emphasis will be placed on HMOs. A competitive market can be described as a social arrangement whereby life is made difficult for providers so that consumers can have access to reasonably priced services.

Some economists feel that cost effectiveness will be observed only if consumers themselves have a direct financial stake in health care. "Co-payment," which is being considered in developing legislation, would require consumers to pay a portion of the costs out of pocket. If this occurs, it will be very important to keep the occupational therapy product defined in such a way that the consumer as well as the third-party payer will be eager to purchase it.

Recognition for Occupational Therapy in Health Care

The strategy in a competitive environment is to streamline efforts and direct them to doing the best job possible. For occupational therapy personnel, this means helping patients acquire the skills they need to function at their maximum level and return to a degree of independence with a choice of acceptable options in performing everyday activities. What occupational therapy does must be very visible and easily marketable. Its services will have to be described as products—for example, Driving Program, Work Evaluation, Seating and Mobility Clinic, and Life Skills Program. These labels will make the services easier to understand and will assist purchasers in understanding the results of the services.

Society is demanding accountability for its dollars. What occupational therapy personnel offer to the health care system is gaining increased recognition for several reasons:

1. The public is more accepting of individuals with disabling conditions.
2. Chronic disease affects nearly 20 percent of the American public.
3. Head trauma has become a social problem, and head trauma rehabilitation requires occupational therapy intervention.
4. The population is aging. Programs are needed to maintain the independence of the elderly and decrease the costs of the long-term management of their health.
5. The change to the Prospective Payment System has raised the consciousness of all providers to the fact that some people do not fit within the norm for care and that society has a responsibility to them.

The Changing Roles of Hospitals

For years it has been known that there are alternative, less costly methods for delivering health care services. Hospitals have been reluctant to support these systems because under the former payment structure, they were paid for services to patients who were hospitalized. The set fees under the Prospective Payment System now make it economically advantageous for hospitals to move patients/clients with long-term problems out of acute care beds and into another type of health care setting as quickly as feasible. Thus, hospitals are organizing in a vertical system as illustrated in Figure 2.

This organization serves the hospital well. Patients can be readmitted for necessary procedures. They and their families sense that the hospital is reaching out to meet their needs. Most important to the hospital is the ability to keep patients in its market by placing them in affiliated systems.

A very skillful economic strategy has created the greatest opportunity

FIGURE 1–2
The Vertical System of Health Care

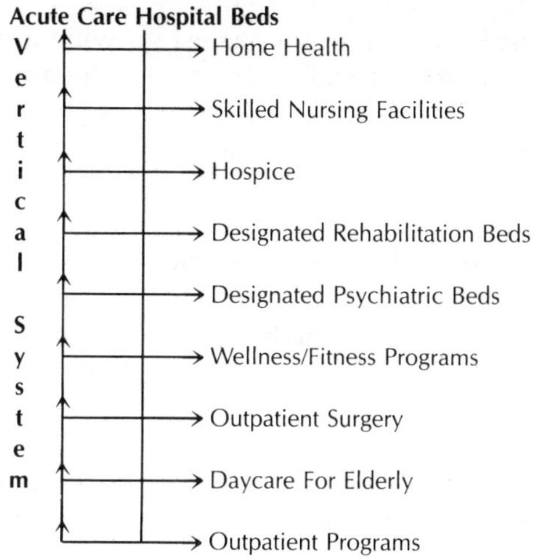

in history for rehabilitation. Nearly every one of a hospital's vertical programs requires the rehabilitation profession's skills to be effective. The challenge to the profession is to provide the human resources to staff the programs. Should occupational therapy not have the personnel, other professionals will expand their roles to fulfill the needs.

Introducing Rehabilitation Services into HMOs

It is important for the HMO to have a good price and a quality service oriented to wellness and low costs. Occupational therapy is one of the rehabilitation services that can be offered in an HMO. Physicians, nurse practitioners, and social workers in HMOs should be oriented to the rehabilitation field's capacity to help them save money as well as promote health. HMO staff should be familiarized with occupational therapy services, such as developmental screenings, patient/client education, arthritis programs, work capacity, hand-related services, and particularly the use of assessments of performance dysfunction as a screening tool. Some HMOs require home health rehabilitation services. Many are eager to develop contractual relationships for a full scope of rehabilitation services. A rehabilitation organization can develop a business arrangement with an HMO to receive a set amount per month per HMO enrollee.

Additional Payment Sources

In the past, rehabilitation organizations and professionals expected their payment from medical insurance. This will continue to be true for chronic medical problems causing disability. However, other disabling conditions are the result of work-related, home, and automobile accidents, which are covered by liability insurance. The insurance industry has recognized the cost-benefit potential of comprehensive models of rehabilitation that help the individual acquire skills to function at a community level and become employed. This recognition gives impetus to occupational therapy personnel to provide their services in systems other than acute care hospitals.

Occupational health is one of the fastest-growing areas of medicine. It will be very important to provide occupational therapy services directly to industry, not only to rehabilitate injured workers but also to assist the industry in organizing and designing the workplace to prevent costly accidents and illnesses.

To control services and costs, the insurance industry is setting up its own rehabilitation programs to manage catastrophic conditions such as head injury and spinal cord injury. Within ten years the major rehabilitation organizations will either be linked contractually to the insurance industry or replaced by facilities managed directly by the insurer.

Competition

With an oversupply of physicians, nurses, and allied health personnel in general, and a government-stimulated competitive environment, there will be more advertising, further expansion of community-based programs (especially by hospitals), and a greater emphasis on cost. Cost will be the determining factor in whether or not services are obtained.

Medicare's shift to the Prospective Payment System has laid the groundwork for all third parties to move into the prospective payment mode. This orientation has major implications for hospital-based care and is having a profound effect on when and where rehabilitation services are delivered. Quality will be assumed, and organizations will seek bids from service providers. It will be very important to develop programs that are cost-effective using qualified but less costly personnel. Certified occupational therapy assistants will play an important role in delivering a cost-effective service. Where possible, aides should be trained for support treatment.

Cost Containment

The competitive market plan guarantees that costs will continue to be the topic of debate in health care delivery. The question will be asked, What can be expected from this expenditure? To provide information on the importance of their services, occupational therapy personnel must integrate quality assurance concepts into daily activities and document program effectiveness. The approach that must be taken to contain costs is the employment of standard and reliable measures to show functional changes in the performance of patients. Mere generalizations about performance will not demonstrate the necessity for services.

Application of Technology

Medical technological changes will alter the roles of occupational therapy personnel in rehabilitation. Likely decreases in stroke, heart disease, and cancer will change the rehabilitation case mix.

Technology also makes it possible to explore other options of patient/client management. The rehabilitation field is just beginning to benefit from major technological advances. As yet, the technology is expensive because of development costs. In the next decade there will be greater acceptance of computer applications, of environmental adaptations, and perhaps of implanted computers to control motions and bodily functions. Occupational therapy personnel must stay informed about and be involved in research on linking technology to human performance. Over the years their roles have evolved; the potential for even greater change is imminent.

OPPORTUNITY

This is a very important time for occupational therapy. The system demands the profession's expertise; the opportunities exceed its current supply of human resources. With the establishment of designated rehabilitation and psychiatric hospitals, the expansion of home health organizations, the increased role of skilled nursing facilities as rehabilitation settings for the elderly, the establishment of comprehensive outpatient rehabilitation facilities, and employers' emphasis on returning the injured person to gainful employment, occupational therapy personnel are in demand. Health care organizations need the profession's services to increase and maintain their market. The profession must respond with the confidence that the people it serves are being given the opportunity to gain meaningful lives. The situation is not unlike when the founders of occupational therapy sought to bring a humanness and a new morality to a system that did not place an acceptable level of effort on supporting human potential.

Occupational therapy's development has not been easy. Participating in the growth and evolution of an organized, complex system never is. The profession is now ready to assume a responsible role in lending support and direction to that system as it struggles to be effective. It is critical that occupational therapy personnel understand why assuming this role is difficult, and know that with specific knowledge and skills, and a strong commitment to what the profession's contribution can be, patients and society as a whole will benefit.

SUMMARY

Because of rising costs, the lack of services to meet specific needs, an imbalance of services for different populations of the society, and advances in medical technology, the health care industry has become the object of scrutiny by the government and the public. In the past the health care system was described in terms of health problems. Today, economic terms prevail. Annual health care costs are over $400 billion, and the federal government's share of the expense is nearly $150 billion.

The basis for much of the government's involvement in health care is the concept of the right to health, which has been present in political thought at least since 1796. Related to this concept is the matter of ethics. Ethical issues have become social issues because of medicine's potential to maintain and prolong life.

The federal government has made many significant contributions to health care since the mid-1940s through support of the construction of facilities, the training of personnel, and the planning of health systems. By the early 1970s it was acutely aware of the need to control costs, and several pieces of major legislation followed. The most recent of these introduced a new system of payment for hospital services to Medicare beneficiaries, which is expected to have profound effects on the health care field.

The health care industry is labor intensive. The field now supports well over two hundred occupations, and new ones are appearing continually. Organizations providing care have also diversified greatly. The freestanding hospital has become vulnerable, and larger health care systems have formed, linking different types of health care facilities. Another notable development of recent years is the health maintenance organization, a prepaid health care plan that began to proliferate in the mid-1970s and is expected to flourish on into the 1990s.

Not all health care services are provided through the medical-industrial complex. Public health is primarily concerned with preventing disease through public programs such as air pollution control, occupational safety, and neighborhood health centers. Increasingly, though, it is having to provide medical care to individual patients/clients because many Americans lack health insurance and are turning to the public health system for the care they need.

Occupational therapy has been a part of the health care system since the early 1900s. Writings on the evolution of its theories and its concepts of occupation provide an important complement to the contemporary picture of the profession. Current trends in the supply and distribution of professional personnel indicate that, building on its dramatic growth during the 1970s, the profession continues to expand, though more slowly. The growth has not kept pace with demand, however. Shortages are evident in certain geographic areas and practice settings. In the last ten years some movement toward employment in community-based settings, schools, home health, HMOs, and private industry has been evident, and this should continue at least for the next three to five years.

For the near future at least, competition will prevail. The strategy in such an environment is to streamline efforts and direct them to doing the best job possible. For occupational therapy personnel, this means helping patients/clients acquire the skills they need to function at the maximum level and return to a degree of independence. What occupational therapy does must be very visible and very marketable.

The new Medicare payment system now makes it economically advantageous for hospitals to move patients/clients out of acute care beds and into another type of health care setting as quickly as feasible. Thus, hospitals are organizing into a vertical system of care. This creates the greatest opportunity for rehabilitation in history. Nearly every one of a hospital's vertical programs requires the rehabilitation profession's skills. Opportunities for occupational therapy personnel will exist as well in health maintenance organizations and industry.

In the competitive environment of tomorrow, cost will be the determining factor in whether services are obtained. It will be very important to develop cost-effective programs using qualified but less costly personnel. It will also be important for occupational therapy personnel to document program effectiveness using standard and reliable measures of patient/client performance.

This is a very significant time for occupational therapy. The profession must respond with the confidence that the people it serves are being given the opportunity to gain meaningful lives. The profession is now ready to assume a responsible role in lending support and direction to the struggling health care system.

References

1. *The Compact Edition of the Oxford English Dictionary*. Oxford, England: Oxford University Press, 1979
2. Chapman B, Talmedge JT: The evolution of the right to health concept in the United States. *The Pharos*, January 1971, pp 30–51
3. Wilson FA, Neuhauser D: *Health Services in the United States*, 2nd edition. Cambridge, MA: Ballinger Publishing Co, 1982, pp 194–196, 200–205
4. Shepp CG: Trends in hospital care. In *Multi-Hospital Systems: Strategies for Organization and Management*, M Brown, B McCool, Editors. Rockville, MD: Aspen Systems Corp, 1980, pp 3–9
5. *HMO Fact Sheet*. U. S. Department of Health and Human Services, Public Health Service, Office of Health Maintenance Organizations, April 1985
6. Wolman A: APHA in its first century. *Am J Public Health* 63(4):319–321; April 1973
7. Lundy JP, Skevant AC: *Issue Brief: Health Insurance Proposals in the 98th Congress*. Library of Congress, Congressional Research Service, Education and Public Welfare Division, 1984
8. Hopkins HL, Smith HD: *Willard and Spackman's Occupational Therapy*, 6th edition. Philadelphia: JB Lippincott Co Inc, 1983
9. Reed KL: *Models of Practice in Occupational Therapy*. Baltimore: Williams & Wilkins Co, 1984
10. American Occupational Therapy Association, Ad Hoc Commission on Occupational Therapy Manpower: *Occupational Therapy Manpower: A Plan for Progress*. Rockville, MD: American Occupational Therapy Association, 1985
11. American Occupational Therapy Association, Strategic Integrated Management System: *Environmental Impact Statement*. Rockville, MD: American Occupational Therapy Association, Strategic Integrated Management System, 1983–1984

Additional Resources

Alford RR: *Health Care Politics: Ideological and Interest Groups—Barriers to Reform*. Chicago: University of Chicago Press, 1975

Drucker PF: *Managing in Turbulent Times*. New York: Harper & Row Publishers Inc, 1980

Ginzberg E: *The Limits of Health Reform: The Search for Realism*. New York: Basic Books Inc, 1977

Greenberg W, Editor: *Competition in the Health Care System*. Rockville, MD: Aspen Systems Corp, 1984

Greenberg, W, Southby RM: *Health Care Institutions in Flux*. Arlington, VA: Information Resource Press, 1984

Johnson EA, Johnson RL: *Hospitals in Transition*. Rockville, MD: Aspen Systems Corp, 1984

Kropf R, Greenberg JA: *Strategic Analysis for Hospital Management*. Rockville, MD: Aspen Systems Corp, 1984

Mechanic D: *Future Issues in Health Care: Social Policy and the Rationing of Medical Services*. New York: Free Press, 1979

Reinhardt UE: Table manners at the health care feast. *National Journal*, May 9, 1981, pp 855–861

Section II

Planning

Section II, "Planning," consists of five chapters: "Strategic Planning," "Program Planning," "Facility Planning," "Financial Management," and "Marketing." All treat some aspect of the primary function of planning—setting goals and objectives. As a concept and as a process, strategic planning (Chapter 2) provides the bridge from the broad health care context of Chapter 1/Section I to the narrower context of the occupational therapy organization, taken up in Sections II–VII. The chapter explains a five-step process that will help occupational therapy managers keep their organization abreast of social, economic, political, and technological trends. Forms for monitoring issues and analyzing their implications, examples of plans to deal with selected issues, and other practical illustrations keep the narrative oriented toward applications.

Chapter 3, "Program Planning," discusses the building blocks of occupational therapy organizations. It explains a thorough process of program development, from the conception of a program idea to its implementation. Accompanying figures illustrate key documents in program planning—the proposal, the statement of scope, and the budget.

Chapter 4, "Facility Planning," deals with the physical environment of the occupational therapy organization, leading a manager through the several phases and the many steps of designing and constructing facilities to house a variety of services and programs. Alternative methodologies for assessing space needs are presented and described, and several figures and tables are included to help a manager visualize work flow and plan the efficient use of space.

Chapter 5, "Financial Management," explains the developments that have made this function so important in health care today and describes its major components: financial accounting, financial management, and budgeting. The multitude of concepts, principles, procedures, and financial statements associated with financial management are explained, and the terms used in them are defined. The chapter also describes and compares cost finding and cost accounting, two helpful tools of financial management.

Five marketing concepts—product, price, place, promotion, and position—and four marketing processes—organizational assessment, environmental assessment, market analysis, and communications—are the subject of Chapter 6. The chapter contrasts the traditional mission-oriented planning cycle of health care organizations with a market-based planning scheme that examines mission in light of the wants and the needs of consumers. Marketing's close relationships to strategic planning and community relations are explained.

Chapter 2

Strategic Planning

Patricia C. Ostrow, MA, OTR, FAOTA

The lessons of the business world can be applied profitably to management of a service-oriented program such as occupational therapy to help it thrive in the new, competitive health care environment. One of these lessons is the need for strategic planning based on systematic thinking and commitment of resources to actions. If the subject seems too foreign, it is well to remember that occupational therapy personnel already have the required skills in problem solving. Patient care requires analytical thinking, decisions regarding ameliorating action, and evaluation of that action. Those same skills are basic to strategic planning. This business-world skill called strategic planning can be useful to occupational therapy managers and a natural extension of their abilities. With it, occupational therapy personnel can ensure the availability of their services to patients/clients who would benefit from them.

THE VALUE OF STRATEGIC PLANNING

"Whatever failures I have known, whatever errors I have committed, whatever follies I have witnessed in public and private life, have been because of action without thought." That comment, attributed to Bernard Baruch, reflects a general belief that quick intuitive responses should be balanced with reflection. Yet fast, incisive behavior is frequently more powerful and effective than slow, carefully planned reactions. How can

---

Since 1982, Patricia C. Ostrow has served as the coordinator of strategic planning for AOTA, along with her duties as director of the Quality Assurance Division. She has given numerous speeches and seminars on strategic planning, and, as a member of the World Future Society and the Issue Management Association, has attended over 100 hours of conference programs on the subject.

appropriate responses to complex and crucial issues be met promptly, yet with full consideration of all the ramifications of the problem? One answer is strategic planning. It provides a springboard for systematic thinking that launches creative and intuitive ideas. Strategic planning allows one to look ahead, anticipate problems, and plan alternative responses. It facilitates thoughtful and timely decisions, and provides the analytic backdrop for quick intuitive responses when they are necessary.

This is an era of transition, a time when fast-paced change is the norm. People, the government, the economy, and technology, as well as the natural environment, are all changing within themselves and in relation to one another. An organization—be it an occupational therapy department, a fire department, a hospital, or an auto manufacturer—needs a way to anticipate and adapt to changes in its environment. Strategic planning offers this opportunity.

When difficult risk-taking decisions face a manager, they may be postponed. Strategic planning is a system that facilitates risk-taking decisions, by sustaining the systematic thinking to choose rationally between a variety of risk-taking courses of action. Many strategic planning systems use structured group decision processes to choose objectives, to generate alternative action plans, and to select one that considers the future impact of present decisions (1).

Strategic planning not only fosters the decisions crucial to survival of the enterprise; it integrates the actions that support them. Results of the actions are evaluated and revised as needed. Strategic planning coordinates time, money, people, and other resources with integrated actions. Projects are monitored and revised on the basis of results. Rigorous staff discussion about goals, plans, and resource allocations occur during strategic planning. This intensified communication supports integrated actions by staff that sustain overall strategies. *Without* strategic planning, short-term budgetary pressure may overshadow strategic goals. *With* strategic planning, strategic goals are formally included in the budgeting process, thus integrating immediate and longer-range objectives.

DEFINITION OF TERMS

Although a full description of the strategic planning process is presented later, it is well to begin by defining terms. A *plan* is a blueprint for arranging, realizing, or achieving something. A *strategic plan* pertains to goals that are essential, basic, or critical to the existence of an organization. For example, sending a fleet across the Atlantic in peace time may require elaborate plans and programs, yet a strategic plan is not needed unless another nation opposes the fleet's progress. The word *strategy* is historically related to military command, so that one meets the enemy under conditions advantageous to one's own force. The strengths and weaknesses of both sides and the opportunities and risks within the environment must be analyzed. A strategic plan for an enterprise, then, is a careful design for achieving a result relative to a crucial issue, based on an analysis of the positive and negative forces in a situation (2).

The term *strategic planning* has a variety of nuances in management literature. George Steiner (3), a professor of management at the University of California, Los Angeles, equates strategic planning with long-range planning, integrated planning, and comprehensive overall planning. He defines strategic planning further by stipulating that it must anticipate the opportunities and threats that lie in the future and deal with the possible ramifications for the future of decisions made today. He emphasizes that strategic planning is a continuous process, from setting overall organizational aims and defining strategies and detailed operational plans to achieve them, to assessing the impact of actions and revising the operation in light of the feedback. Steiner states that strategic planning is also a philosophy that dedicates one to action on the basis of systematic surveys of the future; it is a system that links strategic plans, mid-range programs, short-range budgets, and operating plans (3).

On the other hand, Peter Drucker (4), a New York University professor of management, warns,

> The skill we need is not long-range planning. It is strategic decision-making, or perhaps strategic planning. General Electric calls this work "strategic business planning" . . . the work starts with the question, "What is our present business?" Indeed, it starts with the questions, "Which of our present businesses should we abandon? Which should we play down? What should we push and supply new resources to?" (p 122)

With this example Drucker seems to be cautioning his readers that strategic planning should focus on essentials such as the nature and viability of the primary mission. He goes on, urging readers to make the crucial risk-taking decisions: "It is necessary in strategic planning to *start* separately with all three questions. What *is* the business? What *will* it be? What *should* it be? These are separate conceptual approaches. With respect to 'What *should* the business be?' the first assumption must be that it will be different" (4, pp 122–123).

John Naisbitt (5), a well-known futurist, gives a few examples of how some major corporations have answered these strategic business questions. Singer Sewing Company pinpointed its role of providing the machinery for women to create clothing and other cloth items at home by asking, What *is* our business? Undoubtedly aware of the impact on sales from women's return to the work force (What *will* our business be?), Singer redefined itself as an aerospace company. The skills of its personnel in designing and creating precision machinery were applied to aerospace systems as well as to sewing machines. Similarly, Sears, which is a retailer, has expanded into banking (5).

Drucker (4) reminds readers that strategic planning is not just forecasting, because attempts to anticipate probable futures are fraught with problems. In fact, strategic planning that seeks to create a trend, an innovation, or an event that will change the future, is in his view preferable to strategic planning that just adapts to the future. Singer and Sears made strategic decisions that changed their futures. Drucker's warning that forecasting is not strategic planning is valuable. It is too easy to become totally focused on data-based speculations about the future and overlook or avoid the difficult action decisions crucial to broader strategic planning (4).

Boris Yavitz (6), a professor in the Graduate School of Business at

Columbia University, notes that strategic planning focuses on basic long-term directions, with a statement of where and how the organization wants to move providing direction for short-term plans and integrating all functional plans into an overall scheme. The strategic plan must be realistic (not pie-in-the-sky), action oriented, and thoroughly understood and accepted by all the senior and middle managers directing the organization (6).

By now it should be clear that all strategic plans have basic ingredients in common, although experts emphasize different elements. These ingredients may occur in a formal, continuous, systematic, data-based process involving participation by many people, or in an informal, intuitive, day-by-day process engaged in by one person. A middle ground between these extremes is recommended in this chapter, so that one can harness the trend data and the participation of a group of people to sustain the best creative and intuitive insight for strategic planning.

James Quinn (7), a professor of management at Dartmouth College, offers a definition of strategy that summarizes the major ideas expressed above and adds his own emphasis:

> A strategy is the *pattern* or *plan* that *integrates* an organization's *major* goals, policies, and action sequences into a *cohesive* whole. A well-formulated strategy helps to *marshall* and *allocate* an organization's resources into a *unique and viable posture* based on its relative *internal competencies and shortcomings*, anticipated *changes in the environment*, and contingent moves by *intelligent opponents* (p 7).

Quinn (7) notes that an enterprise may have a strategy that is not verbalized but is a widely held understanding, perhaps not apparent to the players themselves, that results in a stream of decisions. This true strategy, which may disagree with the formal strategy, must be addressed if the strategic posture of the organization is to be understood or changed.

Finally, rounding out this search for the most useful definition of strategic planning, Drucker's (4) is a comprehensive guide: "It is the continuous process of making entrepreneurial (*risk-taking*) *decisions* systematically with the greatest knowledge of their futurity; organizing systematically the *efforts* needed to carry out the decisions; and measuring the results of the decisions against expectations through organized *systematic feedback*" (p 125).

THE PROCESS OF STRATEGIC PLANNING

There is no single process of strategic planning. In the reference list accompanying this chapter, entire books are listed that address the strategic planning process. Those books, in turn, have excellent references within them. The purpose of this chapter is to introduce the subject of strategic planning and to provide the reader with a simple strategic planning system that has been tested and refined. The five-step process described in this chapter reflects the basic steps in any problem resolution: (a) identification of the issues, (b) analysis of the issues, (c) decision making regarding the strategic goals and plans, (d) implementation of the plan, and (e) evaluation of the results (followed by a return to step *c* if the results do not meet expectations or achieve goals).

Organizing for strategic planning need not be complex. Full participation is advantageous because going through the process is as beneficial as the plan itself in bringing everyone to a common understanding of issues, objectives, and actions. For this reason, appropriate participation of all levels of the occupational therapy department is encouraged.

A strategic planning committee is frequently used. Some committees have a few rotating members to bring in various viewpoints. Some form of input to the committee from all staff is advisable.

It is very important that significant leaders support the planning process, or it will be seriously hampered. Therefore, the power structure of the enterprise must be recognized in the strategic planning structure.

One person should be responsible for sustaining and coordinating planning. The occupational therapy manager may assume the planner's role or delegate it to some other significant leader of the team. If the latter is the case, the manager must stay fully identified with the planning process for it to succeed.

The method of introducing planning to the staff is as crucial as the structure. To some, a formal planning system may seem to lessen their own power and autonomy, so the way in which participative planning can enhance their initiatives must be fully explained and demonstrated. Planning should be introduced gradually, with steps added over time. It is crucial to allow enough time for the strategic planning committee to meet, and to be sure the group is not too tired when it meets. A consultant can, in many instances, assist the department with the first two- to four-hour meeting. He or she can also describe the process and help the group identify trends and issues.

Step 1: Identification of the Issues

As noted earlier, Drucker's (4) definition of strategic planning has three main characteristics: risk-taking decisions, systematic effort, and systematic feedback. A process to accomplish these is described in the following paragraphs.

The process begins with the selection of those trends relevant to occupational therapy services. According to Naisbitt (5), the most reliable way to understand the future is to understand the present. Therefore, entrepreneurial decisions—the setting of strategic goals based on Drucker's three questions—should be based on a review of the external and internal environments. One can start with a systematic evaluation of the social, political, technological, and economic environment in which the occupational therapy department exists. There are various ways to do this. Many futurists have written books and articles analyzing current trends and predicting their impact. Newsletters and magazines that focus on the identification of trends are available: *The Bellwether Report*, *John Naisbitt's Trend Letter*, *Health Care Strategic Management*, *The Futurist*, and *The Kiplinger Washington Letter* (8–12). The trend newsletters identify all megatrends, so health care often gets short shrift. When health care is considered, the focus is on trends that affect hospitals and physicians. The strategic planning committee will need to extrapolate the implications for occupational therapy. For example, the trend toward corporate medicine is often discussed, but there is no analysis of its effect on occupational therapy.

It is important to note that futurists fall into different schools of thought. There are pessimistic and optimistic futurists, as well as those in the middle of the road (13). For example, *Future Shock* and *Limits to Growth* point out the pollution, population, and nuclear arms problems that are accelerating exponentially (14,15). On the other hand, *Doomsday Has Been Canceled* and *Critical Path* emphasize that crisis precedes transformation (16, 17). They argue that society has great potential and that the current period of flux has inherent opportunities for remarkable advances.

Between these extremes are those who advance a variety of possibilities and choose a middle road, such as Hawkin and others (18) in *Seven Tomorrows* and Bezold (19) in his survey of four alternative futures for health care. Abstracts of recent futuristic works are available from the World Future Society in an annual publication called *Future Survey Annual* (20). The section on health yields many valuable references.

Other than books, newsletters, and magazine articles written by futurists, it is useful to monitor census reports and newspapers for data relevant to health care. One of the best ways to monitor the present is to select high-impact health journals, such as the *Journal of the American Medical Association*, the *New England Journal of Medicine*, and *Hospitals* (21–23). Monitoring several leading health care journals can yield such valuable reports as Tarlov's "Increasing Supply of Physicians" in the *New England Journal of Medicine* (24), Naisbitt's and Elkins's "Hospital and Mega-trends" in *The Hospital Forum* (25), and Relman's "Future of Medical Practice" in *Health Affairs* (26). These reports contain ideas that may be *emerging trends*, which are of particular value because they are easier to influence. Identification of a significant emerging trend buys one time to carefully plan optional responses to it. Publications that reflect trends in the profession, the community, and the state, as well as in the nation, should be monitored.

For the occupational therapy department that wishes to monitor for trends systematically and continuously, the following system is recommended. The strategic planning committee should make a list of journals and newspapers that it wants to monitor and let members volunteer to assume responsibility for screening one or two. When a member discovers an article of interest, he or she should send a copy of it, accompanied by one or two sentences stating what trend or issue it reflects, to the person who chairs the strategic planning committee. Figure 1 gives an example of an Issue Report Form.

The articles found by reviewers can be grouped and reviewed by the committee when it meets. Environmental scanning is described in more detail by Renfro (27, 28).

The purpose of environmental scanning is to find strategic issues. Asking these questions can help one decide if an issue is strategic:

a. Is it an internal or external development that could affect the organization's performance?
b. Must the organization respond to it in an orderly fashion?
c. Can the organization reasonably expect to exert some influence on it?

FIGURE 2–1
Issue Report Form

Source of Information about the Issue

Periodical ________ Presentation ________

Title ________________________ Book ________ TV/Radio ________

Author ________________________ Conference Proceedings ____ Other ________

Source ________________________ Date ______ Page(s) ____ Vol ____ No. ____

Summary

Rate the importance of this issue by circling one of the following: 5 = High, 4 = Medium-High, 3 = Medium, 2 = Medium-Low, 1 = Low.

Scanner's Comments (Impact on the Profession)

Scanner __________ Location __________ Phone __________ Date __________

Note: Distributed by Lynne Hall at a 1982 Issues Management Seminar. Reprinted, with adaptations, by permission of the author.

Issues have a life cycle that is reflected in the frequency of references to them in the society and its publications. At first there may be only isolated signals in avant-garde publications. Some areas of the country are more apt to consider and test new ideas, such as the indicator states of California, Colorado, Connecticut, Florida, and Washington. [*The Bellwether Report* (8) monitors these states for trends.] As an idea grows it will be found in more publications. Eventually a single event may crystallize the growing sentiment into a full-blown issue.

Knowledge of the life cycle of an issue is a key to strategic planning. An issue's life cycle starts with social expectations. It then becomes a political issue, and legislation and regulations follow. The impact on society is felt as change is enforced. An example is the environmental protection issue. Concern for the environment was of interest to only a few in the fifties. In 1963, Rachel Carson's book, *Silent Spring*, riveted attention on environmental pollution (29). During the 1968 presidential elections, the environment became an issue. In 1970 and 1972, the Clean Air and Clean Water Acts, respectively, were passed by Congress. In the ensuing years, penalties growing out of litigation were imposed on offenders. General Electric, for example, was fined seven million dollars for polluting the Hudson River in 1976. Earlier cognizance of this issue could have saved the company considerable anguish.

In the same way, social concern for cost-effective, but excellent, health care has grown into a major public issue, as yet unresolved. The Medicare Prospective Payment System is only one current solution. Occupational therapy personnel are wisely considering how they can align themselves with these social goals of decreased health care costs and continued availability of quality service.

Internal monitors to assess concerns within an occupational therapy department are also a necessary part of situation assessment. Interviews, surveys, or brainstorming sessions during meetings can accomplish this. The department's overall values, strengths, and weaknesses should also be assessed. The goals of the department, the projected results of present efforts to meet those goals, and possible gaps in the two should be discussed. Similarly, goals and values of the organization/community in which the department functions should be analyzed.

Issues identified from internal and external monitors should be put in order of priority. The strategic planning committee can decide which are the most important, that is, which are most likely to have a significant impact in one to two years, and which in three to five years.

Also, the committee can assess if the occupational therapy department can have a major influence on the issue. It is likely that only fully developed issues will be identified at first. As noted earlier, emerging issues are easier to affect, but it is also more difficult to know when an emerging issue is going to come to full social attention and result in changed laws, practices, and behaviors. Some emerging issues may deserve continued monitoring, with regular reconsideration; others may require immediate action; still others may need analysis for full consideration of all options. In the beginning, only two to four issues should be put in the last category.

Step 2: Analysis of the Issues

When it is time to study the high-priority issues selected for full planning analysis, a subcommittee might be assigned the task with a date to report back. This mutually agreeable deadline is critical. One *must keep a bias for action*, avoiding at all costs what has been termed analysis paralysis—overly detailed, lengthy, highly structured examination of an issue that impedes action (30). A brief but comprehensive description of the issue will facilitate action planning.

A literature review is an essential starting point for issue analysis. It can be time limited, for even a quick review of recent data or developments relevant to the issue can save considerable time and energy in the forthcoming actions. A strategic plan should be built on the best possible information. This is also the time for a telephone survey of other occupational therapy personnel who may have up-to-date information about an issue. The American Occupational Therapy Association staff, state association presidents, and other department heads may have experience with the issue.

Each issue chosen for analysis (versus the issues put on "monitor only" or "immediate action") should be given a title and described succinctly, and the opportunities and risks associated with it should be enumerated. The major environmental forces that make it an issue now and in the future should be reviewed. The assumptions about the future relative to the issue should be spelled out in writing. Vague assumptions lead to vague plans. Furthermore, with explicit assumptions written down for quick reference, it is easy to recognize when the assumptions change, and then review the plan to see if it needs revision or suspension.

Pinpointing the strengths, weaknesses, and values of the organization relative to the issue is another component of the analysis. With this information the challenges (opportunities and risks) to the organization or the department can be described.

The analysis can be accomplished in a variety of ways. The results of the literature search and telephone survey should be reviewed. From this base of data, a small committee could brainstorm the implications of the issue for the department. One way to do this is to put an issue, with a circle around it, in the center of a large blackboard. As people suggest implications resulting from the issue, they are noted on the board, circled, and linked to the issue with a line. Further events that are likely to occur as a consequence of the first implications can be linked to them until a full picture of the issue's possible impact is accomplished.

An example of the implications wheel is shown in Figure 2. The issue is the pending initiation of Medicare's Prospective Payment System in skilled nursing facilities (SNFs). One possible implication of this is that a limited and specified amount of money would be available to treat a diagnosis. If so, hospitals might open SNFs on their grounds or increase the number of beds in the hospital that can be either SNF or acute care. Either course would make the hospital eligible for all of the reimbursement fees. If that were to occur, occupational therapy personnel would need to be prepared to serve the needs of SNF programs. This example shows only one chain of implications to demonstrate the process. Full discussion could fill the wheel.

A word about forecasting seems pertinent here. Extrapolating trends is the most common forecasting technique. Everyone does it when trying to understand the future. Frequently the assumption is made that changes will continue in the same direction and at the same rate or that things will remain as they are. One should be wary of making these assumptions without full consideration of the confidence levels related to them. A dramatic event can change very stable patterns, and trends do not necessarily continue at present rates. Other forecasting methods, such as scenario building, cross-impact analysis, relevance trees, and Delphi, are explained by Cornish (31) in *The Study of the Future*. They can be used along with trend extrapolation, but they are not necessary for initial strategic planning programs.

With the brainstorming session and the visual wheel showing the possible chain of cause-and-effect relationships, a full picture of the situation can be seen. When all implications are displayed, the group should decide which it thinks are most likely to occur. Next, the group should determine which of the issues with high certainty offer the greatest

FIGURE 2–2
Implications Wheel

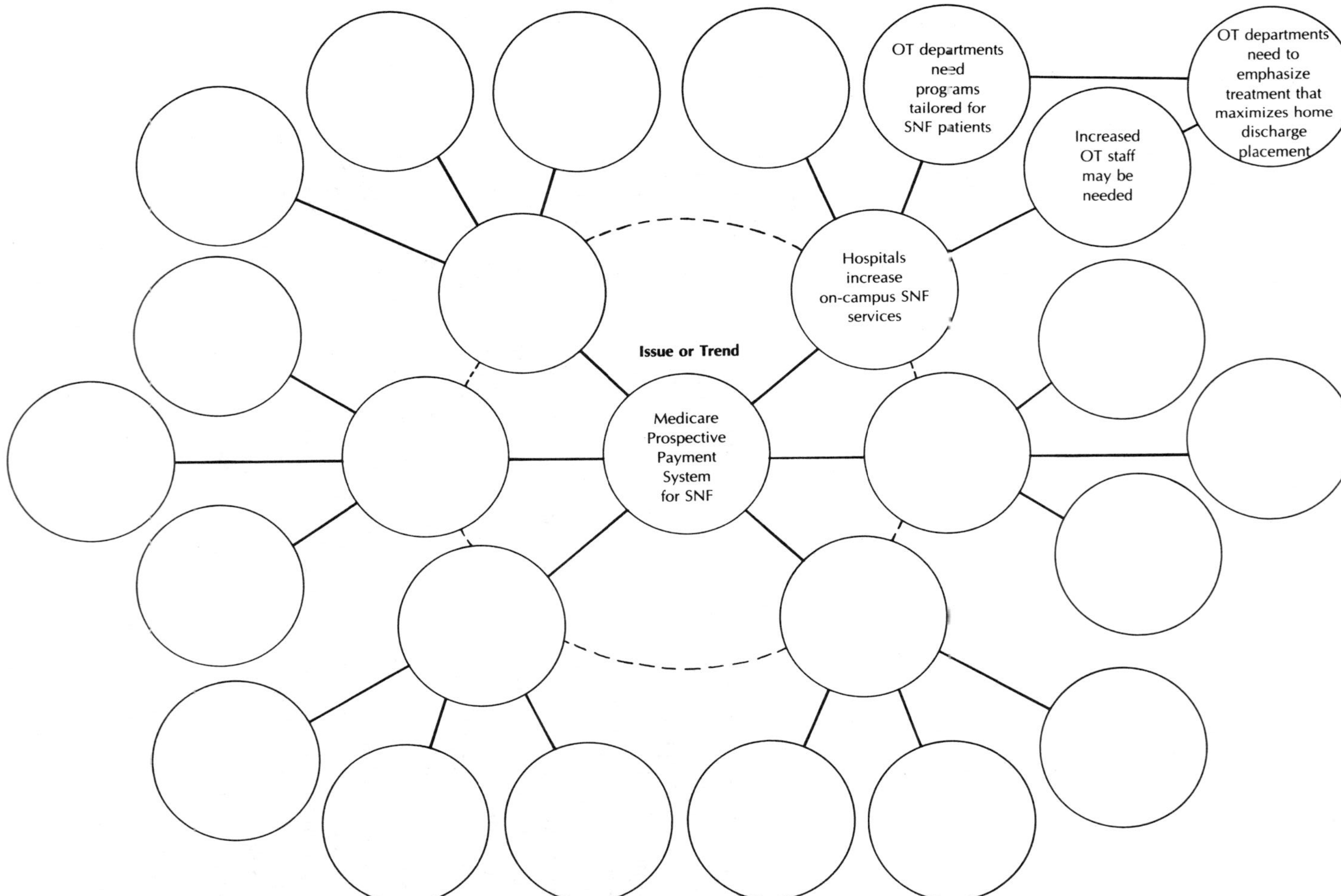

Note: Distributed by Lynne Hall at a 1982 Issues Management Seminar. Reprinted, with adaptations, by permission of the author, Joel Barker, President, Infinity Limited, Inc. St. Paul, MN 55107.

opportunities or risks for the occupational therapy department. Any implications of low certainty and high risk should also be noted. These projected opportunities and threats are included in the written analysis.

An issue that has been carefully analyzed by the American Occupational Therapy Association (AOTA) is related to accountability. Figure 3 shows how input from all segments of AOTA was synthesized in the analysis, which spelled out the opportunities and risks inherent in the issue.

Step 3: Decision Making Regarding the Strategic Plan

With the written analysis of issues and planning challenges in hand, a small committee should brainstorm what strategic action the department could take to reap the opportunities available in the situation and ameliorate the risks. The options for each risk or opportunity might be listed, or a single plan might be proposed. Advantages and disadvantages should then be discussed, considering how the department's strengths, weaknesses, and values create positive or negative forces relative to the plan. Finally, the preferred options should be selected.

When listing possible actions relevant to an issue and its planning challenges, every effort should be made to support creative, fresh ideas.

FIGURE 2–3
Analysis of the Accountability Issue

Issue Title: Demand for both cost and treatment effectiveness and quality care

Issue Definition: Data to demonstrate the beneficial outcomes and efficiency of occupational therapy are called for in response to demands for accountability and cost containment from hospital administrators, consumers, legislators, physicians, and third-party payers.

Strategic Significance:

Opportunities

- The impact of occupational therapy services could be improved by collecting outcome data via quality assurance, program evaluation, and research.
- Professional growth could be enhanced as the feedback of data points out areas for changes in skills, knowledge, or management.
- A strong competitive edge could result for those occupational therapy programs with outcome and cost-effectiveness data.

Risks

- Available occupational therapy services could be underused.
- There could be a loss of quality in care.
- The elimination of services could diminish the accessibility of occupational therapy to patients who need it.

Planning Challenge: To provide resources that help prepare members to meet the new demands for outcome data on benefits and costs, showing how the data can improve the use of occupational therapy.

Note: Adapted from the Strategic Integrated Management System, The American Occupational Therapy Association, Rockville, MD.

The group facilitator can do this in a variety of ways. Brainstorming, nominal group technique, and a process called synectics structure a meeting so that innovation is increased (32–34). At a minimum the facilitator would be wise to break the meeting into two segments: the first to produce a long list of innovative options, and second to assess or refine the options. During the first segment everyone is advised to suspend critical judgment and put forward what he or she wishes would happen, suggesting even radical or unusual ideas. Peters and Waterman (30) quote a senior manager: "Easy communications, the absence of barriers to talking to one another are essential" to the innovative process (p 218). Group members should also try to build on each other's ideas and can ask questions to clarify an idea.

In the second segment of the meeting, the advantages and disadvantages of the options can be discussed. Is the option doable—is there enough time and person power to accomplish it? Is it cost-effective? Will it have a significant impact on the issue? After selecting the best possible options, the committee should plan how to present them to the full strategic planning committee.

The preferred option, that is, the strategic plan, should be selected by the strategic planning committee using the criteria: Is the plan doable and cost-effective? Will it have a significant impact?

When a group is developing a strategic plan, it should be specific about the goal and objectives without bogging down in details. At this point the strategy being discussed is the overall objective—not the specific tactics to accomplish it. The way in which the option is conceived and worded is important. If it is too global and diffuse, or lofty and unattainable, it will not be useful. The strategic plan to "put a man on the moon by the end of a decade" was made in response to Russian breakthroughs in space. That plan was very clear, whereas the statement that "we are going to be a world leader in space exploration" would not have provided enough direction.

Step 4: Implementation of the Plan

After the strategic plan is selected, tactics to implement it must be developed. Implementation is the most common point of failure. Without rigorous care the creep of everyday demands can overwhelm the best-laid plans. This can be avoided by breaking the plan into action steps, setting timetables and responsibilities for each step, and allocating sufficient resources—time, people, and funds—to it. An effective approach is to post the action steps, the timetables, and the names of responsible parties.

The time dimension should be considered carefully. When should the work be started to get results at the appropriate time? With reference to the issue analyzed in Figure 3, if one waits until efficacy data are critical to continued reimbursement and then starts collecting or searching for them, the necessary information will be obtained two years too late.

Systematic and purposeful work on obtaining the objectives must be done. Part of this work Drucker (4) calls "sloughing off yesterday." Resources such as time, people, and funds are usually tied up with routine projects, even though some of these are no longer reaping great benefits. All projects should be reviewed to see how resources may be better spent (4).

One of the most effective ways to keep a plan in action is to break it down into steps that seem pertinent and doable to those responsible for the task. Staff, therefore, must participate in the identification of action steps and assessment of timetables. Figure 4 shows the major projects selected to respond to the opportunities and risks in the accountability issue analyzed in Figure 3. There are many projects in Figure 4 because of the size and scope of the organization that developed them. In a smaller enterprise it would be advisable to select only a few projects—perhaps only one, depending on resources.

Each project can be further analyzed into four or five tasks. The timetables and budgets for them should be prepared by responsible staff to present to the strategic planning committee.

Step 5: Evaluation of the Results

As part of strategic planning, a way to evaluate the impact of the plan is desirable. *Assuming* that action will fulfill the desired results leads to many disappointments. To develop an evaluation process, the strategic planning committee should ask, How will we know when this issue is resolved or improved? For the accountability issue one answer might be,

FIGURE 2–4
Strategic Plan for the Accountability Issue

Issue Title: Demand for both cost and treatment effectiveness and quality care.

Strategic Goal: From both the national and local perspectives, attain and use assessment data about treatment efficacy, cost effectiveness, and quality of occupational therapy services.

Planning Objectives:

1. By 1988, 75% of all fieldwork training centers will involve students in quality assurance and/or program evaluation systems that demonstrate how data on cost and treatment effectiveness are used to improve practice decisions, reimbursement, referrals, etc.
2. By 1986, AOTA will have an ongoing system to collect already-published efficacy data and make it easily accessible to occupational therapy personnel.
3. AOTA will update occupational therapy personnel in effective documentation of patient/client care.
4. By 1988, 75% of occupational therapy academic curricula will teach basic skills and provide experience in the use of program evaluation and/or quality assurance.
5. Treatment modalities will be continuously identified, monitored, and assessed for cost and outcome effectiveness.
6. AOTA will provide human and material resources to the membership to increase the use of program evaluation techniques and quality assurance.
7. Field studies to assess cost and treatment outcomes of occupational therapy services will be conducted.

Note: Adapted from the Strategic Integrated Management System, The American Occupational Therapy Association, Rockville, MD.

when sufficient, up-to-date data on cost and treatment effectiveness have been collected, are available, and have been used successfully by members. How would one measure that? By surveying members, educational programs, state associations, and the American Occupational Therapy Association staff. Have sufficient data been collected and used successfully? Do legislators, third-party payers, and health care administrators need more data? Testing the environment with these questions would assess the impact of the strategic plan and help refine or revise it.

Evaluating the outcomes of every action program undertaken to accomplish a strategic goal may be too time-consuming, but attainment of the goal itself can be assessed. If the action plans are not working, the strategic planning committee should return to Step 3, brainstorm ways to improve the projects, or consider eliminating them and developing new ones.

Evaluation of outcomes is best performed by those responsible for the action. Self-evaluation, where the goal and the measurement of it represent the input and agreement of the individual responsible for the work, contributes to higher morale and motivation. Although strategic planning may take many ideas from war-games theory, it is a suitable idea for a democratic society currently moving away from authoritarian and toward participatory management. In strategic planning, democratic participation is a key to success. Plans made by a select, isolated few tend to be mislaid or waylaid.

STRATEGIC PLANNING PRINCIPLES AND CONCEPTS

Although many of the major principles and concepts of strategic planning have been mentioned in this chapter, a few deserve additional discussion. Two of the guiding ideas offer an interesting counterpoint. One principle is succinctly expressed by Naisbitt (5): "Trends, like horses, are easier to ride in the direction they are going" (pp 88–89). The other guiding principle is, Set trends, don't follow them (4, p 124).

Both of these ideas can be useful. One or the other, or a combination of the two, may be the choice in different situations. In any given environment where change is occurring rapidly, there is greater opportunity to establish a new pattern of behavior, a new "trend." That possibility should be discussed in the planning phase. One could in some instances both ride and set the trend by capturing the energy for change in an evolving system and establishing a new way of doing things. A rider on a runaway horse will not try to bring it immediately to a standstill, but will channel the direction of the charge into safe areas. Similarly, awareness of the needs and beliefs represented in a trend can be the basis for actions that set a new direction.

An example of both riding and setting the trend can be found in recent hospital innovations. Facing the new Medicare Prospective Payment System that curtailed length of stay, hospitals launched many new programs to augment services and make themselves a part of the community, thus increasing the number of patients coming in for care. Advertising hospital services and providing conveniently located, walk-in outpatient clinics were two of the actions taken. These have now become trends.

Another concept, that of discovering emerging trends, should be reemphasized. During the formative stage of an issue, making a positive impact on it is much easier. Those who have followed the legislative process know that suggestions made while legislation is being written meet with greater success than those offered after a law has been enacted. So it is with trends. When new and innovative solutions are needed, suggestions are welcome. Once a system is established, introducing new ideas into it is much harder.

Another important strategic planning principle addresses the relationship between strategic planning and day-to-day decisions. If the strategic plan is not reflected in short-range and mid-range actions and decisions—including budgets and other resource allocations—it will probably never be realized. "Budgets," says Steiner (3), "are integrating methods to translate strategic plans into action. They are guides to action" (p 215). Yavitz (6) concludes, "Allocation of capital hurts or helps strategy implementation. . . . unless resources flow to priority programs, strategy will stagnate" (p 185). All strategic planning specialists agree, the day-to-day decisions about budgets, about time and talent allocation, and about actions determine the success of a strategic plan.

Contingency planning is another concept to consider. In some situations alternative plans of action are desirable. Strategic planning is based on assumptions about the future and predictions about how key actors will behave. Such predictions have degrees of uncertainty. The higher the uncertainty, the greater the need for contingency planning. Contingency plans are also helpful when response time is very short and delay could be ruinous, or when particular conditions are likely, such as rain at an outdoor June wedding. With low uncertainty in the predictions, contingency plans are not necessary. If moderate uncertainty surrounds future expectations, reassessment of progress and reevaluation of the strategy may be necessary to accomplish planning revisions.

When high uncertainty prevails, the strategic plan may progress by zigs and zags, although the goal may remain consistent. Strategic thrusts—actions allowing focused attention on one or two stages of a strategy, with continuous reassessment of the environment—may be the best way to achieve a strategic goal. Sequential moves allow flexibility and modification of the plan as needed. In an environment of very high uncertainty, the strategy may be to concentrate on preparing the enterprise to move swiftly when likely events occur (6).

A strategic plan needs to be controlled. The usual way of controlling efforts is to measure their actual outcomes against a standard (as described in the chapters on program evaluation and quality assurance). In control of strategy, both the target result—the strategic goal—and the predicted result lie in the future. Any corrective action must be taken before results are in hand. Control then requires reviews and updates of predictions based on the latest information about the environment and the progress to date on projects. The latter can be based on actual results compared with expectations. The control system is a steering mechanism, keeping the plan on target and implementing corrective actions in the strategic plan as needed. This process is complicated because the lead time between projects and outcomes may be long, so expectation of short-term results may be unrealistic (6).

A final principle to remember: There are psychological, power-based, and informal relationships crucial to the strategic planning process. They blend with the formal strategic plan described in this chapter. Strategy emerges from formal planning, power-behavioral relationships, internal decisions, and external events flowing together until key people hold a consensus for action. Quinn (7) has called this logical incrementalism. He stresses how organizations probe the future and experiment with incremental (partial) commitments rather than global, total strategies. Logical incrementalism may appear muddled, but carries its own logic (7).

Strategic planning is more than a rational process with special tasks and techniques. It is a social, political, and organizational process. It must be synthesized with the "culture" of the occupational therapy department. Because of this, strategic planning should be introduced in a way that facilitates acceptance in that setting. The stage should be set for it. The process should begin slowly. Major players should be supportive and involved. They must know what strategic planning is and what it will accomplish for them and the department. If they are opposed to it, the effort will never be fully successful. Therefore, the manner in which strategic planning is initiated should be thought out carefully, giving consideration to the organizational culture and political ramifications.

Individuals may have concerns about strategic planning that must be ameliorated. Some may feel they are losing control and autonomy as the planning group considers how to integrate all department programs relevant to strategic goals. Making these points might allay their concerns: (a) There are benefits in sharing creative thinking. (b) Both formal and intuitive planning are needed. (c) The managers responsible for a project will have major input and control. Others in the department may dislike any new tasks or new committee meetings. They may be persuaded to participate by arguments about possible time-saving benefits and satisfactory results of structured group decisions and strategic planning.

EVALUATION OF THE PLANNING SYSTEM

Even as the planning system is being developed, decisions should be made regarding how and when it will be evaluated. A questionnaire for the whole staff to answer anonymously is one possible solution. Questions could address how well (on a scale of 1 to 5) the strategic planning system helped the occupational therapy department develop its basic goals:

- Were future major opportunities recognized?
- Were major risks identified?
- Were department strengths and weaknesses appropriately appraised?
- Did the system clarify priorities?
- Were useful long-range objectives set?
- Did doable program strategies result?

- Did short- and medium-range decisions and actions support strategic plans?
- Was the process effective at sustaining in-depth analysis? Creative thinking?
- Were new ideas welcomed?
- Was the process too complex? Too routine? Too inflexible?
- Did it take an appropriate amount of time?
- Were the staff supportive?
- Did the process improve and facilitate communication throughout the department (7)?

PITFALLS OF STRATEGIC PLANNING

No introduction to strategic planning would be complete without a consideration of the potential hazards of the process. Some form of strategic planning has been practiced by industry for over three decades. There are common pitfalls—taking too much time, generating too much paperwork, bogging down in details, fostering complications in action and communication, forgetting that the purpose of strategic planning is to make better short- and medium-range decisions and actions, using inadequate inputs to planning, expecting too much in the beginning, and expecting plans to be realized without shifting to accommodate to the constantly changing environment.

Steiner (3), wanting to clarify common strategic planning problems, surveyed six hundred companies, both large and small. About a third responded, with 75 percent of the responses coming from strategic planning departments. Fifty typical pitfalls were described. The ten most important ones to avoid were ranked by the respondents:

1. Assuming that planning can be completely delegated to a planner
2. Top managers' spending insufficient time on strategic planning
3. Using unsuitable goals as the basis for strategic planning
4. Involving major personnel inappropriately
5. Not using a manager's contribution to achieving the strategic plan as the basis for evaluating his or her performance
6. Failing to develop a climate congenial to strategic planning
7. Failing to integrate planning into the entire management process
8. Injecting such formality into the system that it becomes inflexible and restrains creativity
9. Top managers' failing to review middle managers' plans
10. Managers' making intuitive decisions that run counter to formal plans (p 294).

With all these problems, what was the degree of satisfaction with the planning system? Seventy-eight percent reported average to very high satisfaction. Fifteen percent had some satisfaction, and nine percent were highly dissatisfied. Those in the latter category reported significant ensnarement in one of the pitfalls. Attention to these common mistakes is essential.

SUMMARY

Strategic planning is based on the assumptions that there are alternative futures; that useful predictions can be made about the alternatives, given a sound picture of present trends; and that people can influence the future that eventually emerges. A skill borrowed from the business world, strategic planning facilitates risk-taking decisions by sustaining the systematic thinking necessary to choose rationally between a variety of actions. Strategic planning not only fosters the decisions crucial to the survival of an enterprise; it integrates the actions that support them. It provides for evaluation and revision, and coordinates time, money, people, and other resources.

A strategic plan is a careful design for achieving a result relative to a crucial issue, based on an analysis of the positive and negative forces in a situation. It asks three basic questions: What is our present business? What will it be? What should it be? There is no single process of strategic planning. Entire books have been written on the subject. This chapter introduces the reader to a simple, five-step system:

1. Identification of the issues. This involves systematic and continuous evaluation of the social, political, technological, and economic environment in which the occupational therapy department exists. The evaluation can be accomplished by scanning books and periodicals that focus on trends, looking for developments that could affect the organization, that it should address in an orderly fashion, and that it can reasonably expect to influence.
2. Analysis of the issues. This should begin with a review of the literature relevant to an issue and a telephone survey of knowledgeable fellow professionals. The opportunities and the risks associated with the issue should be delineated, and the assumptions about the future relative to it should be spelled out in writing. Another component of the analysis is pinpointing the strengths, weaknesses, and values of the organization pertaining to the issue.
3. Decision making regarding the strategic plan. A small committee should brainstorm what strategic actions the department could take to reap the opportunities available in the situation and ameliorate the risks. Advantages and disadvantages of the various possibilities should then be discussed, and a preferred option should be selected.
4. Implementation of the plan. The strategic plan should be broken down into action steps, with responsibilities, timetables, and budgets designated for each one.
5. Evaluation of the results (followed by a return to step 3 if the results do not meet expectations or achieve goals). The framework for an evaluation can be provided by asking two questions: How will we know when this issue is resolved or improved? How do we measure that?

Organizing for strategic planning need not be complex. Full participation by staff is advantageous because going through the process is as beneficial as the plan itself in bringing everyone to a common understanding of issues, objectives, and actions. A strategic planning committee is frequently used. Some form of staff input to the committee is advisable, as is recognition of the organization's power structure in the strategic planning scheme. The method of introducing strategic planning to the staff is crucial. It should be initiated gradually, with full explanations and demonstrations for the benefit of staff members who may feel threatened by it.

Two guiding principles of strategic planning are (a) ride trends in the direction they are headed and (b) set trends, don't follow them. Another important principle is to discover emerging trends, which are easier to influence. Also, strategic plans should be reflected in short- and mid-range actions and decisions, and contingency plans should be developed, especially when high uncertainty surrounds predictions.

A strategic plan must be controlled by measuring outcomes against preset standards. This keeps the plan on target and allows for corrective action if needed.

Strategic planning emerges from formal planning, power-behavioral relationships, internal decisions, and external events flowing together until key people hold a consensus for action. It has pitfalls, such as assuming that planning can be completely delegated and using unsuitable goals as the basis for planning. Nonetheless, satisfaction with the process appears to be very high.

References

1. Wilkinson G: Strategic planning in social service delivery in the voluntary sector. In *Planning and Social Service Delivery in the Voluntary Sector*, G Tobin, Editor. Westport, CT: Greenwood Press, 1985.
2. DeGreene KB: *The Adaptive Organization: Anticipation and Management of Crisis*. New York: John Wiley & Sons Inc, 1981
3. Steiner GA: *Strategic Planning: What Every Manager Must Know*. New York: Free Press, 1979, pp 3, 7, 9, 13–15
4. Drucker PF: *Management: Tasks, Responsibilities, Practices*. New York: Harper & Row Publishers Inc, 1973
5. Naisbitt J: *Megatrends: Ten New Directions Transforming Our Lives*. New York: Warner Books Inc, 1982, pp 2, 88–89
6. Yavitz B, Newman WH: *Strategy in Action: The Execution, Politics, and Payoff of Business Planning*. New York: Free Press, 1982, pp 4–5, 206, 245
7. Quinn JB: *Strategies for Change: Logical Incrementalism*. Homewood, IL: Richard D Irwin Inc, 1980, pp 9, 15–59, 299–303
8. *The Bellwether Report*. Washington, DC: The Naisbitt Group. (Address: 1101 30th Street, N-W, Washington, DC 20007)
9. *John Naisbitt's Trend Letter*. Washington, DC: The Naisbitt Group
10. *Health Care Strategic Management*. Ann Arbor, MI: Chi Systems Inc
11. *The Futurist*. Bethesda, MD: The World Future Society
12. *The Kiplinger Washington Letter*. Washington, DC: The Kiplinger Washington
13. Hubbard BM: The future of futurism: Creating a new synthesis. *The Futurist*, April 1983, pp 52–58
14. Toffler A: *Future Shock*. New York: Random House Inc, 1970
15. Meadows DH, et al: *Limits to Growth: A Report for the Club of Rome's Project on the Predicament of Mankind*, 2nd edition. New York: Universe Books Inc, 1974
16. Vajk P: *Doomsday Has Been Canceled*. Culver City, CA: Peace Press Inc, 1978
17. Fuller RB: *Critical Path*. New York: St. Martin's Press Inc, 1981
18. Hawkin P, Ogilvy J, Schwartz P: *Seven Tomorrows*. New York: Bantam Books Inc, 1982
19. Bezold C: Health care in the U. S.: Four alternative futures. *The Futurist*, August 1982, pp 14–28
20. Marien M: *Future Survey Annual 1981–1982*. Bethesda, MD: The World Future Society, 1983
21. *Journal of the American Medical Association*. Chicago: American Medical Association
22. *New England Journal of Medicine*. Boston: New England Journal of Medicine
23. *Hospitals*. Chicago: American Hospital Publishing Inc
24. Tarlov AR: Shattuck Lecture—The increasing supply of physicians, the changing structure of the health services system, and the future practice of medicine. *N Engl J Med* 308:1235–1244, 1983
25. Naisbitt J, Elkins J: The hospital and mega-trends. Part 1, *Hosp Forum*, May-June 1983, pp 9–13; Part 2, *Hosp Forum*, July-August 1983, pp 52–56
26. Relman AS: The future of medical practice. *Health Aff*, Summer 1983, pp 5–19

27. Renfro WL: The future. *Assoc Manage*, November 1983, pp 140–143
28. Renfro WL, Morrison JL: Detecting signals of change. *The Futurist*, August 1984, pp 49–53
29. Carson R: *Silent Spring*. New York: Fawcett World Library, 1962
30. Peters TJ, Waterman RH: *In Search of Excellence: Lessons from America's Best-Run Companies*. New York: Harper & Row Publishers Inc, 1982
31. Cornish E, et al: *The Study of the Future: An Introduction to the Art and Science of Understanding and Shaping Tomorrow's World*. Washington, DC: The World Future Society, 1977
32. Taylor JW: *How to Create New Ideas*. Englewood Cliffs, NJ: Prentice-Hall Inc, 1961
33. Delbecq AL, Van de Ven AH, Gustafson DH: *Group Techniques for Program Planning: A Guide to Nominal Group and Delphi Processes*. Glenview, IL: Scott Foresman & Co, 1975
34. Prince GM: The mindspring theory: A new development from synectics research. *J of Creative Behav* 9:159–181, 1979

Chapter 3

Program Planning

Gloria Scammahorn, OTR

Program planning is a dynamic process. It begins when an idea for a program is conceived or a need for a program is sensed. A goal is tentatively stated, and the need for the program is formally assessed. With data from the assessment in hand, the goal statement is refined, and the program's scope is clarified. The resources required for the program and the financial implications are identified, and plans for implementation are made. As the planning proceeds, the idea for the program evolves. The following diagram shows the components of the planning process and their interactions:

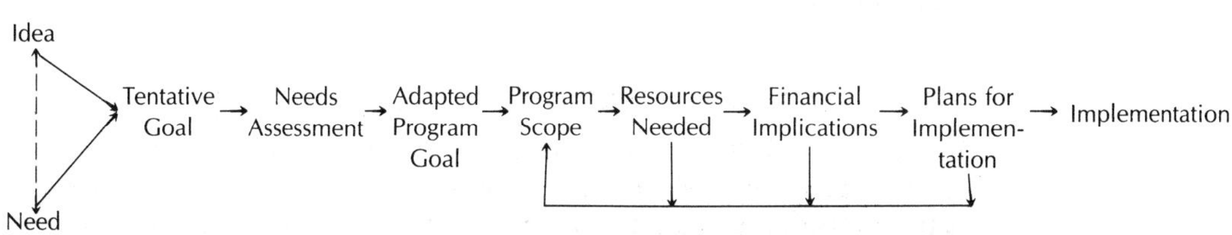

The planning components that are considered in this chapter are as follows:

1. The planners
2. The review and approval process
3. The idea and the need for the program

Gloria Scammahorn is the director of the occupational therapy department at the Research Medical Center in Kansas City, Missouri. The department provides services for Research Health System including program development in home health agencies, nursing homes, hospitals, and public schools.

4. The adapted program goal
5. The scope of the program
6. The resources required by the program
7. The financial implications of the program
8. The plan for program implementation.

THE PLANNERS

A program can be planned by one person or a committee. The choice depends in large part on the financial resources, the time, and the personnel available to plan. Program planning benefits from the diversity of input that a committee provides. "Rationality is achieved from a multiplicity of decision makers pursuing their partisan interests in interaction with others" (1, p 719). Having several decision makers brings the energies, the skills, and the values that are needed to identify the relevant issues and the consequences of alternative approaches to problems. These might be neglected by a single planner (2).

Using a committee slows down the planning process, but the more people who are on the committee, the more support the program will have once it is implemented. "It has been shown that implementation success increases with . . . participation of citizens, experts, and community interest groups . . ." (1, p 711). An example of the makeup of a committee to plan a hospital-based hand rehabilitation program is the occupational therapy manager (the committee chairperson), a staff occupational therapist with expertise in hand rehabilitation, patients/clients, referring physicians, and the physical therapy manager. If funding will come from an outside source, it is wise to have this group represented on the planning committee also.

A committee approach is not always necessary for program planning. The occupational therapy manager or a staff therapist can act as a central planner, and then decide the approach to be used for each step of the planning process.

THE REVIEW AND APPROVAL PROCESS

Every system has its own process for the review and approval of ideas for new programs. Most require a written program proposal, especially if the proposed program has significant financial implications. Figure 1 is a suggested outline. The proposal should address each of the components of the planning process. This will give the people in authority the information they need to make an intelligent decision about the acceptability of the program. The proposal should be brief but cover all pertinent details. If it cannot be kept brief, an executive summary should be included. Diagrams, charts, or graphs make a good impression in a proposal, and a picture may clarify key points. Attaching support documents can be helpful. Letters of endorsement can come from physicians, teachers, patients/clients, or other key people interested in the program's approval. Statistics, brochures from successful established programs, and other such information can provide details for those who want them.

FIGURE 3–1
Outline for a Program Proposal

I. Introductory Summary Statement
- A. Patient/client population to be served
- B. Program's goals and objectives
- C. Services to be provided

II. Findings/Facts
- A. Needs assessment
- B. Other statistics
- C. Benefits to patients/clients, the organization, and the community
- D. Resources needed

III. Finances/Economic Benefit
- A. Revenue projections
- B. Expense projections
- C. Comparison of projects
- D. One year's budget

IV. Implementation
- A. Location
- B. Plan
- C. Schedule

THE IDEA FOR THE PROGRAM

The impetus for an occupational therapy program can come from many sources—for example, growth in the organization in which an occupational therapy department or unit is based, requests from a community agency or consumers, and market research. Medicare's Prospective Payment System has prompted the formation of multi-institutional systems of health care (3). This has resulted in some occupational therapy organizations offering the services of their personnel to hospitals and community agencies on a contractual basis. Also, individual occupational therapists have begun to establish private practices. These developments have come in part as a result of needs in the community.

With the change in health care to a more businesslike approach, many occupational therapists are learning a market orientation (4). They are using data generated by organizational and environmental assessments and a market analysis to make decisions on program development (see Chapter 6 for an introduction to marketing concepts). Marketing is a systematic way to determine needs. Using a marketing approach means going to the consumers of a service to assess demand.

If an idea for a program has been generated through market research, the idea's viability has already been confirmed. If an idea comes from another source, the need for it must be systematically assessed. The first step is to translate the idea into a tentative goal statement that clarifies what must be studied to determine the idea's viability. Following are two examples of a goal statement in first draft:

1. Study the need for occupational therapy services among students in the Kansas City school district.

2. Study the need for occupational therapy services among the hand injury patients of the orthopedic and plastic surgeons at Research Medical Center.

THE NEED FOR THE PROGRAM

Many sources can be tapped to help an occupational therapy organization determine if its services are needed by a system. Local standards and regulatory agencies collect information on health status indicators. From this information, statistics on potential patients/clients—for example, age, diagnosis, and often, unmet health needs—can be compiled. Medical records personnel in health care organizations also gather information that can be helpful.

Interviewing key personnel (consumers) in a target system gives information about what they see as unmet wants and needs. In a nursing home, for example, consumers to interview are the patients/clients, the administrator, the home's contract physician, the head nurse, the activity director, and the designated social service person. In a school, consumers are students, parents, the principal, the special education director, other special services staff, and special education teachers.

The type of information to seek is that which answers the question, Is there a need for occupational therapy among these consumers? Care must be taken during this assessment not to suggest that the program will definitely be established.

The information that is gathered during the needs assessment should be analyzed and reviewed. A decision is then made on the viability of the program idea. It may become clear that proceeding with the program is not wise. Although leaving a program unfinished is difficult, an occupational therapy manager should concentrate on the programs that are most needed.

THE ADAPTED PROGRAM GOAL

If the planners decide that the original program idea should be implemented, the goal statement should be further developed using the information collected. The sample first drafts presented earlier in this chapter might be restated as follows:

1. To provide occupational therapy services to the learning disabled population in the Kansas City school district.
2. To provide occupational therapy services to inpatients and outpatients who have undergone hand surgery at Research Medical Center.

The goal statement is becoming more specific. To determine the viability of this adapted idea, the needs of the consumers who have been identified should be assessed and the benefits of the program to them should be defined. The same key people who helped determine that the original idea was viable can help once more, if necessary, or related health care statistics can be checked. Statistics can come from the organization in which the program will be based or from community agencies. Medical records departments can again be helpful.

Assessing the Need for the Adapted Idea

How this needs assessment proceeds will vary with the type of program that is planned and the system in which the program will be located. This assessment should produce an estimate of the number of patients/clients who will benefit from the program and the competition available to them. Contacting potential consumers to collect data on needs can be done by interview or questionnaire. During this survey, as during the earlier one, care should be taken not to promise that the program will be implemented. In gathering data, "personal interviews, nominal group techniques, and conventional discussion group techniques were more effective (in terms of response rate and participants' motivation in the planning process) than impersonal questionnaires . . ." (1, p 729). If the potential consumer can be seen face to face, better information will be gathered, but a questionnaire may have to be used to save time.

Defining the Benefits

Identifying the benefits of a program further clarifies its compatibility with the organization that will sponsor it. A program will benefit three groups—patients/clients, the organization, and the community—each in a different way. For example, it may improve the living situation of a hospital patient after he or she is discharged by reducing disability or increasing independence. For the hospital, it may generate revenue, provide a service required for accreditation, or boost public support. The community may gain a service not available in the area before, or one that competes effectively with a service already being provided.

The information that has been gathered should be analyzed and reviewed, and once again a decision on the viability of the program idea should be made. Many opportunities exist for new occupational therapy programs. The time it takes to develop new programs should be allocated to those that will be most viable. Showing a need must precede the allocation of resources to a new program (5). In deciding whether to proceed, primary consideration should be given to the benefit to the sponsoring organization. If the proposed program is judged to be a viable concept, further planning can begin.

THE SCOPE OF THE PROGRAM

The planners now need to consider the intended scope of the program. The representation of this on paper will at first be a working draft. Change and clarification will come as the needed resources, the financial implications, and the plan for implementation are considered. Defining the scope involves identifying the patients/clients who will receive services, the proposed objectives of the program, the occupational therapy services that will be delivered, and the expected volume of service.

Identifying Patients/Clients

The idea should become more specific. This means deciding what population to serve (and what population not to serve). The process of deciding is called market segmentation, defined as "dividing a market into smaller homogeneous groups" (6, p 47). For example, a new occupational therapy program in an acute care hospital usually identifies stroke patients as its first market because in such a hospital, of the various diagnoses that occupational therapists can treat, stroke is the most frequent one. The identification of a particular population to serve makes it easier to clarify the objectives of a program and the services that will be provided.

Stating the Objectives of the Program

Once the population to be served has been identified, program objectives should be written. They should state what outcomes are desired and clarify what the program will achieve. Also, they should be compatible with the goals and the objectives of the system sponsoring the program. The objective of a pediatric program in a hospital setting might be stated this way: to provide occupational therapy evaluation and treatment services to ten multiply handicapped children per week. In a school setting the phrasing might be expressed thus: to provide consultative services to the teachers of special education students in three schools so that remediation and compensation techniques used with the multiply handicapped population are integrated into the classroom.

In determining objectives it is helpful to consider other occupational therapy programs that meet identical needs. The American Occupational Therapy Association (AOTA), the local occupational therapy association, or a search in the *American Journal of Occupational Therapy* may be of assistance in finding programs with the same or similar objectives.

Determining the Services

After the patient/client population and the objectives are identified, the range of occupational therapy services that will be provided is determined. To accomplish this task, the needs of patients/clients, the system, and the community are considered. With regard to patients'/clients' needs, reading in *Willard and Spackman's Occupational Therapy* (7), doing a literature search, or discussing possibilities with therapists who have worked with the type of patient/client identified will help develop a list of services that could be provided.

System considerations include whether the system already offers competing services or has policies that need to be considered as services are planned. For example, in an established hospital an occupational therapy department planning a program for stroke patients should first look into the services already being provided by the departments of physical therapy and patient care.

To gather information on current programs offered by the organization, the occupational therapy manager should meet with or survey the people who will be affected. Data gathering for a mental health program in a hospital might include the following activities:

1. Interviewing or sending a questionnaire to staff psychiatrists regarding unmet patient needs.

2. Surveying the nursing, social work, and other departments regarding programs already offered.
3. Auditing medical records to gather statistics on the types of mental health patients historically seen by the hospital.
4. Interviewing hospitalized patients regarding what they feel are unmet needs.

In a school setting similar activities might be appropriate:

1. Interviewing the special education director, key teachers, and parents regarding unmet student needs.
2. Surveying the existing programs in speech therapy and adaptive physical education regarding the services that they offer.
3. Auditing the individualized education programs of special education students to determine the types of functional problems being identified by teachers.

Such information will help the occupational therapy department or unit fit its services to the organization's needs.

Considering Community Needs

If the program being planned will provide services to consumers from the community, the scope of services already being provided by other occupational therapy personnel in the referral area should be considered. At this point the planners must identify how the new occupational therapy program will differ from existing ones. This is known as a service differentiation, which means "distinguishing one's service from other services in the same marketplace" (6, p 45). It requires assessing consumers in the geographic area the program will serve and then distinguishing the new occupational therapy program according to the consumers' needs. An example is provided by an outpatient program that establishes service hours from 7:00 a.m. to 7:00 p.m. to allow patients/clients to come before and after work. This differentiates it from other programs in the area, which are open from 8:00 a.m. to 4:00 p.m.

A potential program's chance for success is very limited if it duplicates existing programs in the community. To differentiate service, information must be gathered on similar programs in the organization and the service area. This can be done through informal means and by checking with patients/clients, physicians, and other referral sources.

Projecting Volume

An estimate of the volume of service that will be provided must now be made. The services provided each month will usually vary, so it is best to project highs and lows. The needs assessment that was done to justify services should give a starting estimate. Its accuracy can then be checked by keeping appropriate statistics each month. This may later help justify new resources for an expanded program.

After all of the foregoing factors are considered, a one-page summary of the scope of the program should be written. Figure 2 offers an example.

FIGURE 3–2
Scope of the Occupational Therapy Hand Rehabilitation Program

Patients/Clients

People who have had tendon repairs, fractures, crush injuries, nerve repairs, or metacarpal phalangeal procedures

Program Objective

To increase by 50 percent the occupational therapy services provided to hand injury patients of the orthopedic and plastic surgeons at the Research Medical Center

Occupational Therapy Services

1. Evaluations: range of motion, sensation, strength, function
2. Treatments: splinting, exercise programs, coordination training, training in activities of daily living

Service Differentiation

1. Clinic hours from 7 AM to 7 PM
2. Patients/clients begun as inpatients and continued as outpatients

Volume Projection

1. One to two inpatients per week
2. Four to six outpatients per week

THE RESOURCES REQUIRED BY THE PROGRAM

The next area for planners to consider is what staff, space, supplies, and equipment will be needed by the new program.

Staff

A new program usually requires new positions, and these must be justified. They may be part time or full time, and they may call for registered occupational therapists (OTRs) or certified occupational therapy assistants (COTAs). In deciding on the type of occupational therapy staff needed, the manager should consider the level of knowledge and skill required to perform the proposed services. The AOTA's delineation of the roles of entry-level OTRs and COTAs offers guidance on this issue (8). Chapter 12 explains some methods of quantifying staffing needs.

Following are questions to consider in deciding how many and what types of occupational therapy staff to request:

1. How many patients/clients are estimated to need treatment?
2. How long will treatment take?
3. How often will patients/clients be treated?
4. Can patients/clients be grouped, or must they be seen individually?
5. Must direct treatment be given, or can an alternative method be used?
6. What documentation is required? How will it be done? How much time will it take?
7. How much meeting time will be required?
8. How much time is needed to transport patients/clients? What type of transport will be used?
9. How much preparation time will the therapists need?

10. What secretarial support is available?

11. If patients/clients will be seen by professionals in other disciplines, how will this affect the scheduling of the occupational therapy staff's time? How much time should be allowed for informal consultation with the other professionals (e.g., to set schedules or update them on an unexpected occurrence)?

12. If student training will be a part of the staff's duties, how much time will it involve?

After considering the various factors, the manager should lay out an ideal schedule for a workweek, including breaks and lunch time.

If new staff will be needed, the following points should be addressed in a request attached to the program proposal (5):

1. The number and the type of staff requested.
2. The reasons for them, clearly stated.
3. Statistical data supporting the need for them.
4. A description of the duties they will perform.
5. The effect of the additional positions on the duties of existing positions in the department or unit.
6. The estimated cost of the positions for the budget year in which they will go into effect.

Calculations and projections for the program may show the need for more than one staff position. If so, the manager might consider filling one at the outset and adding the others as the volume of services increases or as lost services are documented.

Short-term ways of staffing the program and thereby justifying the need for additional staff are to temporarily increase staff's work time or realign their responsibilities, run a pilot test, use on-call help, or contract with outside personnel for services. A pilot test involves running the planned program for a set period (say, three to six months), during which the additional staff are temporary employees. To make their positions permanent, they must meet projected productivity levels. The alternative of using on-call staff is often approved because they are used only as needed and do not receive holiday, vacation, or sick pay.

Besides occupational therapy personnel, some programs require the following staff:

1. A medical director, if the referring physician cannot give medical direction
2. A secretary and/or a receptionist
3. A transporter
4. Someone to do housekeeping and maintenance jobs.

All staff requirements and justifications for them should be documented.

Space

Planning the space for a program that is unfamiliar is a difficult task. Visiting similar programs already in existence is helpful. It decreases the possibility of not having appropriate space for the program being designed. Some programs can be set up in space already available. Others necessitate the acquisition of new space. Space should be accessible, convenient, and pleasant. Chapter 4 treats this subject in greater detail.

Supplies

Supplies are items the program staff will use that must be replaced. Different programs require different types and amounts of supplies. A visit to a similar established program will help the occupational therapy manager determine what supplies are needed. The types usually ordered by occupational therapy organizations are media, office supplies, splinting materials and devices, and evaluation/testing materials.

To ensure that consumable items are available when needed, a system for regularly taking an inventory of supplies must be planned. Monthly inventories give statistics on usage that facilitate projections of what and how much to order on a continuing basis.

Equipment

As with supplies, different kinds of programs require different types and volumes of equipment. Occupational therapy organizations customarily order three types: capital, expendable, and adaptive. Capital equipment usually costs $300–$500 or more and is expected to last over two years. Tables, desks, chairs, file cabinets, kilns, biofeedback equipment, and possibly standardized test kits fall in this category.

Expendable equipment includes items that cost less than $300 and will not last two years because of heavy usage or likely loss. This includes weights, screwdrivers, dishes, scissors, and so forth.

Adaptive equipment can be categorized as expendable equipment or as supplies, depending on the item. It is stocked for use during treatment and may also be sold to patients/clients. If it will be sold, an inventory system must be devised.

A list should be made of the equipment and the supplies that the proposed program will need. Once the list is finalized, the amount of each item to be ordered can be added. Figure 3 illustrates a beginning list for a hand rehabilitation program.

THE FINANCIAL IMPLICATIONS OF THE PROGRAM

In most settings a program's merit is determined by its financial viability. Part of the process of planning for a new program is an analysis of costs and benefits. This includes comparing the expenses and the revenues. The philosophy of the system will determine whether a program may

FIGURE 3–3
A Partial List of Equipment and Supplies Needed for a Hand Rehabilitation Program

Service	Amount	Capital Equipment	Amount	Expendable Equipment	Amount	Supplies
Evaluation	1 each	Cabinet, file cabinet, table, chair				
Range of motion			3	Goniometers	60	Forms
Strength	1	Dynamometer	1	Pinch gauge	60	Forms

be implemented if its design shows it likely to be either profitable, self-supporting, or less than break-even.

Expenses

Expenses will fall into two categories:

1. Direct, or controllable by the program manager
2. Indirect, or not under the direct control of the program manager

In a written program proposal, direct expenses are often presented in a budget format (see Figure 4). Direct expenses include the costs of salaries, supplies, and expendable equipment. These are estimated for a year of operation. The cost of capital equipment is also a direct expense, but is presented as a start-up figure.

The indirect cost of the program—heating, lighting, housekeeping, rent, and so forth—is not always presented. The budget director or the organization's administrator can tell the occupational therapy manager what indirect expenses, if any, should be presented in the program proposal.

Salaries and benefits. The largest expense of any occupational therapy program is the salaries of the staff. The cost of salaries is determined by multiplying the personnel estimate by the salaries of staff in similar non-occupational therapy (health care) positions in the organization sponsoring the program. If salary scales are not available, contacting the AOTA, the local occupational therapy association, or local health care organizations can be helpful in indicating averages or ranges. The cost of employee benefits (e.g., holidays, vacations, sick days, overtime, insurance, retirement, and Social Security) should also be estimated. Further, the expense of salaries for on-call staff during times of high load, illness, and vacation should be considered.

Supplies. The cost of supplies should be estimated. This includes all

FIGURE 3–4
Hand Rehabilitation Program Expenses for One Year of Operation

Salaries		
One staff therapist		$24,000
Benefits		
25% of salary		6,000
Supplies		$7,400
Splinting materials	4,000	
Forms and office supplies	400	
Adaptive equipment	3,000	
Start-up expenses		5,000
Expendable equipment	2,000	
Capital equipment	3,000	
Continuing education		200
Promotion of the program		600
Repair of equipment		50
TOTAL		$43,250

the consumable items—craft supplies, splinting materials, office supplies, and so forth. The manager can determine the cost by looking at the resources required to run the program. Both the start-up cost and the cost per month thereafter should be calculated. The manager should consider budgeting some supplies on a quarterly basis because bulk purchases decrease the cost per item.

Equipment. The cost of equipment can be estimated by looking through equipment catalogs. The initial expense will be the greatest. Periodic replacement of some equipment will be necessary, and additional equipment may be required as the patient/client load increases.

Capital equipment is budgeted each year as a one-time expense. In estimating, the manager should consider the cost of the following items (5):

1. The equipment itself, plus a percent increase to compensate for inflation by the time the equipment is actually purchased
2. Freight/shipping
3. Installation
4. New space needed for the equipment, or alterations in existing space
5. Service contracts
6. The depreciable life of the equipment (the length of time until it will have to be replaced)
7. Materials needed to operate the equipment.

Other expenses. The expense of continuing education for the staff should be budgeted. Continuing education costs include registration, travel, room and board, and books. The amount will depend on the availability of training facilities in the system and workshop offerings in the locale. Other factors to consider are whether senior occupational therapy staff can be freed to train new graduates and whether audiovisual equipment is available to operate rented training videotapes.

Additional expenses that should be estimated, if appropriate, are mileage reimbursements and parking fees for staff who travel for the program; the costs of promoting the program and recruiting staff; and charges for repairing and servicing equipment.

Revenue

Revenue projections are based on the expected volume of service. Estimating over a three-year period is best because establishing a new program often takes that long. Revenue is estimated by multiplying the expected volume (in units of service) by the unit charges for services. It is wise to be conservative in revenue projections. In most situations, revenue should cover expected expenses within a short time (six months). If it does not, fees should be reevaluated.

Establishing a fee schedule. The manager should determine if, and how, charges will be assessed. An organization's financial department can give guidance on whether the program's fees should cover direct expenses, cover direct and indirect expenses, or generate a profit. Surveying other programs in the organization that charge for services, or other occupational therapy programs, will give a starting point for designing a fee system.

Fees can be charged for each unit of time or each service. Consideration should be given to fees for evaluation, treatment, consultation, group work, splinting, adaptive equipment, treatment outside the facilities, and transportation. AOTA's uniform terminology (9) may be helpful in establishing categories. The manager should work closely with the organization's business office and with third-party payers to clarify the type of documentation required for payment.

Payment for services. Third-party payers vary in their coverage of occupational therapy services (see Chapter 18 for specific information about payment systems). Their documentation requirements for payment also vary. Checking with AOTA, the local occupational therapy association, state and federal agencies, and major insurance companies can help an occupational therapy manager gain familiarity with local policies.

Comparing Expenses and Revenue

After a proposed program's expenses and revenues are estimated, the two should be compared. The outcome will show that the program will either make a profit, just cover its costs, or run at a loss. As noted earlier, which of these is acceptable depends on the sponsoring system's philosophy. At this point the program may need to be revised to ensure final approval. Financial viability is often a deciding factor in the outcome of the approval process.

THE PLAN FOR IMPLEMENTATION

A time line for implementation should be set up. In the process the manager should consider staffing requirements, resources, policies and procedures that need to be written, promotion that should occur, and the content and the implementation of plans to evaluate the success and monitor the quality of the program.

Staffing Requirements

The time line must consider the planning for staff needs. Job descriptions for the staff should be developed or adapted, and the organizational structure of the department or unit should be revised to reflect the new positions. Staff orientation and continuing education programs must be planned. The supervisory staff must recruit and select staff with the required skills. They must also determine how staff will be evaluated and compensated. A system to measure the staff's productivity should be designed and implemented (10). Chapter 12 discusses these subjects in greater depth.

If the program consists of staff services to another organization, there should be a contract to specify the scope of work; the contract period; the staff to be provided, their availability, and their reporting relationships; the space to be allocated; the responsibility for providing supplies; the cost and payment schedule; liability; and conditions for termination.

Resources

The time line should include when to purchase equipment and supplies so as to have them available at the program's start-up time. In laying out the time line, the manager should recognize that the delivery may take much longer than desired. Consideration also needs to be given to the space layout—where services will be offered, how patients/clients will be served, and where storage areas are needed.

Policies and Procedures

The mechanics of the program should be planned. Written procedures and standards will decrease the risk of liability. Procedures are especially helpful if students or inexperienced staff will be carrying out aspects of the program. Guidelines are even more important when team interaction is required. The guidelines should include program scope, medical direction, safety policies, administrative direction, and the program's relationship with other departments. The standards of regulatory agencies and the conditions of third-party payers may have a bearing on the policies and procedures of the program. Chapters 18 and 19 treat this subject. For example, in a hospital, policies and procedures should reflect the requirements of Medicare, the Professional Review Organization, Blue Cross/Blue Shield and other insurance carriers, the Joint Commission on Accreditation of Hospitals, and the state licensing board.

Promotion

A plan should be written to promote the program. The characteristics of the program that make it beneficial and attractive to the consumer should be highlighted. The success of a program depends on the sponsoring organization's in-house resources, the cooperation received from referral sources, the way in which the program is introduced, the manner in which it is publicized, and ultimately the satisfaction of the patient/client. Chapter 16 offers a detailed discussion of promotion.

Evaluation

The success of the program will be evaluated in terms of its efficiency, the quality of its services, its acceptance by the community, and its financial stability (1). The objectives set forth as the program is being developed will state expected outcomes or goals. In evaluating the results, a comparison of expected outcomes and actual results is important to determining success. Chapters 13 and 14 explain the purposes and the methods of some widely used evaluation strategies.

SUMMARY

Program planning is a dynamic process. It begins when an idea for a program is conceived or a need for a program is sensed. A goal is tentatively stated, and the need for the program is formally assessed. The goal statement is refined, and the program's scope is clarified. Resources required and financial implications are identified, and implementation is planned. As the planning proceeds, the idea for the program evolves.

A program can be planned by one person or a committee. Planning benefits from the diversity of input that a committee provides. The more people who are on the committee, the more support the program will have once it is implemented.

For review and approval of the new program, a written program proposal will probably be necessary. It should address each of the components of the planning process.

The idea for a program can come from many sources—for example, growth in the organization, requests from consumers, and market research. Usually the need for a program idea must be formally assessed. The first step is to translate the idea into a tentative goal statement that clarifies what must be studied to determine the idea's viability. Next, planners can tap many data sources to determine if occupational therapy services are needed by a system—for example, local standards and regulatory agencies and medical records departments in local health care organizations. Also, interviewing key personnel in a target system gives information about what they see as unmet wants and needs.

The information that is gathered should be analyzed and reviewed. If the planners decide that the original program idea should be implemented, the tentative goal statement should be further developed, and the viability of the resulting adapted program goal should be assessed. Further, the benefits of the program to three groups–patients/clients, the sponsoring organization, and the community–should be defined.

The planners now need to consider the intended scope of the program. This involves identifying the patients/clients who will receive services, the proposed objectives of the program, the occupational therapy services that will be delivered, and the expected volume of service. A one-page summary of this information should be written.

The next area for planners to consider is what staff, space, supplies, and equipment will be needed by the new program. New positions must be justified. This may be done in writing, with documentation of the need, and it may also be done by staffing the program on a short-term basis (e.g., by temporarily increasing existing staff's work time or running a pilot test). Estimating needed space and supplies is aided by visiting similar established programs. Equipment will fall into one of three categories: capital, expendable, and adaptive.

Part of the process of planning for a new program is an analysis of costs and benefits. This includes estimating expenses and revenues and comparing them. Expenses include direct ones, such as salaries, supplies, and equipment, and may include indirect ones, such as heating and lighting. Revenues should be projected over a three-year period because establishing a new program often takes that long.

When the program is approved, a time line for implementation should be set up. This should allow time for staffing the program (e.g., developing job descriptions and planning staff orientation), obtaining resources, writing policies and procedures, developing a promotion plan, and setting up an evaluation system.

References

1. Van de Ven AH: Problem solving, planning and innovation, Part 1, Test of the program planning model. *Human Relations* 33:711–740, 1980
2. Van de Ven AH: Problem solving, planning and innovation, Part 2, Speculations for theory and practice. *Human Relations* 33:757–779, 1980
3. Schramm CJ: American health care delivery: A system in transition. *The Coordinator*, November 1984, pp 1–3
4. Olson TS: Health care marketing. In *Willard and Spackman's Occupational Therapy*, 6th edition, HL Hopkins, HD Smith, Editors. Philadelphia: JB Lippincott Co, 1983, chap 42
5. *Budget Manual*. Kansas City, MO: Research Medical Center, May 1983
6. Clark RW, Shyavitz L: Strategies for a crowded marketplace. *Health Care Manage Rev*, Summer 1983, pp 45–51
7. Hopkins HL, Smith HD, Editors: *Willard and Spackman's Occupational Therapy*, 6th edition. Philadelphia: JB Lippincott Co, 1983
8. American Occupational Therapy Association: Entry-level role delineation for OTRs and COTAs. In *Reference Manual of the Official Documents of the American Occupational Therapy Association*. Rockville, MD: American Occupational Therapy Association, 1983
9. American Occupational Therapy Association: Uniform terminology for reporting occupational therapy services and occupational therapy product output reporting system. In *Reference Manual of the Official Documents of the American Occupational Therapy Association*. Rockville, MD: American Occupational Therapy Association, 1983
10. Bair J, Gwin CH, Editors: *A Productivity Systems Guide for Occupational Therapy*. Rockville, MD: American Occupational Therapy Association, 1985

Chapter 4

Facility Planning

Pamella Leiter, OTR

Since the implementation of the Medicare Prospective Payment System, many health care organizations have been experiencing a decreasing length of stay for patients/clients receiving general medical-surgical services. This has created a need for them to develop new markets, emphasizing specialty programs such as home health, rehabilitation, mental health, substance abuse, and cardiac rehabilitation (1). Because occupational therapy is usually offered within these programs, expansion and diversification of occupational therapy services may become necessary, and occupational therapy managers may be expected to plan the renovation of existing facilities or the construction of new ones.

Facility planning can be both challenging and rewarding. It involves analyzing the present and future program objectives and visit trends of the occupational therapy department. Relationships within the organization, the equipment and the construction required by the new services, the need for the new facilities to be accessible to people with disabilities, and the needs and the desires of the staff all become considerations. These must be communicated to a hospital space planner, a consultant, or an architect to effect a result that will be efficient, safe, comfortable, and esthetically pleasing. Along the way, constraints imposed by design

---

In her position as the director of rehabilitation administration at Michiana Rehabilitation Institute in South Bend, Indiana, Pamella Leiter has participated in space planning for an occupational therapy clinic, a technical aids center with offices, and a rehabilitation engineering laboratory. She is currently involved in the design of an off-site outpatient rehabilitation facility, a 30-bed inpatient rehabilitation unit, and a 49-bed freestanding rehabilitation hospital.

elements, the budget, or the physical environment may necessitate compromise and the setting of priorities.

Putting the necessary time into preconstruction planning is important because of the large amount of capital that is being invested and the difficulty and expense that will be involved in making changes after construction has been completed. Also, many problems with facilities today are the result of "cumulative, short-term, interim solutions to individual problems, implemented in an uncoordinated manner" (2, p 99). Ellerbe, Inc., a planning consulting firm in Minneapolis, "recommends a 12-month cycle for this process, but the cycle's length may vary depending upon the size and the type of the . . . project, . . . the level and accuracy of available data and prior planning, and the extent of staff participation built into the planning process" (2, p 97). Other firms, such as Hansen Lind Meyer of Iowa City, think that twelve months is quite generous given the health care market and the cost of financing projects today. They find that once initial approval is obtained, the traditional design process takes only six to eight months, depending on the scope of the project (Warren Hendrickson, written communication, November 1984).

Facility-planning skills may be required in only a few instances in an occupational therapy manager's career. The first time a manager is called on to plan facilities, one of the most useful, yet most informal methods of becoming familiar with various alternatives is to visit as many occupational therapy facilities as possible and discuss their merits and problems. Learning from others' experiences can increase one's chances for success.

Preconstruction Planning

The preconstruction phase of facility planning involves several steps, each important to the smooth execution of the total project:

1. Considering organizational factors
2. Analyzing functional and space needs
3. Allocating space
4. Writing a proposal
5. Planning the detailed use of space
6. Working with the architect.

Considering Organizational Factors

On initiation of planning, the occupational therapy manager should review the project with organization administrators, occupational therapy staff, physicians, and consultants, if any, to develop a concept of future program needs. The emphasis on planning and the amount of market information that is routinely collected differ across organizations. The manager should use whatever information is available for predicting trends. The organization's planning department may have previously studied the program needs of the occupational therapy department, and that may have provided the impetus for the expansion. If so, the data from the study can be used to determine which occupational therapy services should be offered. If no preplanning has occurred and there is sufficient time, the organization's marketing department might contract with a consultant to conduct a market research study of previous and current consumers' needs and their opinions of the department's services.

Obtaining a complete view of the long-range program objectives enhances a manager's ability to plan for the future, because work stations and equipment are affected by such objectives. Flexibility in the finished facility is important, however, because the health care market is changing rapidly. Program objectives may have to be modified as new opportunities arise.

One method of coordinating planning is through a user group, a committee comprising a cross-section of personnel who represent various areas of competence important to planning and building. Several types of users can offer helpful input to the project. Administrators with a knowledge of the organization's long-range objectives will have ideas about the role and functions of occupational therapy within the rehabilitation program. Occupational therapy staff who use the clinic areas can contribute information and views about work stations, equipment, work flow, and arrangement of clinic space. Physicians or medical directors who are key referral sources may have specific recommendations for the expansion of services. Consultants can function as impartial third parties. They may have valuable suggestions from their experience with other projects and can be instrumental in evaluating the needs of other committee members and developing alternatives.

With this method, planning becomes participatory. The occupational therapy manager should play a major role in setting priorities and evaluating alternatives, but the committee can help the manager review options and develop criteria for evaluating them. A decision can then be reached that is satisfactory to all or most of the committee members, as well as the manager. Meetings of the committee should continue as the preliminary working drawings and the design documents are being developed, to provide numerous opportunities for input and review (Warren Hendrickson, written communication, November 1984).

A major project may cause uncertainties and some inconvenience among occupational therapy staff, particularly those not on the planning committee. To alleviate this, the staff should be provided with regular status reports. These will help develop appropriate expectations of what will be accomplished, encourage a realistic view of the time frame for project completion, and facilitate the staff's adjustment to the new facility.

Analyzing Functional and Space Needs

When a new facility is being proposed, its feasibility must be established at various levels, that is, with the organization's internal decision makers, such as the administration or the board of directors, and possibly through the state's Certification of Need (CON) process, usually controlled by the state department of health. Collection of objective data is the first step in establishing need, usually followed by justification of project cost. A written proposal using a convincing methodology to determine functional and space deficiencies and needs may be necessary to establish feasibility and to provide information for a CON review, if one is required (3).

Determining the need for additional space may be the responsibility of the occupational therapy manager or the planning department. Roles and responsibilities in this regard vary across organizations. If the planning department is responsible, it will determine the methodology to be used and write the proposal, and the occupational therapy manager will assist by providing information such as statistics, program objectives, and equipment needs. In later phases the manager will be involved in reviewing plans and in setting priorities if compromises need to be made. This chapter assumes that the occupational therapy manager will be involved in much of the planning and provides information on how to plan effectively with or without a planning department.

Using space need methodologies. Experts in facility planning have developed numerical formulas, or space need methodologies, to describe the amount of space required for hospital departments. Regulatory agencies have adopted guidelines using such methodologies for evaluating proposals for hospital renovation, expansion, and new construction. Each of the methodologies possesses inherent shortcomings. Although the use of a methodology or a guideline may be required and may facilitate comparison, caution must be observed in interpreting the results (3). None of the methodologies described in this chapter are universally accepted.

> Planners and regulatory bodies have been eagerly searching for the most appropriate measure and distribution of space for years, only to give up in futile dismay. Most of this confusion with numerical equations is a universal definition of terms. When we discuss "square feet" are we talking about net square feet or gross square feet? Another dilemma is to establish a criteria for measurement. Will the criteria be square feet per bed, square feet per procedure, square feet per person, etc. (4, p VII–1)

In this chapter no attempt is made to solve these problems. However, the occupational therapy manager should describe the methodology used, to indicate that the assertion of need is based on more than opinion. Project reviewers will thus have less basis to dispute the assessment (4).

In approaching a functional and space needs assessment, the method recommended by Cynthia Hayward, a registered architect with Chi Systems in Ann Arbor, Michigan, "is based on a detailed examination of departmental function and a quantified analysis of the workload, staffing, equipment, and various other 'space generators' within the department" (3, p 7). This method suggests that the functions that consume space must be considered before any methodologies are employed. Such in-depth planning at the outset can determine which space can be shared between departments, how it can be shared, how efficiency can be increased by locating related departments in proximity to each other, how many work stations will be required as a result of the number of patient/client visits and the hours of operation, how much space will be necessary to accommodate the level of staffing, and what major pieces of equipment will be needed (3). After these functional requirements are determined, they should be compared with the results of the space need methodology, and alterations should be made. A department's needs and objectives are best met through this approach. It is most easily used in new construction or in institutions with ample space to house their services.

In many organizations the planning department may initially work with preliminary space need information when applying for the CON and later determine a location for the occupational therapy department. The strategy in this approach is to determine how many square feet of space are necessary for the program to operate efficiently and to make an estimate of project cost for the purpose of the CON application. After CON approval, a location is assigned and the actual planning of the use of the space occurs. The location and its configuration may then determine how the space can be used. All needs may not be met, and some program objectives may have to be compromised. This approach may be used in organizations wishing to expedite a CON approval or in situations in which a decision to expand occupational therapy services has preceded a commitment to a facility or organizational space plan.

A space need methodology from the U. S. Department of Health, Education and Welfare (5) that has been used by some facility-planning consultants requires data on the number of departmental gross square feet (DGSF), the number of visits that occur in the occupational therapy department annually, and the number of hours that the department is open weekly. DGSF is defined as "the total area assigned to a specific department including partitions and internal corridors . . . whereas departmental net square feet (DNSF) is defined as "total useable space assigned to a specific departmental activity excluding partitions and internal corridors . . . (4, p VII–1). The methodology provides the planner with a *utilization factor,* defined as the number of visits per square foot. The utilization factor describes how much use a particular space is getting. Although a norm is not available, this factor can be helpful in predicting trends in space use (see Table 1).

TABLE 4–1
Utilization Factor

$$\frac{\text{Annual number of visits}}{\text{DGSF}} \times \frac{40}{\text{Weekly hours of operation}} = \text{Visits per square foot}$$

Comparing **results obtained from space need methodologies with standard estimates** is often useful. A table of preliminary space estimates for occupational therapy has been developed by Chi Systems:

Total Annual Visits	Space Range
7,500 or less	400–1,000 sq. ft.
7,500–15,000	1,000–1,750 sq. ft.
15,000–25,000	1,750–2,500 sq. ft.
25,000 or more	2,500 plus

Note: From Chi Systems, Inc. Source is unpublished updated version of material from *Evaluation and Space Programming Methodology for Physiotherapy, Occupational Therapy, Speech Pathology, and Audiology Departments*, Ottawa, Ontario, Canada: Department of National Health and Welfare, Health Services and Promotion Branch, November 1978, p 97.

The U. S. Department of Health and Human Services recommends guidelines that are similar, but oriented toward larger occupational therapy units (see Table 2).

Other guidelines available include the following:

1. The Northern Indiana Health Systems Agency in its *Criteria and Standards for Acute Inpatient Facilities and Services* recommends a standard guideline of 4–8 square feet per bed (6, p 81). In other words, if a hospital has four hundred beds, the recommended size of the occupational therapy department would be somewhere between 1,600 and 3,200 square feet.
2. *Cost Containment and Financing of Hospital Construction* (7) recommends that physical medicine departments be allocated 12.36 square feet per bed. So, in the earlier example of the four hundred-bed hospital, this methodology would recommend 4,944 square feet for occupational therapy, physical therapy, or any other rehabilitation service considered a part of the physical medicine department. The problem with methodologies based on square feet per bed is that the amount of space consumed by the outpatient program is not considered.
3. California Department of Health Services regulations (8, p III–2) state, "The minimum floor area for occupational therapy service shall be 28 square meters (300 square feet), no dimension of which shall be less than 4 meters (12 feet)."

The occupational therapy manager should investigate whether guidelines such as these are available in his or her state or locale. A resource that may be helpful in the search is the state health agency or the state department of health.

Considering trend statistics. In analyzing the results of the methodology used, adjustments should be made in the figures to reflect visit trends, that is, the amount of increase or decrease in the number of visits each year. The occupational therapy manager must judge whether these trends will continue for the next three to five years. If they are expected to change significantly, it is important to plan for them, adding to or subtracting from the number of square feet determined by the methodology. It is also important to consider whether new services are to be added in the new space. The new services may cause an increase in

TABLE 4–2
U. S. Department of Health and Human Services Guidelines

Annual Total Visits	Space Range
15,000–25,000	1,750–2,500 sq. ft.
25,000–35,000	2,500–3,500 sq. ft.
35,000 and over	3,500–5,000 sq. ft.

Note: As cited in Boyd/Sobieray Associates Inc: Charleston Area Medical Center, General Division, Medical Rehabilitation Unit, Certificate of Need Application, Case File No. 83-3-1008-H, December 1983, p C-17.

patient/client visits, which should be allowed for in the expected total of square feet. This analysis is a critical step in planning.

Allocating Space

Regardless of the methodology used to determine square footage needs, location will affect the final proposal.

Locating near related services. In a hospital setting, an occupational therapy clinic should be located near the inpatient hospital units that it serves or where transportation of patients can be accomplished as efficiently as possible. Being located close to other rehabilitation services is also helpful. This allows patients who have multiple referrals to schedule appointments one after another and be escorted from service to service. An example is a patient who has been referred for both physical therapy and occupational therapy. Locating near other rehabilitation services can be conducive to the sharing of areas such as reception rooms, offices, conference rooms, and restrooms, thereby allowing more space for patient/client treatment (9). Areas that can be considered for sharing are designated in Table 3.

Creating an impression of convenience. Recently, as competition and consumer choice have begun to affect the health care system, convenience has assumed a new importance. Factors that can create an impression of convenience include parking facilities near the building; short, uncluttered hallways from the parking area to the information desk; and the use of clear directional signs and symbols leading the patient/client to the occupational therapy clinic. It has been determined that when given a choice between two hospitals offering the same services, a potential patient is more likely to choose the hospital with more convenient facilities (10).

Considering special needs. The manager of an occupational therapy department needs to evaluate its program objectives to determine if new services will require the following:

1. Privacy during the teaching of dressing or bathing activities
2. Special ventilation when using craft supplies such as turpentine that may have noxious fumes
3. Soundproofing and isolation from treatment areas, as in the case of a workshop for fabrication of adaptive equipment.

Such needs place certain restrictions on the location of the department (11).

If a community-based occupational therapy clinic is being considered, visibility to potential consumers may become an important factor. If possible, a location should be sought near a community agency or a physician's office serving similar types of patients/clients. Convenient parking and clearly marked signs may also assist in attracting patients/clients.

Writing a Proposal

Administrators may request a written proposal to determine the project's consistency with the organization's long-range plan and to evaluate its financial feasibility. The proposal may also be used in the CON review.

TABLE 4–3
Occupational Therapy Space Allocation

	(NSF)
Primary Activity Areas	
* **Assessment/consultation room	(120)
*Heavy activity area work station	(120)
Light activity area work station	(80)
**ADL kitchen/dining area	(140)
**ADL "kitchenette" unit	(60)
**ADL laundry area	(60)
**ADL bathroom	(80)
**ADL bedroom	(140)
Support Areas	
**Splint room	(120)
Equipment storage (minimum) (10% of the NSF for heavy and light activity areas with 40 NSF minimum)	(40)
*Waiting area (minimum) (15 NSF per person)	(80)
*Reception/control area (minimum) (workstation per clerk)	(80)
*Patient toilet	(50)
**Male patient lockers (minimum) } 8 NSF (full-length) or	
**Female patient lockers (minimum) } 5 NSF (half-length) per locker	
*Stretcher/wheelchair alcove	(25)
*Janitor's closet	(30)
Administrative Areas	
**Director's office	(120)
* **Chief therapist's office	(100)
* **Therapist work area (minimum)	(100-60)
* **Clerical area (minimum) (per person)	(80)
* **Male staff lockers/changing area (minimum) (per person) (8 NSF full length or 5 NSF half length per locker)	
Toilet	(30)
Shower	(20)
* **Female staff lockers/changing area (minimum) (per person) (8 NSF full length or 5 NSF half length per locker)	
Toilet	(30)
Shower	(20)
* **Staff lounge (minimum)	(90)
* **Staff toilet	(30)
* **Conference room (minimum)	(120)
* **Classroom (minimum)	(150)
* **Residents' area (per FTE student)	(50)
* **Students' area (per student)	(35)

* Shared
** Optional
NSF: net square feet, total usable space assignment to specific departmental activity, excludes partitions and internal corridors; ADL: activities of daily living; FTE: full-time equivalent.

Note: From Chi Systems Inc. Source is unpublished updated version of material from *Evaluation and Space Programming Methodology for Physiotherapy, Occupational Therapy, Speech Pathology and Audiology Departments*. Ottawa, Ontario, Canada: Department of National Health and Welfare, Health Services and Promotion Branch, November 1978, p 97.

The development of the proposal may be the responsibility of the planning department, a consultant, or the occupational therapy manager. The proposal should include the following:

1. A brief description of the current occupational therapy program and its objectives.

2. A statement of the need for the project: (a) a brief description of the services to be added or eliminated over the next three to five years; and (b) a chart of past and present visit trends, and trends projected over the next three to five years.

3. An estimate of the amount of gross square feet affected or required. A chart of the existing gross square feet assigned to the occupational therapy department compared with the projected need in gross square feet over the next three to five years would be helpful. The methodology used to determine the need should be explained.

4. An estimate of the cost of the project. This can be figured by multiplying the estimated amount of gross square feet by the estimated cost per square foot. The latter figure varies by geographic location and the amount of renovation necessary. The organization's facility planner, architect, construction manager, or administrator can probably provide it.

5. A list of considerations relating to location.

Planning the Detailed Use of Space

Once approval has been received and a location has been assigned, the next step is planning the best use of the space. The assigned space may not be as large as was requested, its configuration may not be ideal, or its location may not be as accessible as was desired. As a result, compromises may have to be made.

Determining functional areas. A list of the desired functional areas, the equipment to be located in them, and the activities to take place in them should be developed at this time. Desirable functional areas for an occupational therapy program depend on its objectives—for example, whether it is a hospital-based physical disabilities program, a rehabilitation hospital, a mental health program, a private practice, a hand therapy service, a pediatric service, or a service attached to a physician's office. Functional areas to be considered and their importance in four types of programs are indicated in Table 4.

Analyzing the work flow. A well-planned work area will increase efficiency and provide for privacy and comfort. Logical arrangement of the functional areas depends on a thorough analysis of the flow of activities. The work flow of a typical occupational therapy department is diagrammed in Figure 1. This system allows for the smooth movement of patients/clients and staff through the department and decreases confusion and congestion. It also allows for separation of reception, staff activity, and treatment areas.

Placing equipment. Once the functional areas have been determined, making a list of the activities expected to take place in each area will assist in determining the equipment needed and the building implications. A method that can be used to elicit this information is shown in Table 5, using the example of a laundry.

TABLE 4–4
Functional Areas in a Hospital, a Rehabilitation Hospital, a Community Mental Health Agency, and a Pediatric Agency*

Primary Activity Areas	Clinical Setting: Hospital	Rehabilitation Hospital	Mental Health Agency	Pediatric Agency
Activities of Daily Living				
Kitchen and dining area	1**	1	1	3
Housekeeping area	2	1	3	3
Laundry	2	1	1	3
Bathroom	2	1	3	3
Bedroom	3	1	3	3
Fine motor area	1	1	3	2
Sensorimotor/perceptual area	1	1	2	1
Neurodevelopmental activities	1	1	2	1
Wheelchair mobility	2	1	3	2
Hand splinting	1	1	3	2
Group activities	2	3	1	2
Light crafts	2	2	1	3
Power tools	3	1	2	3
Noxious media	3	2	1	3
Evaluation	1	1	1	1
Prosthetics	2	1	3	2
Driving evaluation (may use sensorimotor/perceptual area)	2	1	3	3
Car (for transfers, wheelchair placement)	2	1	3	3
Administrative Areas				
Director's office	1	1	1	1
Supervisor's office	2	2	2	2
Occupational therapy personnel work area	1	1	1	1
Clerical area	1	1	1	1
Staff changing area with locked area for valuables				
Male	3	3	2	3
Female	3	3	2	3
Staff restroom				
Male	1	1	1	1
Female	1	1	1	1
Staff lounge	2	2	2	2
Conference room	1	1	1	1
Classroom	2	2	2	2
Support Areas				
Equipment storage	1	1	1	1
Adaptive equipment fabrication	1	1	3	1
Waiting area	1	1	2	1
Reception	1	1	1	1
Visitors' restroom	1	1	1	1
Patient/client lockers, coat closet	1	1	1	1
Stretcher/wheelchair storage	1	1	3	1
Janitor's closet	1	1	1	1

*The importance of functional areas varies from setting to setting depending on program objectives. These ratings are meant to be used only as guides.

**1 = very necessary; 2 = may be necessary; 3 = may not be necessary

FIGURE 4–1
Flow Diagram for Typical Occupational Therapy Department

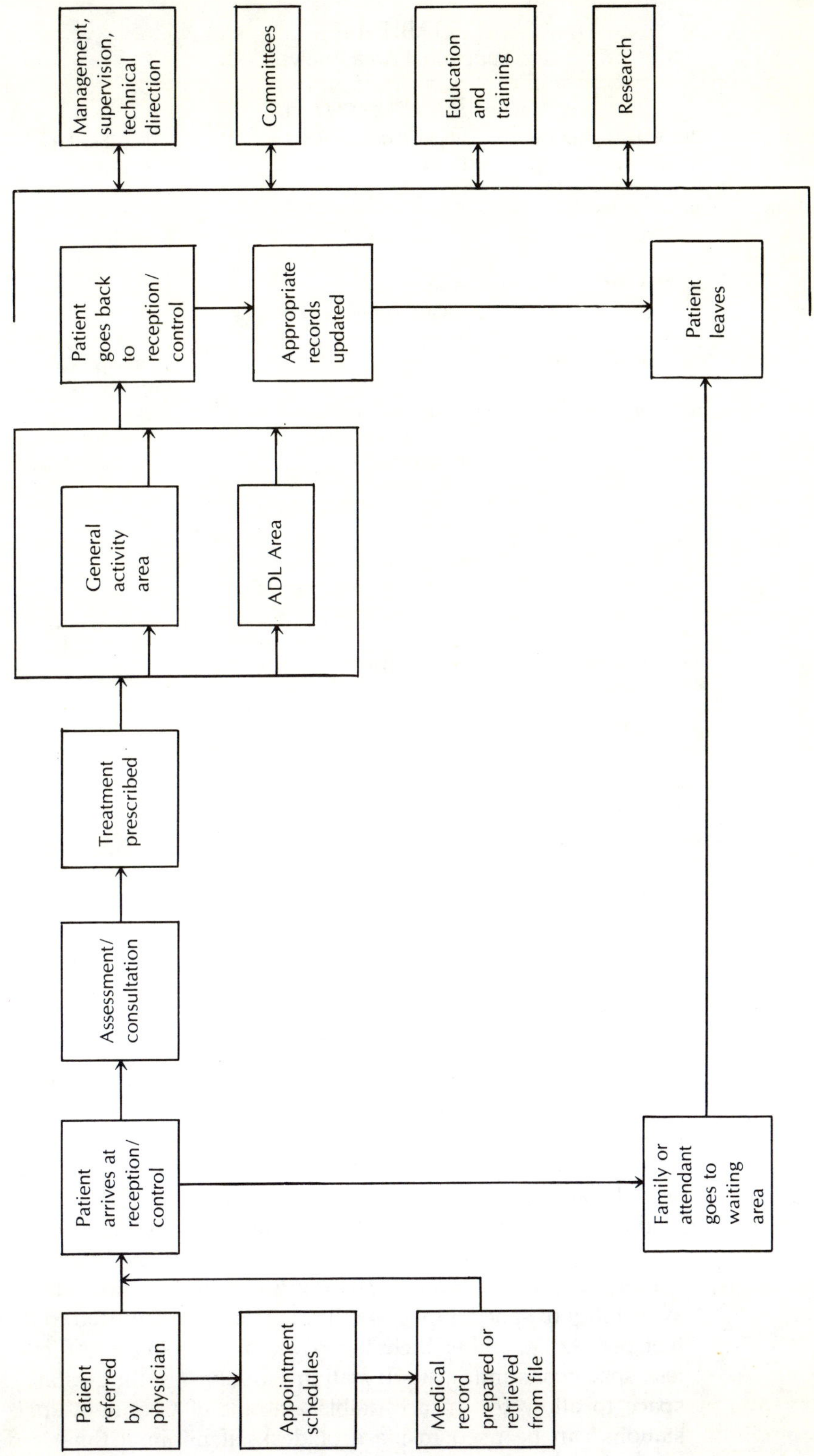

Note: From Chi Systems Inc. Source is unpublished version of material from *Chi Space Planning Workbook*, Ann Arbor, Mich, 1978.

TABLE 4–5
Functional Area Analysis

Example: Laundry

Typical Activities	Characteristics of the Activity	Implications on the Building	Possible Area Contents
Washing Drying Ironing Airing Cleaning	use of electrical equipment	power	trough washing machine dryer clothes horse basket/trolley iron ironing board display facilities storage: • clean and dirty clothes • cleaning agents • cleaning equipment
	use of water	plumbing surface finishes and flooring	
	variable noise level	acoustics	
	indoor/outdoor drying	topography and land surface area relationships: • direct access to outdoor area • ready access to other ADL areas • relationship to: sun, wind and potentially polluting areas	
	potential hazards: • equipment • environment • personal	safety requirements	

Note: From KB Crawford, Editor, *Manual for Planning Occupational Therapy Facilities*, Victoria, Australia: Victorian Association of Occupational Therapists, 1982, p 27. © 1982 by Victorian Association of Occupational Therapists. Reprinted by permission of the publisher.

Equipment to be used by people in wheelchairs will require space around it for wheelchair maneuverability. At least five feet should be allowed for a wheelchair to turn around, pass, and pull up to objects (12).

One way to plan for efficient use of space and placement of equipment is to draw a scale diagram of the rooms, and make paper models of the equipment that will occupy them and the patients/clients and staff who will use them. The equipment models can be arranged within the assigned space to conceptualize the effect of placement (13). Rough sketches of the equipment arrangements will assist in explaining the proposed floor plan to the planning committee and/or the architect.

Designing work stations. The design of work stations depends on the availability of space. Options ranging from one hundred to thirty square feet per staff member include private offices, shared offices, desks, or less space-consuming work stations. In some settings staff share desk space to allow for an acceptable amount of treatment space. Writing stations can be used in place of desks if minimal time is devoted to paperwork, reading, or research and space is required only to complete brief notes. Private or separated writing space tends to improve efficiency because it lessens the opportunity for discussion during work time. It can also assist in alleviating some of the stress often found in a busy occupational therapy department.

Considering safety factors. Safety considerations fall into two categories: structural and organizational (11). Structural considerations are as follows:

1. Tables or mats folding down from the wall must be anchored securely.
2. Electrical outlets must be properly grounded.
3. Sharp corners on upper storage cabinets and tables should be padded and designed to avoid danger of injury.
4. Flooring should be nonslip, particularly around areas that may become wet.
5. Securely anchored grab bars should be provided in bathroom areas used by patients/clients.
6. Emergency call systems should be installed in any isolated clinical areas.

Among the organizational considerations are these:

1. Work areas such as the kitchen should be organized to minimize the distances over which hot containers and substances must travel, from sink to stove, stove to table, sink to oven, and so forth.
2. Work areas should be arranged so that patients/clients are easily visible if a staff member should need to step away.
3. Telephones or other communication systems should be readily accessible in treatment areas for emergencies.
4. An intercom system should be designed to allow for communication without interrupting patient/client treatment.

Designing interiors. The interiors budget includes items such as flooring, wall covering, furniture, and paintings. Making selections in the early stages of planning will allow sufficient time for delivery. Consideration should be given to the atmosphere one is attempting to create. *Calming, safe, organized, homey, clinical,* and *institutional* all might describe the interior design of an occupational therapy clinic. The design may have to conform to an organizational standard that allows little opportunity for uniqueness. However, when possible, the design should appeal to the types of patients/clients treated in the clinic. For example, if a large portion of the caseload is pediatric, a juvenile decor may be desirable.

If consultation with an interior designer is within the budget, this service can be quite helpful. The occupational therapy manager may need to inform the interior designer about accessibility standards (e.g., for table heights) and stress the importance of functional equipment. Durability, ease of cleaning, ease of storage, comfort, safety, and flexibility are important factors.

Working with the Architect

At this point in planning, the occupational therapy manager will most likely be working with an architect. The range of services offered by architectural firms varies. Usually one can expect the architect to develop preliminary working drawings, complete design documents, and produce final drawings. The manager can provide the architect with all the information that has been gathered to date and any preliminary sketches that have been done. The information should include special considerations based on the patient/client population, as well as accessibility standards, particularly if the architect has had no previous experience in designing for people with disabilities (12, 14, 15).

The architect should be aware of federal, state, and local regulations that affect construction and renovation projects. The organization's engineering or maintenance department should have access to information on fire codes, building codes, and state department of health regulations. Organizations that receive federal funding must comply with section 504 of the Rehabilitation Act of 1973, which requires that facilities be accessible to people with disabilities. Standards for barrier-free facilities are incorporated in *American National Standard Specifications for Making Buildings and Facilities Accessible to and Usable by Physically Handicapped People* (16). This manual includes information on clearances, wall and floor textures, heights of water fountains and grab bars, and so forth. Hospitals accredited by voluntary accrediting bodies (e.g., the Joint Commission on Accreditation of Hospitals) must conform to the standards that apply to buildings and safety.

Creating preliminary working drawings. The architect will try to incorporate all ideas into preliminary working drawings, sometimes referred to as a schematic design. An attempt will be made to accommodate all of the needs within the assigned space and to develop a functional arrangement. Opportunities should be provided for careful input and review. If the manager is not accustomed to reading blueprints and interpreting drafting symbols, he or she may want the architect to explain the drawings in detail. The manager should understand thoroughly every aspect of the drawings and make recommendations for modifications before construction begins, because afterward, changes are more difficult and more expensive to make.

Developing a design. During design development the architect will conduct an intensive room-by-room analysis of the physical elements that must be incorporated into every room for it to function at its optimum—elements such as plumbing, lighting, power, acoustics, temperature control, ventilation, flooring, and surface finishes. The result will be a highly detailed set of design documents that quantify and locate every item going into a specific room. These documents will also require careful review.

Producing final working drawings. The information generated in the previous stages will be translated into final working drawings or construction documents. In complex projects the high level of detail from the design development stage may be incorporated through overlay drafting and computer graphics systems. Once again, careful examination will be required to be certain that all the changes have been made (16) (Warren Hendrickson, written communication, November 1984).

Reevaluating cost. Usually an accurate estimate of the facility's cost cannot be made until this time. It should be compared with the estimate in the written proposal, and final approval should be obtained. If the project is in excess of the budget, it will be necessary to put options in order of priority and reevaluate the need for them.

CONSTRUCTION

Once the architect's final working drawings are approved, the project will most likely be supervised by a construction manager. The occupational therapy manager will have little involvement at this time, except to check periodically on progress and communicate all concerns to the construction manager. A timetable for completion of the various stages of the facility should be established and available for review. An agreement should be reached on how to handle any changes, that is, whether the construction manager should be notified of the need for changes as problems are discovered, or whether all requests for changes should be submitted after the construction is completed. To avoid cost overruns, most construction managers prefer as few changes as possible. Each possible change should therefore be considered carefully before a request is made.

When the facility is finished, a list should be made of any aspects of the work that are defective or have not been completed as outlined on the blueprint. This final review must be thorough because it may be the manager's last opportunity to request any changes.

SUGGESTIONS FOR CONSERVING SPACE

If the assigned space does not meet the occupational therapy department's needs and no alternative locations are available, several options should be considered. Placing storage cabinets at higher levels and installing shelves and hooks can help make the maximum use of floor and wall space. Stackable or movable furniture and work stations may also help. For example, a mobile splinting cart that stores splinting supplies and a heating device can be moved as needed to areas where space is available and even be wheeled to a bedside for convenient splinting. Doors that slide require less space than doors that swing open. In some states, however, fire codes may prohibit sliding doors. In many situations, mats or tables can be folded down from a wall for appropriate uses and then folded back up to make space for gross motor activities, group therapy, or conferences.

Decisions can be made as to the appropriateness of multipurpose versus specialized use of space. If necessary, treatment space can be shared by various professional groups. For example, an occupational therapy evaluation room might also be used for speech therapy treatment, or a pediatrics treatment room might be used by both the physical therapy and the occupational therapy department (9). Sharing can pose problems, such as scheduling conflicts. Before such problems interfere with daily operations, it is advisable to develop a system agreeable to the various departments involved.

Another method of conserving space is to perform treatment outside the clinic when feasible. If the setting is realistic, this can often enhance the value of the therapy. For example, a cafeteria or a restaurant can be a site for teaching the social aspects of eating skills once a patient/client has reached an appropriate level of rehabilitation. A homemaking evaluation can be performed in a patient's/client's home, and wheelchair mobility skills can be taught on the sidewalk or in an institution's gift or coffee shop. Ideally, such creative service delivery will be used because of its potential for improving the quality of treatment rather than because of insufficient treatment space. The occupational therapy manager should be aware that this type of programming can negatively influence staff productivity, given the travel and preparation time involved.

Some organizations are leasing off-site space for outpatient programs and using on-site space for growing inpatient programs. The advantages of this approach include the following:

1. A need for additional treatment space can be met without embarking on a building project.
2. A lease is temporary, allowing time to evaluate the growth of a new program before making structural changes.
3. Off-site locations may provide closer parking for patients/clients, sparing them a walk through long institutional corridors.
4. The location-marketing advantages of a community-based clinic are available. The outpatient facility might be strategically located in a part of the community providing convenience and visibility to a target market group. An example would be leasing space for an outpatient orthopedic rehabilitation clinic adjacent to a health club. Patrons of the health club may remember the clinic if they need therapy, and patients/clients of the clinic may want to join the health club as their rehabilitation program progresses.

The disadvantages of this approach include the cost of duplicating work stations and equipment in two locations and the problems encountered in staffing two sites. If the sites are very far apart, staff coverage for absences becomes difficult.

SUMMARY

Planning a new occupational therapy facility involves a number of carefully integrated phases and steps and the participation of many individuals, each having an area of expertise. The occupational therapy manager is asked to embark on an unfamiliar project using a combination of analytical planning, management, and visualization skills, with a result that is permanent and capital intensive.

In preconstruction planning, organizational considerations such as an organization's long-range goals, existing program objectives, consumers' needs, and physicians' referral patterns influence the objectives of the new services, which in turn affect the design of work areas. Space-need methodologies may be used to determine the number of square feet the facility will require and to make a preliminary estimate of the facility's cost. The results obtained from a methodology should be adjusted to reflect trends in patient/client visits. A committee representing various interest groups and different areas of competence might be developed to provide input and assistance in monitoring the project.

The location of an occupational therapy facility depends on factors such as the relationship of the occupational therapy department to other rehabilitation and clinical departments. Convenience, accessibility to the patient/client population, and marketing possibilities are all important. A special consideration in locating a community-based clinic is visibility to potential consumers.

A written proposal may be necessary to gain formal approval of the project. It should describe the current program and objectives, establish the need, provide estimates of the cost and the number of square feet involved, and discuss considerations related to location. Organization administrators may use this document to evaluate the project's consistency with the organization's long-range plans, and its financial feasibility.

In planning the use of space, program objectives determine the types of functional areas that will be needed. All occupational therapy programs require primary activity areas, administrative areas, and support areas. Once the functional areas are identified, equipment needs and building implications are analyzed. The design must take into account work flow, accessibility, staff work areas, and safety considerations. Interior design must be functional and appealing.

The architect will translate the needs expressed by the planning committee and the information compiled by the occupational therapy manager into a series of plans. Preliminary working drawings will be completed, and an opportunity will be provided for review and comment. The comments will then be integrated into design development. Final working drawings will bring planning to a close, and the facility will be ready for construction.

A construction manager will most likely handle the construction. The occupational therapy manager will want to check the timetable periodically and communicate requests for changes, if any, to the construction manager. After construction is finished, a final review of the facility will occur, and a list should be made of any defective work or necessary changes.

When space must be conserved, several strategies may be considered: elevated storage compartments, flexible equipment, sharing of space with other rehabilitation services, and off-site locations for treatment.

References

1. Moore BW: CEOs plan to expand home health, outpatient services. *Hospitals* 59(1):74–77, 1985
2. Hanson EG: Preconstruction planning: A frame for development. *Hospitals* 58(21):97–99, 1984
3. Hayward C: Hospital space planning: What happened to all the magic numbers? *Health Care Strategic Manage,* April:4–12, 1984
4. Boyd/Sobieray Associates Inc. *1980–1985 Summary, Memorial Hospital of South Bend Long Range Plan.* Indianapolis: Boyd/Sobieray Associates Inc, undated
5. American Association for Hospital Consultants. *Health Resources Survey Form* (draft), June 1978
6. Northern Indiana Health Systems Agency Inc: *Criteria and Standards for Acute Inpatient Facilities and Services,* adopted April 22, 1981. South Bend, IN: Northern Indiana Health Systems Agency Inc, 1981
7. *Cost Containment and Financing of Hospital Construction.* Philadelphia: South Jersey Metropolitan Area Summary Report, Hospital Survey Committee, 1974
8. California Department of Health Services, Rehabilitation Supplement Service, Licenses. How to start a rehabilitation unit in your hospital. *California State Regulations,* Division 5, Title 22, Section 3, pp 1–4
9. Buller B: Consolidation raises staff productivity. *Hospitals* 58(17):49–50, 1984
10. MacStravic RES: *Marketing by Objectives for Hospitals.* Rockville, MD: Aspen Systems Corp, 1980
11. Crawford KB, Editor: *Manual for Planning Occu-*

pational Therapy Facilities. Victoria, Australia: Victorian Association of Occupational Therapists, 1982
12. U. S. Architectural and Transportation Barriers Compliance Board: Minimum guidelines and requirements for accessible design. *Federal Register*, August 4, 1982
13. Hickock RJ: *Physical Therapy Administration and Management*, 2nd edition. Baltimore: Williams & Wilkins Co, 1982
14. *Handbook for Design: Specially Adapted Housing*, pamphlet No. 26-13. Veterans Administration, April 1978
15. Cary JR: *How to Create Interiors for the Disabled*. New York: Pantheon Books, 1978
16. *American National Standard Specifications for Making Buildings and Facilities Accessible to and Usable by Physically Handicapped People*, publication No. ANSI A117.1-1980. New York: American National Standards Institute Inc, 1980

Additional Resources

Clipson CW, Wehrer JJ: *Planning for Cardiac Care: A Guide to the Planning and Design of Cardiac Care Facilities*. Ann Arbor, MI: Health Administration Press, 1973

Coppa & Avery Consultants: *Architectural Design for Hospitals: Hospital Planning, Ward Design and Efficiency, Out-Patient, Accident and Emergency Departments*, Architecture Series, bibliography No. A-148. Monticello, IL: Vance Bibliographies, 1979

Directory of Architects for Health Facilities. Chicago: American Hospital Publishing Co, 1983

FitzPatrick TK: *Selected Rehabilitation Facilities in the United States: An Architect's Analysis*. US Government Printing Office, 1971

Guidelines to Functional Programing, Equipping, and Designing Hospital Outpatient and Emergency Activities, US Department of Health, Education and Welfare, publication No. (HRA) 77-4002. US Government Printing Office, 1977

Hoover RM: *General Architectural Principles for Rehabilitation Facilities: A Rehabilitation Unit in a General or Special Hospital: The Comprehensive Rehabilitation Center*. Tallahassee, FL: State Department of Education, Rehabilitation Facilities Section, Florida Office of Vocational Rehabilitation, undated, Ideal Services Series, vol 1

Hospital Design Checklist. Chicago: American Hospital Association, 1965

Hospital Equipment Checklist (Group I—Built-in), rev edition. US Department of Health, Education and Welfare, Public Health Service, Division of Hospital and Medical Facilities, 1963

Koncelik JA: *Designing the Open Nursing Home*. Stroudsburg, PA: Dowden Hutchinson Ross Inc, undated. (Address: 523 Sarah Street, Stroudsburg, PA 18360)

Minimum Requirements of Construction and Equipment for Hospital and Medical Facilities, US Department of Health, Education and Welfare publication No. (HRA) 79-14500. US Government Printing Office, 1978

Porter DR: *Hospital Architecture: Guidelines for Design and Renovation*. Ann Arbor, MI: AUPHA Press, 1982

A Portfolio of Architecture for Health. Chicago: American Hospital Association, 1977

Quarve-Peterson J, Webb LE: *Product Inventory of Hardware, Equipment and Appliances for Barrier-Free Design*, 2nd edition. Minneapolis: National Handicap Housing Institute Inc, 1981

Rea J, Frommelt JJ, MacCoun MD: *Building a Hospital: A Primer for Administrators*. Chicago: American Hospital Publishing Co, 1978

Rehabilitation Units: Minimum Criteria and Guidelines. Lansing, MI: Michigan Department of Public Health, Bureau of Health Facilities, June 1973

Salmon FC, Salmon CF: *Rehabilitation Center Planning: An Architectural Guide*. University Park, PA: The Pennsylvania State University Press, undated

Selected References on Functional Programing, Equipping, and Designing Health Care Facilities, US Department of Health, Education and Welfare publication No. (HRA) 75-4008. US Government Printing Office, 1974

Selection of Architects for Health Facility Projects. Chicago: American Hospital Publishing Co, 1975

Standards Manual for Facilities Serving People with Disabilities. Tucson, AZ: Commission on Accreditation of Rehabilitation Facilities, 1985

Chapter 5

Financial Management

Sandra Macey Laase, MM, OTR/L, FAOTA

The objective of this chapter is to provide the occupational therapy manager with an understanding of the financial environment in which health care organizations operate and a foundation in financial accounting, financial management, and budgeting.

THE FINANCIAL ENVIRONMENT OF TODAY'S HEALTH CARE SYSTEM

Three major issues in the health care industry have had a tremendous impact on financial management: cost, reimbursement, and competition.

Cost

As noted in Chapter 1, Table 1, health care expenditures are currently about $400 billion annually and consume about 11 percent of the gross national product (GNP). That table also shows the steady increase in health care's share of the GNP since 1965. Another method of illustrating the growth is to compare increases in health care expenditures with increases in the Consumer Price Index (CPI). For example, between 1950 and 1978, personal health care expenditures rose 1,443 percent while the overall CPI increased 171 percent (1).

Figure 1 shows the actual and projected health care expenditures for

---

Currently the treasurer of The American Occupational Therapy Association, Sandra Laase was a management consultant for one of the big eight accounting firms for about five years. Earlier she held various administrative and supervisory positions.

FIGURE 5–1
Actual and Projected National Health Care Expenditures in Percents, Selected Years 1965–1990 by Provider

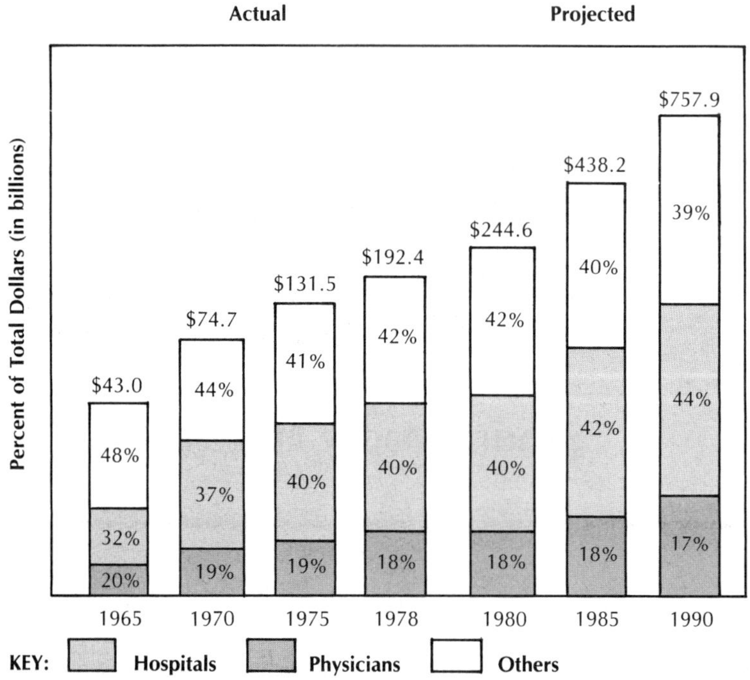

*Percents have been rounded to whole numbers.

Note: Data from BB Longest, Jr: Management Practices for the Health Professional, 3rd edition. Reston, VA: Reston Publishing Company Inc, 1984, pp 8, 10–11. © 1984 by Reston Publishing Co, Inc. Reprinted, with adaptations, by permission of the publisher.

selected years from 1965 to 1990 and the percent according to provider—hospital, physician, and other. The escalation in health care costs has generally been attributed to inflation, increased use of services, and greater intensity of care. Longest (2) cites changes in the system as another causative factor. Beck (3) believes that historically, two-thirds of annual hospital cost increases have been due to normal inflation and one-third to new and better services required to treat more acutely ill patients.

In Figure 1 it can be seen that approximately 60 percent of all health care expenditures go to hospitals and physicians, with about two-thirds of that for hospital care and one-third for physicians' services. This fact accounts for efforts in the past decade by government, insurance carriers, and business to contain hospital costs, encourage less expensive but appropriate alternative care, and limit the growth in physicians' fees. Medicare now pays for inpatient hospital care on a prospective basis; that is, hospitals receive a predetermined fixed amount for each discharged patient, according to a schedule of 470 Diagnosis Related Groups (DRGs). At least one Medicaid program has adopted the concept of prospective payment, and other Medicaid programs and some insurance companies are considering it. Several states have enacted rate-setting legislation that requires the disclosure, the review, or the approval of hospital rates and/or budgets. Prospective payment systems and rate-setting legislation increase the financial risks that hospitals assume and create a strong incentive for them to determine and control their costs of providing patient care services.

Insurance companies have revised incentives in their policies to promote the use of lower-cost providers and decrease unnecessary care. Some have established health maintenance organizations (HMOs), contributing significantly to the rapid growth of the HMO industry in recent years (4).

Business has launched a three-pronged offensive to decrease the cost of health care. On a local level, business leaders have become trustees of hospitals. On a regional and national level, business has stimulated the development of coalitions to combat the cost problem, for example, by gathering data or exerting influence. These coalitions variously comprise representatives from business, labor, government, health planning agencies, third-party payers, and the health care industry. Also, employers have spawned preferred provider organizations (PPOs), whereby they and health care providers have entered into contracts covering services, conditions of service, and price (Chapter 18 describes PPOs in more detail). The issues for financial management here are knowing the true costs of providing services and avoiding violations of the Sherman Antitrust Act.

Reimbursement

To appreciate the complexity of reimbursement, one has to understand cost shifting. "Cost shifting occurs when a hospital must increase prices charged to all payers [billed charges] to make up for shortfalls in reimbursement from some payers" (5, p 101). Approximately two-thirds of health care expenditures are paid for by third parties—government (Medicare and Medicaid), Blue Cross/Blue Shield, commercial insurers, and so forth. The remainder comes directly from individuals, that is, self-payers (2). Medicare and Medicaid pay for "reasonable" costs, which are not the hospital's billed charges, that is, the prices the hospital charges for its services. In essence, the government "commands a 'discount'" (5, p 101) because of its buying power and influence as the largest third-party payer. The effect of cost shifting is felt only by those who pay billed charges—primarily commercial insurers and self-payers (3).

In many cases Blue Cross and even some HMOs with a major share of the market receive hospital discounts (5). Cost shifting is significant when one considers that the government and Blue Cross account for more than one-half of third-party payments (2).

Figure 2 illustrates the magnitude of cost shifting by the government from 1975 through 1982, during which time cost shifting increased 427 percent. Those who pay the billed charges have complained that the cost shifting is, in effect, a hidden tax, and one that increases in indirect

FIGURE 5–2
Cost Shifting by Government

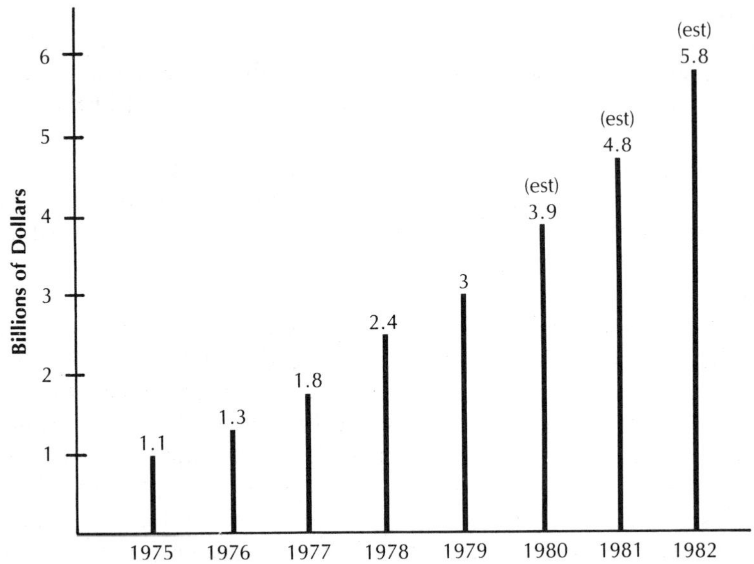

Note: Data for 1975 through 1981 reported in JA Meyer, WR Johnson, S Sullivan, *Passing the Health Care Buck: Who Pays the Hidden Cost?* Washington, DC: American Enterprise Institute for Public Policy Research, 1983, p 8, © 1983. Reprinted by permission of the publisher. Data for 1982 reported in HW Long: The future of financing decisions in the health care industry, in *Health Care Financial Management in the 1980s*, JB Silvers, WN Zelman, CN Kahn III, Editors, Ann Arbor, MI: AUPHA Press, 1983, p 44.

proportion to their share of a hospital's market (6). Johnson and Aquilina (5) discuss how this practice results in a series of cost shifts that ultimately affect almost everyone (see Figure 3). The concept of cost shifting can be applied to comparable reimbursement situations in health care organizations other than hospitals.

One measure of a hospital's financial success is its ability to maintain an adequate cash flow. This has become increasingly problematic as commercial insurers have extended their payment times.

Hospitals have responded in a variety of ways to the cost-shifting dilemma. Price increases have generally been driven by the aim of obtaining as much reimbursement as possible. Many hospitals have employed reimbursement specialists or contracted for such expertise. Efforts have been made to reduce costs and increase productivity without jeopardizing the quality of care. A more effective popular strategy has been independent corporate reorganization or affiliation with a multihospital system (3). The purposes are to maximize reimbursement, to protect a hospital's assets, to increase access to capital markets, and to decrease expense, risk, and exposure of marketing plans (3). Multihospital systems also benefit from reduced costs because of economies of scale.

FIGURE 5–3
The Cost-Shifting Chain

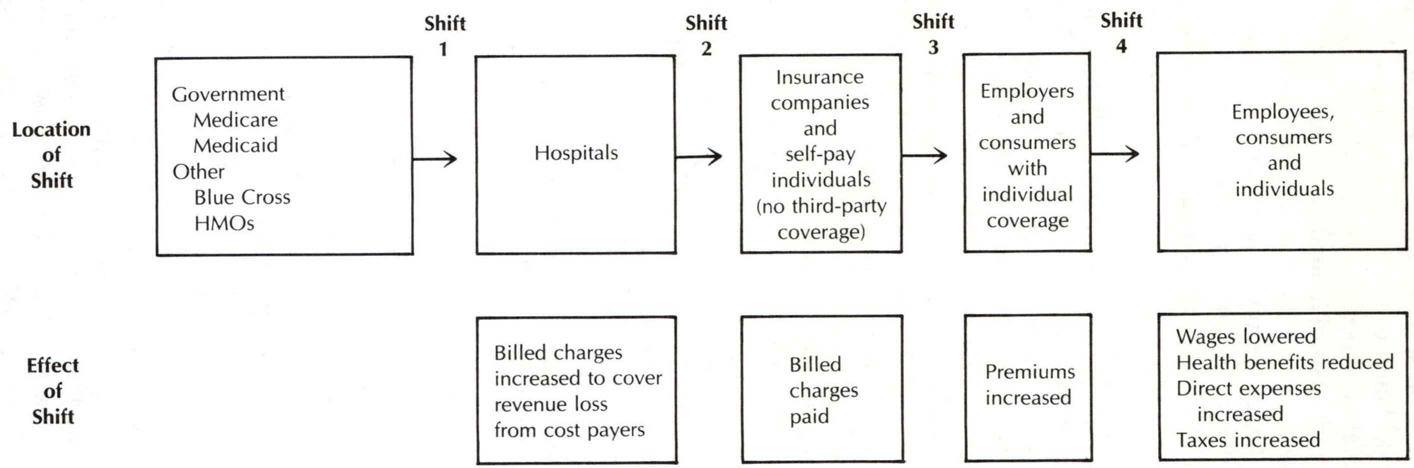

Shift 1: Government, Blue Cross, and HMOs pay less than charges and shift costs to hospitals.

Shift 2: Hospitals shift costs to other payers, that is, insurance companies and consumers with no third-party coverage.

Shift 3: Insurance companies shift costs to employers and consumers with individual coverage. Self-pay individuals pay more than cost payers or are unable to pay and contribute to hospitals' bad debt.

Shift 4: Employees, consumers, and individuals actually bear the burden through—
- Lower wages (employers pay more for insurance and have less available for salary increases)
- Reduced health care benefits
- Increased out-of-pocket expenses (because of greater coinsurance, higher deductibles, and higher prices)
- Increased taxes to support Medicare and Medicaid.

Note: From AN Johnson, D Aquilina: The cost shifting issue, *Health Affairs* 1(4), 1982, p 103. © 1982 by the People-to-People Health Foundation Inc. Reprinted, with adaptations, by permission of the publisher.

Although Medicare reimbursement for hospital inpatients has changed from a retrospective to a prospective basis, the effects of cost shifting remain because the calculation of the fixed amount per DRG uses historical cost data. Therefore, hospitals are faced with additional challenges: to control the unit costs of individual services and to control the length of stay and the use of ancillary services for acute inpatient care (7). Meeting these challenges requires financial officers to determine the cost and the profitability of product lines. This entails intensive interaction between financial officers and managers of clinical departments.

Competition

Competition manifests itself in a multitude of ways that are not mutually exclusive. On one level there is competition for patients/clients. Mistarz (8) contends that hospital diversification is an economic necessity, if hospitals are not to be left with only inpatient care, an increasingly costly service. Depending on the nature of their diversification, hospitals compete among themselves and with a variety of alternative providers for ambulatory care (e.g., ambulatory surgery centers, emergency care centers, and ancillary service group practice), aftercare (e.g., home health agencies and hospices), and health promotion programs (e.g., nutrition and exercise centers and smoking clinics). These competitors influence patterns of service delivery (hospital referrals and admissions) and may ultimately affect the financial status of hospitals.

How hospitals diversify also varies. Some plan and implement new or expanded health services that may or may not involve corporate reorganization. Others develop a network of cooperative relationships with other hospitals and/or alternative providers (8). Joint ventures between hospitals and physicians have become increasingly popular. Other hospitals have joined or been acquired by multihospital systems, either not-for-profit or investor owned. From 1970 to 1980 there was a 204 percent increase in the number of these systems (9).

On another level there has been increased competition for scarce resources, including personnel, philanthropic contributions, and capital. Shortages of professional personnel have contributed to the growth of contract management. With regard to philanthropic contributions and capital, hospitals compete not only with each other and alternative health care providers but also with non-health-industry entities. Not-for-profit health care organizations are using sophisticated marketing techniques and computer technology to gain a share of the philanthropic dollar. Not only is capital limited and less available from traditional sources, but also it is expensive (2). There is a growing fear among not-for-profit hospitals that they will not have access to capital.

Still another level of competition comes from alternative delivery systems, such as HMOs and PPOs. Hospitals' referral and admission patterns may be affected. However, these alternative delivery systems can take many forms. For instance, HMOs may be hospital sponsored or insurance company sponsored, and PPOs may be offered through commercial insurers, Blue Cross/Blue Shield, individual hospitals, or groups of hospitals and physicians.

Increased competition has stimulated a thrust to decrease costs and improve productivity, ideally without sacrificing quality of care. The objective is to price services competitively and gain a larger share of the market. In the case of hospitals competing for ambulatory services, for instance, this is crucial but difficult because of hospitals' past policies of pricing ancillary services to subsidize inpatient care (8). Consequently, many hospitals find their ambulatory services overpriced.

To cut costs, some hospitals have contracted management to a management firm or a larger hospital. This arrangement provides access to specialized resources not otherwise available. Hospitals have also contracted for support services (e.g., laundry, dietary, housekeeping) and clinical services. From 1980 to 1981 the number of contracted inpatient occupational therapy departments increased 45 percent, from 278 to 402 (10).

The health care industry as a whole has become increasingly business oriented. Sloan and Vraciu (9) attribute this to more demand for capital, less reliance on philanthropy, more attention to competition, and a greater understanding of the necessity for profit margins in the long-term financing of any organization. Given that health care organizations have traditionally operated on a small margin of profit, if any (1), managers with business skills can make significant contributions to the health care industry.

Another issue related to competition is the role of the proprietary organization in health care. Supporters of proprietary organizations point to such strengths as a more efficient use of resources and a stronger financial status. Critics charge that they provide only profitable services, do not treat their share of nonpaying patients, and may not adequately deal with quality-of-care issues. At least one study (9) has found that ownership (investor owned versus not-for-profit) is not relevant to a hospital's scope of services, treatment of nonpaying patients, and economic performance. This may very well be a value issue.

EVOLUTION OF FINANCIAL MANAGEMENT

"Hospital finance has evolved from a primitive function of bookkeeping/accounting to a role in which it exerts a major influence in the management of hospital assets and the allocation of scarce resources" (11, p 1). The historical perspective that follows is adapted from Beck (11). Prior to the late 1960s, when Medicare and its requirement for cost reports were introduced, hospital finance was not very sophisticated and did not need to be. Successful fund-raising drives and philanthropy were prevalent. Prices were raised annually by the administrator.

Medicare and a series of other government initiatives to control hospital costs changed this situation. Medicaid also required cost reports. Although states administer their own programs, they are generally based on Medicare reimbursement principles. In 1972 the Economic Stabilization Act imposed wage and price controls on health care as well as other industries. In 1977 President Carter proposed the Hospital Cost Containment Act. Although it was not passed, it facilitated the American Hospital Association's Voluntary Effort campaign, which urged hospitals to reduce costs and control price increases.

The next federal government proposal, System of Hospital Uniform Reporting (SHUR), was also rejected on the basis that standardizing hospital financial accounting and reporting would be costly and, because of institutional differences, would still not enable comparisons among hospitals. In the meantime many states passed cost containment and rate-setting legislation. Then, in April 1983, the Social Security Amendments (Public Law 98-21), mandating the Medicare Prospective Payment System (PPS) for hospitals, were signed into law.

As a result of the increasing complexity of health care finance, hospitals began to establish the position of chief financial officer. The chief financial officer reports directly to the chief executive officer and is responsible for managing financial operations. His responsibilities include assessment of reimbursement case mix, length of stay, diagnostic categories treated, services provided, and related areas. As the principal financial advisor to the CEO, the CFO must fully understand the hospital's mission and goals, and facilitate their achievement. The qualifications of the CFO differ from those of earlier counterparts, the controller or chief accountant. The CFO needs a broader perspective and diverse skills and experience in order to provide the leadership and cooperation that is required to meet the demands of the position successfully. Development and oversight of the budget is often considered the chief financial officer's most important function (1). To accomplish this, the chief financial officer coordinates the work of the department or division directors and other administrators to ensure that the organization meets its mission and goals in a cost effective manner. This task is complicated because, as Beck (11) points out, many decisions in health care organizations involve social, political, and humanitarian—as well as economic—considerations. Table 1 illustrates both the nature of financial planning activities and the close relationship among finance, strategic planning, and marketing. The CFO also directs patient accounting and financial accounting and establishes internal controls that ensure the reliability of the organization's financial

TABLE 5–1
Financial Planning in the Strategic Planning Process

Strategic Planning Tasks	Financial Planning Tasks and Analyses
1. Preparation of initial mission statement	Develop initial financial goals
2. Internal analysis	Evaluate financial position against initial goals • Rate of return on equity and/or growth in assets • Internal sources and uses of capital
3. External analysis	Evaluate external financial environment • Financial position and objectives of competing and complementary organizations • Growth and availability of sources of revenue • Growth and availability of external sources of capital

4. Assessment of present position	Assess current financial position • Comparative financial performance • Share of available revenue received • Access to and use of available capital
5. Revision of mission statement and development of goals	Revise financial goals
6. Development and evaluation of alternative strategies	Determine financial impact of alternative strategies • On financial goals • On the use of capital To do this, • Estimate capital and operating budgets • Estimate impact on utilization, revenues, and expenses
7. Setting of strategies and objectives	Set financial objectives • Determine what movement toward achieving the financial goals should occur each year • Set targets for the acquisition and use of working and long-term capital
8. Development of contingency plans	Develop a financial contingency plan • Set financial "trigger points" • Determine financial consequences of alternative strategies • Investigate alternative sources of working and long-term capital
9. Development and implementation of program and operational plans	Develop program and operational budgets • Develop a capital budget • Evaluate working capital needs • Prepare departmental and program budgets • Develop a financing plan • Set rates and estimate reimbursement
10. Development of evaluation, monitoring, and control system	Establish a financial control system • Implement management by objectives • Determine and evaluate program and department budget variances • Monitor achievement of financial objectives • Monitor capital budgets
11. Revision and implementation of contingency plans	Revise financial plan and implement contingency plan • Reassess assumptions about the external financial environment • Evaluate achievement of financial objectives

Note: From R Kropf and JA Greenberg, *Strategic Analysis for Hospital Management*, Rockville, MD: Aspen Systems Corp, 1984, pp 260–261. © 1984 by Aspen Systems Corp. Reprinted by permission of the publisher.

records and protect the organization's assets. The CFO may be responsible for financial data processing and admitting.

RELEVANCE TO THE OCCUPATIONAL THERAPY MANAGER

As a member of the management team, the occupational therapy manager has a responsibility to perform the functions of planning, organizing, directing, controlling, evaluating, and communicating. Knowledge of financial management is important to successful performance of these functions for three reasons:

1. Certain financial tools and techniques, such as budget preparation and variance analysis, are needed to plan programs and monitor performance.
2. A knowledge of the organization's financial health is critical in program planning and budget preparation and justification. It is also necessary for responsible operations.
3. A mind-set must be developed for both quality of care and cost/reimbursement considerations.

Financial management must be an integral part of the occupational therapy manager's repertoire of skills. Following are examples of questions the manager should raise:

- Are occupational therapy programs in concert with organizational goals and objectives?
- Are occupational therapy resources allocated in the best possible way to address both quality of care and cost factors?
- Are there more cost-effective ways of doing things?
- What are the risks involved (financial and nonfinancial) in alternative courses of action?

BASIC ACCOUNTING[1]

The ability to relate plans to budgets, and budgets to performance, is critical in today's environment. To do so, the occupational therapy manager must be able to communicate in the language of finance and accounting.

Accounting and financial management differ. Accounting is "the art of collecting, summarizing, analyzing, reporting, and interpreting, in monetary terms, information" about an organization (1, pp 7, 9). Financial management is "the art both of obtaining the funds which [an organization] needs in the most economic manner and of making the optimal use of those funds" to achieve the organization's short- and long-term objectives (1, p 9). Financial management tools and techniques are used to determine the cost implications of both capital investment and operating decisions. Information generated by the accounting system is used in making financial decisions. Therefore, it is important to understand the accounting principles that guide the collection and the presentation of financial data.

[1]Material in this section is adapted from Berman HJ, Weeks LE, *The Financial Management of Hospitals*, 5th edition. Ann Arbor, MI: Health Administration Press, 1982.

A distinction needs to be made between financial accounting and managerial accounting. Financial or general accounting provides financial statements or reports for external use, for example, by government agencies, bankers, and third-party payers. These financial statements must conform to generally accepted accounting principles.

Managerial or management accounting uses information from the financial accounting system and other cost information to prepare reports for specific decision-making purposes internal to the organization. These reports assist managers in operating more effectively and efficiently, making nonroutine decisions, and formulating major policies and plans. Managerial accounting is totally responsive to the internal needs of an organization.

Basic Financial Accounting Concepts[1]

The following basic accounting concepts apply to both for-profit and not-for-profit organizations.

Entity concept. For accounting purposes a business or an organization is an entity capable of taking economic action. An entity is assumed to be a going concern that will continue to function indefinitely.

Transactions concept. All transactions of an entity must be included in accounting records and reports so that financial statements accurately reflect the entity's financial condition. Summarizing transactions is an acceptable practice. To the extent possible, accounting transactions should be based on objectively determined facts (e.g., documents).

Cost valuation concept. An item's historical cost, or the price paid to acquire it, is the basis for valuation of an asset or a liability. This is in contrast to its replacement cost or market value.

Double entry concept. Accounting records should reflect each transaction, that is, the changes in assets, liabilities, and/or equity. Every transaction requires at least two entries. Debit entries must balance credit entries.

Conservatism concept. When opinion and judgment are used in valuing assets or estimating income, conservative estimates should be made.

Consistency concept. Consistent accounting principles should be used so that current accounting reports can be compared with those of prior years. This does not preclude changes to improve or update accounting principles; prior years' reports can be restated to reflect these changes.

Full disclosure concept. Significant data must be accurately and completely reflected in accounting reports. Information that could influence the decisions of the users of financial statements should be included and stated clearly.

Materiality concept. Accounting reports should reflect significant activities so that the effort and the cost of recording them are justified. Materiality depends on the relative amount of a transaction, its importance to the total operation, and the effects of its exclusion (e.g., incorrect or misleading conclusions).

[1]The material in this section is drawn from two sources (1, 12).

Accounting Principles and Definitions[1]

Accrual basis of accounting. Generally accepted accounting principles require that financial statements be prepared on the accrual basis. Revenue, deductions from revenue, and losses are recorded in the period in which they are realized (earned), and expenses are recorded in the period in which they are incurred, regardless of the flow of cash. This permits an accurate assessment of net income or excess of revenue over expenses for each accounting period.

Revenue. The *revenue* of a health care organization consists mainly of the value of all the services rendered to patients/clients. Revenue is identified by the organizational unit (department) that produced it.

Deductions from revenue. There are three basic types of *deductions from revenue* (resulting in payment of less than full charges): charity service (a requirement of the Hill-Burton Act or a matter of organizational policy), bad debts (uncollectable amounts), and contractual allowances (differences between charges and contractual rates, as with Medicare and Medicaid). In addition, as a matter of policy, organizations may reduce charges for employees and not bill immaterial amounts if the cost of doing so would exceed the revenue received.

Expenses. *Expenses* are expired costs that have been incurred in exchange for a good or a service that will not produce future revenue. Expenses are charged to the organizational unit (department) that incurred them.

Matching revenues and expenses. Expenses related to a particular service are matched against revenues derived from it in each accounting period. Also, deductions from revenue are matched against gross revenue. This enables each organizational unit to evaluate its performance and to plan and control its activities more effectively.

Capital assets. Acquisitions or improvements that cost over a certain amount and have an expected life of more than one or two years are *capital assets*. These include buildings, fixed and major movable equipment, land, and land improvements. All except land can be depreciated.

Depreciation. *Depreciation* enables the use of capital assets to be allocated to a particular reporting period for purposes of matching revenues and expenses. There are three methods of depreciation: straight line, sum-of-years' digits, and double declining balance. The latter two are often referred to as accelerated depreciation, because a higher allocation of costs is taken in the early years. Depreciation is usually "booked"; it does not involve an outflow of cash. However, third-party-payer requirements or incentives cause many health care organizations to "fund" depreciation, that is, to transfer cash to a restricted account (1, 13).

Fund accounting. Fund accounting requires an organization to segregate its resources, obligations, and capital balances into separate accounts, or funds, based on legal restrictions and administrative and organizational requirements. Each fund has its particular purpose and its own self-balancing accounting records (i. e., debits equaling credits). Interfund transfers are handled as if they involved separate entities. An organization's financial statements generally do not show individual fund

[1]The material in this section is adapted from several sources (1, 11–16).

accounts. However, changes are reflected in the statement of changes in fund balances.

Fund accounting is common in government and not-for-profit organizations and is recommended by the American Hospital Association (AHA) for hospitals. There are two basic types of funds: unrestricted and restricted. The unrestricted fund is called the general or operating fund and is used to account for the resources, the obligations, and the capital of day-to-day operations. The AHA categorizes restricted funds as follows: endowment fund, plant replacement and expansion fund, and specific-purpose funds (12).

Chart of accounts. A chart of accounts is a listing of the titles of all asset, liability, capital, expense, and revenue accounts, each with a corresponding numeric code. Its purpose is to facilitate the recording and the reporting of financial information about an organization.

The AHA no longer recommends that hospitals adopt a uniform chart of accounts because of the variety of their organizations and different needs. The AHA methodology, which is still a useful guide, enables financial reports to be generated by responsibility centers (e.g., an occupational therapy department) and functional areas (e.g., rehabilitation services that may include occupational therapy, physical therapy, and speech pathology). Each responsibility center has a natural classification of expenses as subaccounts: salaries and wages, employee benefits, professional fees, medical and surgical supplies, nonmedical and nonsurgical supplies, purchased services, utilities, other direct expenses, depreciation, and rent (12, 15). A responsibility center is the organizational unit(s) over which a manager has control.

Financial Statements[1]

Generally accepted accounting principles require that organizations annually prepare three financial statements: a balance sheet, an income statement (a statement of revenue and expenses), and a statement of changes in financial position. The general principles governing the preparation of these statements are the same for not-for-profit and for-profit entities, but format and terminology differ somewhat. If an organization uses fund accounting, it may also prepare a statement of changes in fund balances or, in some cases, issue a combined report, statements of revenue and expenses and changes in fund balances.

All financial statements are prepared using data from the same accounting system and are therefore interrelated. Financial statements measure either levels (financial status on a particular date) or flows (changes in financial activity occurring during a specified period) (13, 16). The balance sheet is a level statement that reports the status of each account of the organization on a particular date. The income statement is a flow statement that shows the movement of revenue and expenses into and out of the organization during a specified period, usually 12 months. The statement of changes in financial position, also a flow statement, summarizes all of the balance sheet changes arising from the flow of resources into and out of the organization during a specified period,

[1]Material in this section is drawn from references 13, 14, 16–18.

FIGURE 5–4a
The T-Account

Debit side	Credit side

FIGURE 5–4b
T-Accounts Showing Purchase of Equipment

Cash		Equipment	
	$20,000	$20,000	

FIGURE 5–4c
T-Accounts Showing Purchase of Equipment

Cash		Short-Term Loan Payable		Equipment	
	$10,000		$10,000	$20,000	

usually 12 months (17). Annual reports are prepared using the organization's fiscal year, which may or may not correspond to the calendar year.

The numbers that are entered in the balance sheet and the income statement are the result of numerous accounting transactions. These transactions can be depicted using T-accounts, which show debits on the left side and credits on the right side (see Figure 4a). An increase in assets is entered on the left side. A reduction in assets is entered on the right side. Likewise, an increase in liabilities and fund balance (or equity) is entered on the right side, and a decrease on the left. Therefore, a *debit* represents either an increase in an asset account or a decrease in a liability or fund balance (or equity) account. A *credit* represents either a decrease in an asset account or an increase in a liability or fund balance (or equity) account.

For example, an organization purchases a $20,000 piece of equipment with cash. Figure 4b illustrates how the T-accounts reflect this transaction: Equipment is debited and cash is credited. If the organization financed the purchase with $10,000 in cash and a $10,000 short-term loan, the effect on the relevant T-accounts would be as shown in Figure 4c: Equipment would be debited and cash and short-term loan payable would be credited. In both these transactions the total of debits equals the total of credits. Each accounting transaction involves at least one debit entry and one credit entry. These two elements characterize *double-entry bookkeeping.*

Balance sheet. The balance sheet is a statement of an organization's assets, liabilities, and fund balance. In for-profit organizations the fund balance section is replaced by shareholders' or owners' equity. The total

FIGURE 5–5
Balance Sheet
As of December 31, 1990
(in thousands of dollars)

Assets			Liabilities and Fund Balance	
Current Assets			**Current Liabilities**	
Cash		$ 900	Accounts payable	$ 300
Accounts receivable (net)		1,250	Short-term loan payable	500
Inventories		50	Mortgage payable, current	200
Prepaid expenses		100		
Total current assets		2,300	**Total current liabilities**	1,000
Fixed Assets			**Long-Term Liabilities**	
Land and buildings	6,000		Mortgage payable, long-term	2,800
Equipment	2,000			
		8,000	**Total Liabilities**	3,800
Less accumulated depreciation		2,500	**Fund Balance**	4,000
Total fixed assets		5,500		
Total Assets		$7,800	**Total Liabilities and Fund Balance**	$7,800

amount of the section remains the same, but the accounts differ. The date on the balance sheet is the last day of the period covered by the income statement. Often the prior year's figures for the same date are included for comparative purposes.

Figure 5 illustrates the format and some representative accounts on the balance sheet of a not-for-profit organization. As the name implies, there is a basic accounting equation: assets = liabilities + fund balance (or equity). Usually assets are presented on the left side of the balance sheet, liabilities and fund balance (or equity) on the right. Assets are financed either by sources outside the organization (that is, liabilities) or by the organization itself (that is, fund balance or equity) (13).

Current assets are those that are expected to be converted into cash within a year. Current asset accounts include cash, short-term investments, accounts receivable, inventories, and prepaid expenses. *Cash* represents funds on hand in cash and in savings and checking accounts. Cash and *short-term investments* (e.g., government securities and high-grade commercial paper) are sometimes combined into one account. *Accounts receivable* represent the amounts due from customers for prior services or goods. In the health care industry the bulk of accounts receivable is derived from patients/clients. Other sources may include rents from a physician's office building and fees from a parking facility. Contractual allowances and allowances for doubtful accounts are contra accounts to accounts receivable and contain reserves for charity, courtesy, contractual allowances, and bad debts. A *contra account* is always paired with a parent account. It is always presented as a reduction from the asset or equity parent account. In Figure 5, the net amount of accounts receivable is shown; it is derived from gross accounts receivable minus contractual allowances and allowances for doubtful accounts. *Inventories* include medical, surgical, nonmedical, and nonsurgical supplies. *Prepaid expenses* are expenditures made for future services, for example, insurance.

Fixed assets, also called *property, plant, and equipment*, are permanent or capital assets of an organization. In Figure 5, they are shown at their historical cost less *accumulated depreciation* (a contra account). Net fixed assets are shown at $5.5 million, their *book value*.

Current liabilities are obligations to be paid by an organization within one year. Current liability accounts include accounts payable, notes payable, current maturities of long-term debt, and accrued expenses. *Accounts payable* represent the amounts an organization is obligated to pay for the goods and the services it has received. *Notes payable* include short-term debt obligations. *Current maturities of long-term debt* represent the amount of principal, not the total amount of payment (principal and interest), that will be paid on long-term debt within the year. *Accrued expenses* are obligations that result from prior operations, for example, vacation pay, rent, and interest. An organization's *working capital* is its current assets minus its current liabilities.

Long-term liabilities are obligations that extend longer than one year. They include *mortgages, bonds,* and *capital leases.*

Fund balance represents the difference between assets and liabilities. Increases in this account usually result from *contributions* or *earnings* (18). In not-for-profit organizations a distinction is usually not made. The fund balance consists of the excess-of-revenue-over-expenses figure from the income statement and donated funds (endowments, grants, etc.). In for-profit organizations, *equity* accounts include *retained earnings, common stock, preferred stock,* and *paid-in capital*. The *retained earnings* account contains the after-tax earnings of prior years, minus dividends paid. The other equity accounts reflect contributions.

The fund balance or equity account is not synonymous with or related to cash available (16, 18). In fact, fund balance and equity accounts represent claims on assets and reflect past transactions; they do not contain any funds. In most cases the cash balance will be much less than the fund balance (14).

Income statement. The income statement shows revenue and expense flows and net income earned during a specified period. That is, it explains how an organization's financial position changed through operations. In for-profit organizations this statement is also known as a profit and loss statement. Not-for-profit organizations may refer to it as a statement of revenue and expenses. In such organizations, net income is called excess of revenue over expenses, or surplus (or deficit).

The accounting conventions governing the recognition and the matching of revenues and expenses are used in preparing this statement. Only resource inflows (revenues) and resource outflows (expenses) are shown on the income statement. Exchanges in types of assets or between assets and liabilities are not reflected (13). For example, collection of an accounts receivable is an exchange of an accounts receivable asset for a cash asset. Payment of a short-term loan is an exchange of a reduction in a cash

FIGURE 5–6
Income Statement
For the Year Ended December 31, 1990
(in thousands of dollars)

Operating Revenue		
Gross patient revenue		
Inpatient	$1,400	
Outpatient	900	
		$2,300
Deductions from revenue		200
Net patient revenue		2,100
Other operating revenue		300
Total operating revenue		2,400
Operating Expenses		
Salaries and wages	1,400	
Supplies	300	
Depreciation	160	
Interest	40	
Other	100	
Total operating expenses		2,000
Income (loss) from operations		400
Nonoperating Revenue		
Contributions	40	
Investment income	100	
Total nonoperating revenue		150
Excess of Revenue over Expenses		$ 550

asset for a reduction in a short-term loan payable liability. These transactions are reflected in the balance sheet.

Figure 6 illustrates the format and presents a representative income statement of a not-for-profit hospital. In hospitals, *operating revenue* comes from two sources: patient care and other services that occur in the provision of patient care, for example, cafeteria sales to employees, silver recycling sales, and parking fees from employees and visitors. The corresponding accounts for these two sources are *gross patient revenue* and *other operating revenue*. Gross patient revenue shows inpatient and outpatient revenue. *Deductions from revenue* (e.g., contractual allowances) are subtracted from gross patient revenue to yield *net patient revenue*. Other operating revenue is added to net patient revenue to obtain the *total operating revenue*.

The *operating expenses* consist of assets that are consumed and liabilities that are increased in the provision of services related to hospital operations. The difference between total operating revenue and *total operating expenses* indicates the hospital's *income (loss) from operations*.

Nonoperating revenue is derived from activities that are not related to patient care and normal hospital operations. Figure 6 shows two sources: contributions and investment income. The contributions are unrestricted. Restricted contributions are taken directly into the fund balance because they are not freely available to finance operations (14, 18). Gains or losses on disposal of capital items, and rental of facilities not used in operations are other sources of nonoperating revenue.

The income from operations plus *total nonoperating revenue* equals the *excess of revenue over expenses*. The hospital in Figure 6 shows a surplus of $550,000, which is recorded in the fund balance on the balance sheet. If this were a for-profit organization, it would be added to the retained earnings account on the balance sheet.

Statement of changes in financial position. The statement of changes in financial position, also called the funds or funds flow statement, explains the sources of the funds obtained and the ways in which these funds were used during a specified period. Funds are usually defined as working capital. In fact, the statement is sometimes called a statement of changes in working capital.

This statement is not to be confused with the cash flow statement that summarizes the receipt and the disbursement of cash and measures an organization's ability to meet its short-term cash needs. A statement of changes in financial position shows how an organization obtained and used all financial resources, not just cash, during the reporting period. It is used to analyze an organization's basic financial strengths and weaknesses and to help management in planning.

Figure 7 illustrates the format of a statement of changes in financial position. It is developed using information from the balance sheet, the income statement, and other sources. Details of the methodology are beyond the scope of this chapter.

In Figure 7, sources of funds are income-related sources, sale of assets, and debt financing. Note that depreciation and loss on sale of equipment are added back, because they do not reflect an outflow of funds. Uses of funds are purchase and construction of fixed assets, debt retirement, and increases in working capital. This statement is in a balanced format; total sources equal total uses of funds. Additionally the statement identifies changes in working capital. For purposes of brevity, individual changes in current asset and current liability accounts are not included. (See also refs. 17, 18.)

Accounting decisions. Accounting is not a mechanical discipline; it requires judgment and interpretation. Generally accepted accounting principles reflect the prevalent professional judgment at the time they are applied, but they are subject to different interpretations that may also be acceptable.

Organizations can provide more detail in financial statements than audit guides require. The level of detail reflects what an organization wants others to know (13). Decisions in several areas affect financial operations and the nature and extent of information provided on financial statements—for example, when to recognize revenue as earned, what method of computing depreciation to use, and how to price inventory (13, 14).

FIGURE 5–7
Statement of Changes in Financial Position
For the Year Ended December 31, 1990
(in thousands of dollars)

Sources of Funds	
From operations	
Excess of revenue over expenses	$ 550
Add: Depreciation	160
Loss on sale of equipment	40
Funds provided by operations	750
From sale of building and equipment	205
From increase in mortgage payable	500
Total sources of funds	$1,455
Uses of Funds	
To purchase fixed assets	$ 240
To construct new facilities	700
To retire long-term debt	100
To increase working capital	415
Total uses of funds	$1,455
Changes in Working Capital	
Increase (decrease) in current assets	$ 680
(Increase) decrease in current liabilities	265
Increase in working capital	$ 415

Financial Analysis

Financial analysis consists of assessing an organization's overall financial performance through ratio analysis, comparison with industry norms, and review of the statement of changes in financial position (13).

Ratio analysis. Ratio analysis looks at four critical areas of financial management: profitability, liquidity, asset management, and long-term solvency (13). The information needed for ratio analysis, with the exception of principal debt payments, is obtained from the balance sheet and the income statement. Ratio analysis facilitates comparison of a single organization's performance over time or among similar organizations at a given time.

Because financial statements of health and human service organizations lack uniformity, the value of using ratios to compare performance among organizations or with industry norms is limited. The most valid use of ratio analysis in health care is to evaluate an organization's performance over time. Plotting selected ratios can provide another tool to monitor financial trends. A word of caution is in order, however. If major accounting principles and/or financial accounting decisions are changed by an organization, the results of the ratio analyses may be affected.

Industry norms. Although efforts have been made to establish industry norms for the health care field, particularly for hospitals, Young (13) cautions health care managers to be skeptical of them. Some of his more compelling reasons are the lack of uniformity in health care reporting, regional variations, the fallacy that a norm is the right level, and changes in the environment since the norms were established (e. g., significant decreases in philanthropy).

Statement of changes in financial position. The statement of changes in financial position indicates how management has financed the organization's operations and managed its assets during a specified period. It therefore provides insights into an organization's financial management strategies.

SELECTED CONCEPTS AND TECHNIQUES OF FINANCIAL MANAGEMENT

This section addresses selected financial management concepts and techniques that occupational therapy managers will find helpful: cost classifications and factors that affect costs; cost finding; and cost accounting. The treatment is in no way comprehensive. References appear at the end of the chapter. In addition, the financial staff of an organization can often be very helpful in financial planning and problem solving because they have knowledge of the organization's practices as well as general financial expertise. In approaching financial staff for assistance, it is important for occupational therapy managers to demonstrate some understanding of finance. Financial staff are apt to be more receptive to someone who has made an effort to learn the basics.

Cost Classifications[1]

Whereas financial accounting is concerned with revenue and expenses, managerial accounting is concerned with other types of costs. Understanding their behavior enables the manager to identify and control the cost of health care services and meet specific decision-making needs.

Costs can be classified into four categories:

- Their traceability to the object being costed: direct or indirect
- Their behavior in response to volume: fixed, variable, semifixed, or semivariable
- Their controllability by management: controllable or uncontrollable
- Their relevance in decision making: sunk, discretionary, avoidable, incremental, or opportunity (18).

These categories are not mutually exclusive. In fact, used in combination, they more accurately describe the nature and the behavior of costs.

Direct and indirect costs. *Direct costs* are those that are clearly traceable to one cost objective or one cost center. Examples in an occupational therapy department or program are salaries of all personnel (professional, technical, and support) and medical and nonmedical supplies used in treatment.

[1]Material in this section is adapted from references 13, 15, 18, 19.

Indirect costs are those that are not clearly identified with one cost objective or one cost center. Examples are employee benefits and costs of other departments (e. g., housekeeping and security).

There are two ways to assign indirect costs to cost centers. Indirect costs can be accurately measured and attributed to each cost center, and thereby be converted into direct costs. For example, many organizations assign employee benefits by department. This method can be expensive to implement. It is often used when a substantial increase in cost reimbursement is expected.

The second and more commonly used method assigns indirect costs to cost centers by formula as equitably as possible. For example, housekeeping costs are assigned on the basis of square feet per department.

An easy way of distinguishing direct and indirect costs is this: If a cost center were closed, all of its direct costs would be eliminated. Its indirect costs, however, would remain and would have to be reassigned to other cost centers.

It is important to recognize that the same costs may be direct for one department and indirect for another. Housekeeping personnel costs are direct for the housekeeping department but contribute to the occupational therapy department's indirect costs.

Fixed, variable, semifixed, and semivariable costs. The relationship of costs to volume is an important concept for managers to grasp and apply in controlling costs. *Fixed costs* are those that remain at the same level for a given period despite variations in volume, that is, in the number of units of service delivered. Examples of fixed costs are depreciation, insurance, rent, and minimum staffing. Figure 8a shows fixed cost behavior.

Total fixed costs do not change with volume. However, as the number of patients/clients or treatments increases, the average fixed cost per patient/client or treatment decreases. Figure 8b illustrates why this occurs. That is, the fixed costs are being divided among a greater number of patients/clients or treatments. This concept has ramifications for pricing.

Fixed costs never fluctuate as a function of volume. In different periods, changes may result from increases or decreases in such items as plant and equipment expenditures, depreciation, and discretionary costs, which are explained later in this section.

Variable costs change in direct proportion to changes in volume. If the number of treatments increases by 5 percent, variable costs, such as those for supplies, will also increase by 5 percent. Figure 9 graphically depicts the relationship between supply costs and volume. The steeper the slope of the line, the greater the variable costs per unit.

Although many variable costs are direct, not all direct costs are variable. For example, the cost of equipment used in treatment is direct but not variable; its price does not depend on how much it is used.

Semifixed costs change in response to variations in volume, but not proportionally. Supervisors are a good example of semifixed costs. They are added at intervals as staff increases warrant, for example, one for every five to seven therapists. These costs are also called *step costs*, referring to the nature of their cost curve as seen in Figure 10. Semifixed

FIGURE 5–8a
Fixed Cost Behavior

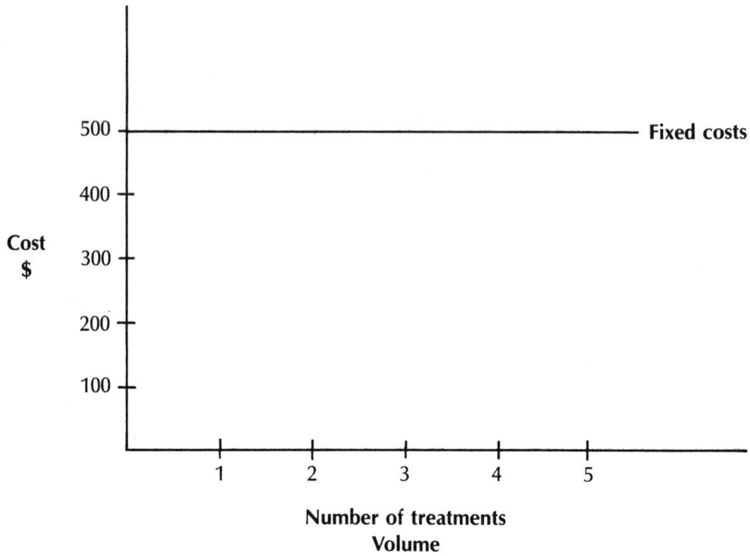

FIGURE 5–8b
Average Fixed Cost per Treatment

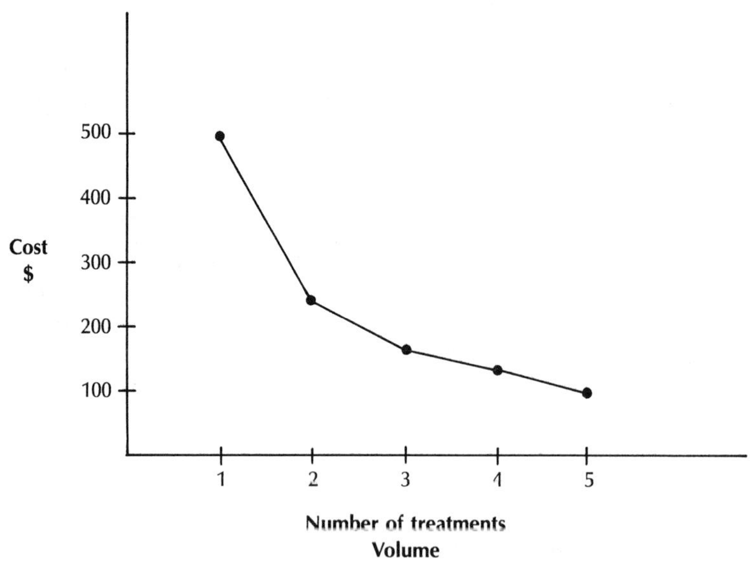

FIGURE 5–9
Variable Cost Behavior

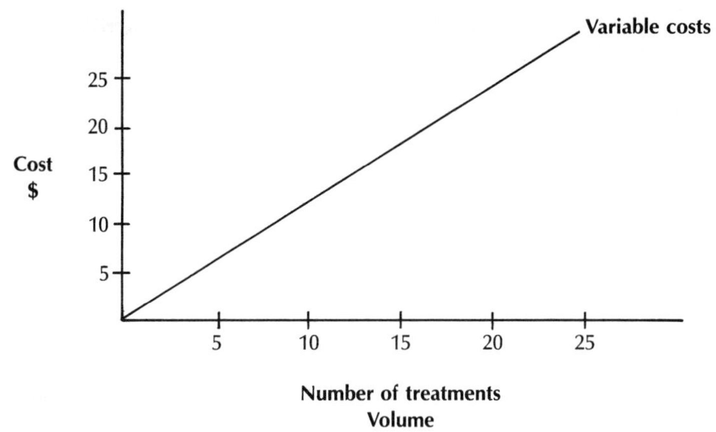

costs can be considered variable or fixed, depending on the size of the steps and the volume.

Semivariable costs are costs that have both fixed and variable elements. Utilities, for instance, have a basic monthly minimum charge (fixed) and another that is directly proportional to the number of units used (variable). Figure 11 illustrates the semivariable cost curve. For purposes of determining the composition of total cost, semivariable costs are separated into their fixed and variable components. Figure 12 depicts the total cost for a department or a program, which consists of all fixed, variable, direct, and indirect costs.

FIGURE 5–10
Semifixed (Step) Cost Behavior

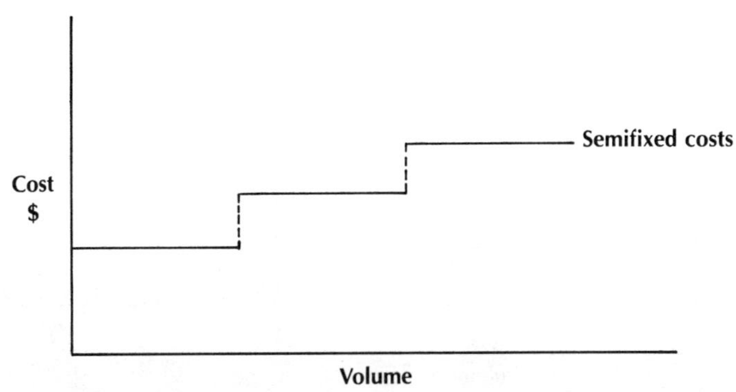

FIGURE 5–11
Semivariable Cost Behavior

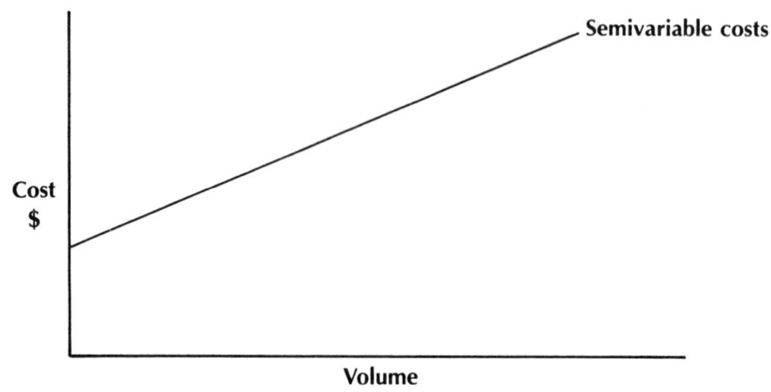

Controllable and uncontrollable costs. Because control is one of the main purposes of cost information, identifying controllable and uncontrollable costs is critical. *Controllable costs* are those over which a manager has a reasonable measure of influence. Examples include department or program salaries and supplies.

Uncontrollable costs are those associated with a department or a program, but over which the manager has little or no control. Once capital expenditures are made, associated depreciation is an uncontrollable cost.

In the health care industry three approaches are generally used to designate controllable costs (18). First and least desirable, all department or program costs are defined as controllable. In most situations this greatly overestimates the amount of costs over which the manager can realistically exercise control. Viewed as inequitable, this situation can have a negative impact.

FIGURE 5–12
Total Cost for a Department

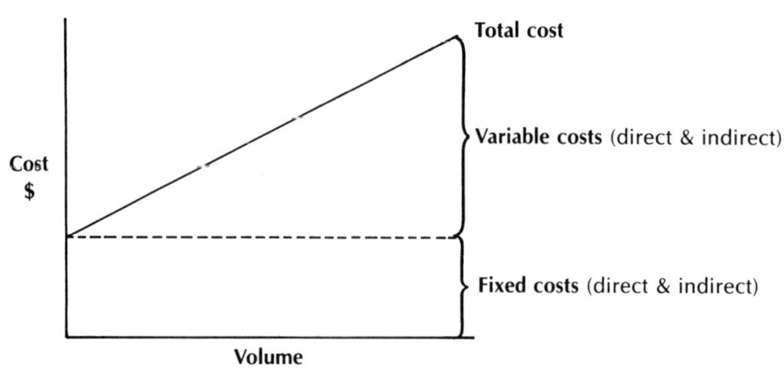

FIGURE 5–13
Approaches to Designating Controllable Costs

	Variable	Fixed	Semifixed	Semivariable
Direct	1 2 3	1 2	1 2	1 2
Indirect	1	1	1	1

KEY: 1 — Controllable costs under first approach
2 — Controllable costs under second approach
3 — Controllable costs under third approach

Second, only direct costs are classified as controllable costs. In this case some direct fixed costs, such as equipment rentals, are not controllable by the manager. On the other hand, the manager can control some indirect variable costs, such as employee benefits.

Third, sometimes only direct variable costs are considered controllable. This is a very restrictive definition of controllable costs and could exclude many costs that are influenced by the manager. Under this approach cost control efforts may be inadequate.

Figure 13 shows which costs are controllable under each of these three approaches.

Costs relevant in decision making. Several cost concepts are useful in decision making. *Sunk costs* represent those that are not affected by the decision under consideration. They have already been incurred and, once committed, are fixed. The book value of an asset is a sunk cost (13, 20).

Discretionary costs are a category of fixed costs. They are designated as fixed by management, but can be changed in different reporting periods by management decision. Therefore, all fixed costs are not sunk costs. Examples include insurance, legal and audit fees, training expenses, and research expenses.

Avoidable costs are those that will be affected by the outcome of a decision. They can be eliminated or saved if an activity is discontinued or volume is reduced. Sunk costs are not avoidable.

Incremental costs are the changes in total costs resulting from a new activity or an increase in volume.

Opportunity cost is the value of the best alternative use of a limited resource that is foregone by its use in a particular way (1, 18).

Factors That Affect Costs

Costs are incurred when an organization's resources are used. Resources can be categorized very broadly as land, labor, and capital. In this sense, capital includes supplies, which are consumed in a year or less, and equipment and facilities, which have a longer life. The health care industry has always been labor intensive, but its long-term capital outlays have also greatly increased because of rapid advances in technology.

Four major factors affect the use of resources: volume, case mix, cost, and improvements in operations. Volume is the most significant factor. Although decreases in volume lower variable costs, hospitals and some other types of health care organizations still have high fixed costs and must closely monitor their occupancy rates and service capacity.

Case mix is another important determinant of costs. Patients'/clients' diagnoses and levels of acuity affect staffing needs, the use of supplies and ancillary services, and the average length of stay or duration of service. Under the Prospective Payment System, hospitals have an incentive to decrease length of stay. This may mean higher costs per patient day but lower costs per hospital stay.

Total costs and unit costs are also affected by any changes in the cost of resources, for example, labor and supplies. Leasing, contracting services, and shared service arrangements are some of the options being exercised to reduce costs.

Improvements in operations can increase productivity, reduce costs, and maintain or even improve the quality of care provided. Clinical and administrative areas whose costs constitute sizable portions of a hospital's budget are under particular scrutiny.

Other important factors include the size and the age of the facility, the types of services offered, the nature and the extent of education and research activities, and seasonal and geographic factors.

Although these factors are not all-encompassing, they provide a basis for thinking about the effects of operations on the use of resources.

Cost Finding

Familiarity with cost finding is essential because many third-party payers (e.g., Medicare, Medicaid, and Blue Cross) require providers to submit cost (finding) reports. Hospitals must continue cost reporting for Medicare payment for at least two years after full implementation of the Prospective Payment System (3).

Cost finding is the process of allocating the costs of the non-revenue-producing, or service cost centers to each other and to the revenue-producing centers on the basis of statistical data that measure the amount of service rendered. (In this section we assume that a cost center is a department.) The financial accounting system collects only direct costs and revenue (if applicable) for each center. Cost finding enables an organization to identify the full costs (direct and allocated indirect) of operating each revenue-producing center. Given that cost finding is separate from and supplemental to financial accounting, its results are neither recorded in the financial accounting system nor included in the financial statements.

The objectives of cost finding are as follows:

1. To provide full cost information as a basis for establishing rates for services and for assessing the adequacy of existing [and proposed] rates
2. To provide information for use in negotiating reimbursement contracts with contracting agencies, and in determining the amount of reimbursable cost

3. To provide information for reports to hospital associations, governmental agencies, and other external groups
4. To provide information for use in managerial decision making in areas other than rate setting (21, p 2).

Cost finding plays a role in the first three objectives, but it has limitations. Because of requirements by third-party payers (e. g., definitions of allowable costs), the full costs determined by cost finding do not represent the actual costs of providing health care services. Cost finding, furthermore, establishes total departmental costs and not individual rates for specific treatments or procedures. Therefore, cost finding can provide only a general guide to rate setting.

Although cost finding creates cost awareness, it was never intended to be used for cost control (21). It is an after-the-fact allocation of costs that is performed as needed. Cost accounting, part of the ongoing financial accounting and management control systems, has broader applications. It enables the organization to identify specific costs and cost behavior within departments and to control them. Therefore, management decisions should be based on cost-accounting data and not cost-finding reports.

Cost finding is predicated on having a current organizational chart with revenue-producing and service cost centers clearly identified; a chart of accounts that reflects the current organizational structure; and a financial accounting system that accumulates accurate financial and statistical data by revenue-producing and service cost center.

Cost finding consists of four steps:

1. Collecting accounting and statistical data
2. Reclassifying cost centers, if necessary (costs may be classified differently for cost finding than for financial accounting)
3. Allocating service centers to revenue-producing centers
4. Preparing the cost report.

Generally speaking, cost centers that provide the most service to the greatest number of other centers and receive the least amount of service from other centers are allocated first. Centers that provide less service to fewer centers and receive the most service from other centers are allocated later. Therefore, the order of allocation may vary among institutions and within an institution over time.

The four methods of cost finding are based on different methods of allocating costs: direct apportionment, step-down method, double distribution, and algebraic apportionment. In *direct apportionment* the costs of the service cost centers are allocated to only the revenue-producing centers. This method is not accepted by most third-party payers (including Medicare), because it ignores the fact that service centers render services to each other and it does not recognize different levels of service rendered by service centers to revenue-producing centers (1). It also does not produce the full costs of the service centers.

The *step-down method* involves the distribution of costs of service centers to other service centers and finally to revenue-producing centers. The name comes from the staircase-like look of the work papers as the costs of the service centers serving the most centers (revenue-producing and service) are distributed first; the service center serving the second largest number of centers, second; and so on. Once the costs of a service center have been distributed, it is closed out; that is, costs of subsequently allocated centers cannot be charged to it. This results in the criticism that the step-down method does not fully allow interdepartmental charges between different service centers and therefore does not identify their full costs. However, this method is acceptable to most third-party payers (1).

Double distribution or *double apportionment* entails two distributions and corrects the major criticism of the step-down method. In the first distribution all direct and indirect costs of all cost centers are distributed to the various centers using appropriate bases of allocations—for example, costs of housekeeping and purchasing on the basis of square footage and costs of laundry according to pounds used. After the first distribution is done, the costs allocated to the service centers are then redistributed to the revenue-producing centers using the same bases of allocations as before. This method produces the full costs of both types of centers.

Algebraic or *multiple apportionment* entails multiple algebraic distributions of expenses among service centers and then finally to revenue-producing centers. This method is the most accurate, but requires a computer. Of the manual methods, double distribution is the most accurate, followed by the step-down method (1).

Although cost finding is constrained by the requirements of third-party payers, it is driven by the desire to maximize reimbursement. Therefore, any permitted flexibility in methodology, cost objectives, bases of allocation, and sequence of allocation should be carefully considered. Given this fact, comparisons among institutions and specific cost centers should be viewed cautiously. Differences may reflect reimbursement strategies and not resource consumption.

Cost Accounting

The health care field is beginning to recognize the value and the power of cost accounting. The impetus for this recognition can be traced to the Prospective Payment System. Hospitals now receive a fixed amount per DRG, so they have a critical need to know and control the actual costs incurred in the care of each case. A cost accounting system can provide that information and enable a hospital to measure its cost containment efforts. It can also aid in—

1. Determining prices and formulating pricing policies
2. Maximizing a hospital's revenue
3. Negotiating with HMOs, PPOs, and other third-party payers
4. Preparing flexible budgets
5. Monitoring productivity and physician performance (efficiency)
6. Strategic planning (22).

A cost accounting system can provide information on full costs and variable costs per procedure, admission, and DRG; fixed and variable costs at procedural, admission, DRG, and cost center levels; standards at the case-volume (physician-controlled) and volume-cost (department-controlled) levels; and areas in which the hospital is particularly cost competitive (22).

Definitions. *Cost accounting* is the "quantitative method that accumulates, classifies, summarizes, and interprets information for three major purposes: (1) operational planning and control, (2) special decisions, and (3) product costing" (20, p 967). The principal objective of cost accounting is to measure as accurately and as efficiently as possible the resources used to produce a particular good or service (13, 15).

Cost objective refers to "any activity for which a separate measurement of costs is desired" (20, p 967). The selection of appropriate cost objectives depends on several factors: (a) whether the amount involved is material; (b) whether the benefit to be derived is worth the cost; and (c) whether the data can be easily collected. Organizations should take a cost-benefit approach to gathering cost information. In other words, management should ask, How much will the additional cost information help us achieve our objectives compared with the costs involved? Some examples of cost objectives are a particular DRG, a day of routine care, an admission (all of the costs associated with a patient's length of stay), and an occupational therapy evaluation.

Macro-costing and micro-costing are two types of product costing approaches (22). *Macro-costing* determines costs using the ratio of cost to charges. For example,

$$\frac{\text{Total department costs}}{\text{Total department charges}} = \text{Ratio of cost to charges (RCC)}$$

$$\text{Charge of specific department procedure} \times \text{RCC}$$
$$= \text{Cost of specific department procedure}$$

The costs derived using the ratio of cost to charges methodology are accurate to the extent that charges reflect actual use of resources. However, charges generally have been influenced by reimbursement and market considerations.

Cost refinements that use standard output measures (e.g., relative value units—RVUs), fixed and variable cost factors, engineering standards, and job order costing are called *micro-costing*. Micro-costing is more complex than macro-costing and requires a greater financial and time commitment. An excellent article describing micro-costing of occupational therapy services has been published in *The American Journal of Occupational Therapy* (23).

Costs are assigned to *cost centers*, which are the "smallest segments of activity or areas of responsibility for which costs are accumulated" (20, p 967). Generally, cost centers are departments. However, some departments may contain more than one cost center. In health care, cost centers are categorized as either revenue-producing or non-revenue-producing (service) centers. *Revenue-producing* cost centers generate reimbursement for the services they render, whereas *non-revenue-producing* costs centers do not. Because reimbursement exists for occupational therapy services, the occupational therapy department is a revenue-producing cost center, or has the capability to be one.

An organization can determine the cost of cost objectives using the process method, the job order method, or a combination thereof. *Process costing* is used when an organization's units of output (products or services) are relatively homogeneous. The average cost of each unit is calculated by dividing the total costs by the number of units produced. Per diem charges are the result of process costing.

Job order costing is used when the units of output vary considerably. Although it may include elements of averaging, it identifies the costs of specific resources used to produce each different output. An example of job order costing is the calculation of the costs of a patient's hospital stay, including per diem plus the costs of additional services the patient received. Because job order costing is more time-consuming and expensive than process costing, its benefits must outweigh the cost and the effort.

Full costing. *Full costing* is the process of allocating the overhead or indirect costs of operating an organization to revenue-producing cost centers. *Overhead* is any cost of doing business other than the direct costs associated with the production of outputs (goods or services) (15). The basic concept behind full costing is that a health care organization must recover all costs, both direct and indirect, incurred in the provision of patient/client services.

Simply, full costing entails the following:

1. Determining patient/client and service cost centers
2. Determining and collecting appropriate allocation statistics for service cost centers
3. Determining the direct costs of all cost centers
4. Assigning indirect costs to appropriate cost centers
5. Allocating service center costs to revenue-producing centers to determine the full cost of each revenue-producing center.

The assignment of indirect costs and the selection of bases of allocation for service centers are a function of a number of considerations, including the need for increased accuracy, the cost of increased precision, the available technology and manpower to devote to the effort, and management's purposes for the data (e.g., pricing, reimbursement, and use of resources) (13).

The step-down method, discussed previously in detail, is the most commonly used method for allocating service center costs to revenue-producing centers (13). *Service center costs* may be categorized as *patient/client support* or *non-patient/client-related* (15). Examples of the former are housekeeping, laundry, maintenance, and dietary. Examples of the latter are administrative and general, personnel, admitting, and data processing. The costs not associated with services rendered by patient care or patient support departments are sometimes referred to as *indirect overhead* or *burden* (15). In health care organizations indirect costs may constitute 50 percent or more of the cost of services (19).

Figure 14 shows the full cost components of an ancillary service.

Differential cost analysis. *Differential cost analysis* is used in decision making to determine the costs and the revenues that will change as a result of various alternatives being considered (13, 19). The following types of decisions require a differential cost analysis:

1. To add or discontinue a service or a product
2. To provide services in house or contract out for them
3. To accept or reject an external proposal that affects the organiza-

FIGURE 5–14
Full Cost Components of an Ancillary Service

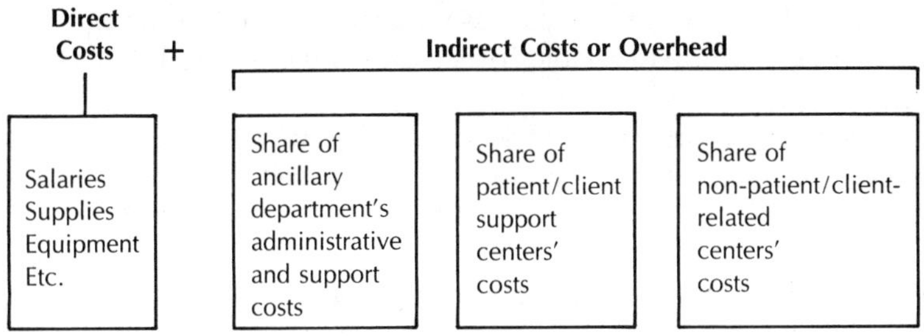

tion's resources (e.g., a proposal from a nursing home to rent an empty hospital wing for an adult day-care program that would be run independently or as a joint venture with the hospital)

4. To sell obsolete capital equipment

5. To offer reduced rates for short-term increases in volume (e.g., screening examinations at less than billed charges for all the children in a school district, in order to detect developmental delays) (13, 19).

Full costs are not used in making these decisions. If they were, the analysis would be inaccurate and could result in the selection of more costly alternatives. As health care organizations generate or are confronted with new options for services and service delivery, managers will increasingly use differential cost analysis.

Each decision-making opportunity is unique and has to be evaluated on its own merits. Because differential analysis focuses on how costs will be affected in the future, the first step is to determine the set of assumptions that will be operational for that period. For example, a set of assumptions may include a 10-percent increase in the volume of a service, no rate increase, and no change in indirect costs. Full costing uses historical data that may or may not be correct depending on the assumptions.

After the assumptions are established, the differential costs are identified. To reiterate, full costs are not used. Instead, one determines which fixed and variable costs (and revenues) will change and to what extent. The analysis requires a careful review of the nature of the decision and its impact. Determining how changes in the assumptions would affect the results is also important. Further, managers should ask, Which set of assumptions has the highest probability of being correct? and How much risk is the organization willing to assume?

When differential costing involves indirect costs, the analysis is further complicated (13). Because indirect costs are not allocated on the basis of actual use by cost centers, cost savings in a particular cost center may or may not effect a reduction in indirect costs to that cost center. Likewise, if certain indirect costs remain constant and the criteria on which allocations are based are reduced in one cost center, the subsequent allocation will redistribute the amount of the reduction to the other cost centers.

The results of differential cost analysis can be reported in terms of either profit (loss) or contribution to indirect costs (revenue minus direct costs) (13). (This is not to be confused with contribution margin, which is gross charges minus variable costs expressed either in total, as a ratio, or on a per-unit basis.)

Unless all of an organization's patients/clients pay charges, the analysis is not yet complete. The effect of cost-based patients/clients must be factored in. Therefore, any reduction in costs must be further reduced by the percent of cost-based reimbursement in order to reflect the organization's savings (13). For example, if an organization can reduce its costs by $15,000, but its reimbursement is 60-percent cost based, the actual savings to the organization would be only $6,000, because the revenue would also be reduced by $9,000 ($15,000 × .60). In this example total health care expenditures are reduced by $15,000, but the organization benefits by only $6,000. This illustration highlights two points: (a) the importance of factoring payer mix into the decision-making process and (b) the role of incentives or disincentives to contain costs, depending on one's perspective (provider or third-party payer). If the cost savings to a provider is relatively small considering the risk involved, the provider will probably not adopt the alternative being considered, even though its adoption would reduce total health care expenditures.

BUDGETING

Of all accounting and financial activities, occupational therapy managers have the most involvement in, and responsibility for, developing and monitoring their budgets. In the current health care environment, department or program managers may be evaluated on their demonstrated skill in budgeting and their effectiveness in monitoring and taking corrective action as needed.

Budgeting is the process whereby an organization's plans for a given period are translated into financial terms. It frequently has a negative connotation associated with restrictions in spending. A more productive attitude is to regard a budget as an organization's best projection of the optimal allocation of resources to meet its objectives.

An organization prepares a master budget, which consists of (a) an operating budget, a pro forma or projected statement of revenue and expenses; (b) a capital budget, a plan for the acquisition of fixed assets; and (c) a cash budget, a summary of the sources and the uses of funds along with a pro forma or projected balance sheet and statement of changes in financial position. Occupational therapy managers prepare operating budgets for their departments or programs and contribute information to the preparation of the organization's capital budget. When the term *budgeting* is used in this chapter, it generally refers to the operating budget, although both operating and capital budgets are mentioned.

Purposes and Benefits of Budgeting

Budgeting is generally associated with the financial operations of an organization. Its usefulness as a management tool extends beyond the financial arena, however. The budgeting process not only contributes significantly to management functions, but it also can exert a positive influence on behavior.

Meaningful budget preparation is based on sound planning. "Planning is the catalyst that changes budget preparation from an arithmetic exercise to a substantive management activity" (1, p 459). Although planning is considered important, it is easily postponed when more pressing, though not necessarily more important, operational concerns arise. Budgeting compels management to plan. Horngren (20, p 132) believes that "this forced planning is by far the greatest contribution of budgeting to management."

The plans represented by the budget reflect expected performance and provide direction for the organization. Because the organization's internal and external environments constantly change, planning and budgeting are continuing, dynamic processes. Used as planning and controlling tools, budgets also give organizations the capacity to anticipate, and adapt to change. This helps organizations function more smoothly, react faster to developing situations, and avoid crises.

Budgeting not only ensures financial coordination; it also improves coordination of operations. Budgeting forces managers to be more aware of organizational goals and objectives; to examine the relationship between their departments or programs and others and the organization as a whole; and to identify problems in the organization related to communication, responsibility, and working relationships (20). Programs and services that are consistent with organizational objectives are the ones that will be funded.

The budget is a powerful tool for monitoring and controlling operations. It provides a standard against which performance can be measured and evaluated. In the budgeting process certain quantitative and financial goals are established. Subsequent performance reporting provides the feedback that enables one to determine progress toward the achievement of those goals. When actual performance differs from that which is budgeted, it must be analyzed. If deviations exceed tolerance levels set by the organization or the manager, corrective action must be taken.

To be successful, the manager must address both technical and behavioral aspects of budget preparation and administration. Much attention must be directed to paperwork, but at least equally as important is the continuing involvement of staff in budget formulation and management activities.

Managers need to involve their staff through communication, education, and meaningful participation at an appropriate level. They cannot delegate their responsibility, but they can discuss organizational goals, elicit and use information and ideas from their staff, provide feedback on actual performance versus budgeted expectations, and work with staff on strategies for corrective action when indicated. This type of interaction between managers and their staff increases motivation and commitment, because it is based on participative goal setting, realistic expectations, regular feedback regarding attainment of objectives, and joint problem solving.

In today's health care environment, staff must understand that *not-for-profit* refers to an organization's tax-exempt status (24). It does not mean that such an organization should break even (have revenues equaling expenses) or operate at a loss. All organizations need net income (profit, or excess of revenue over expenses) to support program expansion and ensure replacement of their facilities. Knowledge of this can help staff appreciate their organization's need for revenue and its reliance on the performance of its revenue-producing centers, such as the occupational therapy department.

Finally, budget preparation and requirements relating to it may also be mandated by federal and state legislation. Hospitals, extended care facilities, and home health agencies participating in Medicare must meet certain planning and budgeting requirements. State rate-setting agencies frequently require health care facilities under their jurisdiction to submit budgets.

The Budgeting Process

Each organization has its own process for developing an operating budget. Table 2, which is drawn from several sources (1, 11, 24), outlines the major steps. The budget director (or the controller) is usually responsible for coordinating the preparation of the budget. The entire process may take three to six months to complete (24), longer if one includes the total planning cycle. A budget committee composed of senior management works closely with the budget director. The period for which the budget is developed is usually twelve months.

An organization's budgeting philosophy influences its budgeting process. Some common budgeting philosophies are program budgeting, incremental budgeting, zero-base budgeting, and management by objectives. Most organizations are using an approach that draws on one or more of these philosophies. *Program budgeting* is a technique whereby an organization's budget is prepared in terms of its major programs—for example, inpatient, outpatient, ancillary services, general services, and administrative and general. At the departmental level, budgeting is done in the traditional manner. However, management coordinates the allocation of resources among programs in a macro sense. This type of budgeting suits top management's needs, but it is inadequate for making detailed decisions about the allocation of resources. Of necessity, it is associated with other budgeting approaches, for example, incremental budgeting and zero-base budgeting.

Incremental budgeting occurs when the expense budget is based on last year's costs plus an inflation factor. Only the incremental portion, the increase over the previous year's level, needs to be justified. The current level of spending is implicitly approved. The major weakness of this approach is the assumption that the previous year's spending level is an appropriate base without any evaluation of current needs, programs, and expenditures.

Zero-base budgeting requires all expenditures to be evaluated and rank-ordered in a structured manner. The department or program manager prepares a decision package for each current or proposed activity or function. The decision package includes the resources needed to accomplish that activity at different funding levels—minimum (e.g., 70–80 percent of the existing level), existing, and increased—and the benefits

TABLE 5–2
The Budgeting Process

Planning	Long-range planning • Approve organizational strategy • Approve operating plan
Budgeting	Development of budget format and guidelines • Prepare economic forecasts (e.g., inflation factors, new developments that may affect the organization, impending government regulations) • Determine budget format and timetable • Establish preliminary assumptions regarding rate increases and net income requirements Distribution of approved budget package, including assumptions, forms, schedules, and historical data Communication: general and technical budget meetings with line management; technical assistance rendered when necessary Forecasting of volume (e. g., patient/client days, outpatient visits, and cost center activity levels) Preparation of preliminary revenue budget, personnel budget, operating expense budget (including budgets for new and expanded programs) Holding of departmental budget hearings Preparation of tentative operating budget (containing projections of revenue, expenses, contractual allowances, bad debts, vacancy allowances, depreciation, interest expense, and insurance) • Determine desired net income, scale and salary increases, rate increases • Approve new programs and new and upgraded positions Approval of budget, first by budget committee, then by full governing board
Monitoring and Controlling	Distribution and implementation of approved budget with regular feedback

to be derived at each. The manager than rank-orders all decision packages. The activities that are most beneficial to the organization, regardless of whether they are current or new, are funded. This approach is very difficult and time-consuming to implement. Its major benefit is that it forces managers to evaluate continuing activities and new alternatives in light of current needs.

The application of *management by objectives* (MBO) in a health care organization requires department managers to negotiate with top management measurable objectives that will improve departmental performance and be accomplished by a specific time within the budget period. The department agrees to achieve the goals, and top management agrees to provide the needed resources and support. After MBO is functioning between top management and department managers, it can be used between the latter and their first-line supervisors, and on down. MBO can be especially useful in coordinating and evaluating departmental and individual progress toward the accomplishment of objectives, in reducing conflict, and in increasing motivation. However, its benefits will be limited if it is mechanically applied or if it does not allow meaningful participation in the objective-setting and budgeting processes. If the program is not managed properly, there is also a danger of avoiding appropriate goals that cannot be quantified and approving departmental objectives that are relatively easy to attain but not particularly germane to the organization's goals and objectives.

Budgeting is a part of the management control process, which depends on variance analysis, responsibility accounting, and performance reporting. Discussion of these subjects is beyond the scope of this chapter; coverage of them is provided in such courses as managerial accounting and financial management.

Managers can improve the financial performance of their departments or programs by understanding the financial ramifications of their decisions and the nature of their operations. Budgeting is an important aspect of this function of management. (For a fuller treatment, see refs. 1, 11, 19.)

SUMMARY

Three major issues in the health care industry have had a tremendous impact on financial management: escalating health care expenditures in the United States, efforts by health care organizations to maximize reimbursement, and greater competition among hospitals, and between hospitals and alternative providers, for patients/clients and scarce resources. All three developments have brought about great pressures and numerous measures in the public and private sectors to contain costs.

Financial management now exerts a major influence on the uses of a health care organization's assets and resources. It must be an integral part of the occupational therapy manager's repertoire of skills.

Accounting and financial management differ. Accounting involves "collecting, summarizing, analyzing, and interpreting, in monetary terms, information" about an organization. Financial management, which builds on accounting, entails "obtaining the funds which [an organization] needs in the most economic manner and making the optimal use of those funds" to achieve objectives.

Financial accounting provides financial statements for external use whereas managerial accounting is used to prepare reports for internal decision making. A number of basic concepts, principles, and procedures govern financial accounting—for example, the double entry concept, which holds that every accounting transaction should reflect at least two entries and that deficit entries must equal credit entries. Generally accepted accounting principles require that organizations annually prepare three financial statements: a balance sheet, which reports the status of each account on a particular date; an income statement, which shows the movement of revenue and expenses into and out of the organization during a given period; and a statement of changes in financial position, which summarizes all of the balance sheet changes arising from the influx and outflow of resources during a given period.

The major components of a balance sheet are current assets (e.g., cash and accounts receivable), fixed assets (e.g., land and buildings), current liabilities (e.g., accounts payable and short-term loans payable), long-term liabilities (e.g., mortgage payable, long-term), and fund balance or, in for-profit organizations, equity. An income statement reports operating revenue (gross patient and other), operating expenses, nonoperating revenue (e.g., contributions and investment income), and excess of revenue over expenses. A statement of changes in financial position summarizes an organization's sources of funds (e.g., from operations, sale of buildings and equipment, and increases in mortgage payable), uses of funds (e.g., to purchase fixed assets, construct new facilities, retire long-term debt, and increase working capital), and changes in working capital (increases and decreases in current assets and liabilities).

Financial analysis consists of assessing an organization's overall financial performance through ratio analysis, comparison with industry norms, and review of the statement of changes in financial position. The most valid use of ratio analysis in health care is to evaluate an organization's performance over time. Industry norms in health care should be viewed with skepticism. Therefore, comparisons with them have limited utility. On the other hand, a statement of changes in financial position yields useful information about an organization's financial management strategies.

Occupational therapy managers will find several financial management concepts and techniques helpful: cost classifications and factors that affect costs; cost finding; and cost accounting. Costs are classified according to their traceability to the object being costed (direct and indirect), their behavior in response to volume (fixed, variable, semifixed, and semivariable), and their relevance in decision making (sunk, discretionary, avoidable, incremental, and opportunity). Used in combination, these classifications accurately describe the nature and the behavior of costs. An organization incurs costs when it uses its resources. Four major factors affect its use of resources: volume, case mix, the cost of the resources, and improvements in operations.

Cost finding is the process of allocating the costs of the non-revenue-producing or service cost centers to each other and to the revenue-producing centers on the basis of statistical data that measure the amount of service rendered. There are four methods of cost finding: direct apportionment, step-down method, double distribution, and algebraic apportionment. Direct apportionment is not accepted by most third-party payers. Algebraic apportionment is the most accurate method, but requires a computer. Double distribution is the most accurate manual method.

Unlike cost finding, which is an after-the-fact allocation of costs, cost accounting is a part of the ongoing financial accounting and management control systems. It is defined as the "quantitative method that accumulates, classifies, summarizes, and interprets information [for] operational planning and control, special decisions, and product costing." Costs are assigned to cost centers, which are the "smallest segments of activity or areas of responsibility for which costs are accumulated." Full costing is the process of allocating the overhead or indirect costs of operating an organization to revenue-producing cost centers. The basic concept behind full costing is that a health care organization must recover all costs, both direct and indirect, incurred in the provision of patient/client services. Differential cost analysis is used to determine the costs and the revenues that will change as a result of various alternatives being considered, for example, whether to add or discontinue a service or a product. Full costs are not used in differential cost analysis.

Of all accounting and financial activities, occupational therapy managers have the most involvement in, and responsibility for, developing and monitoring their budgets. Budgeting is the process whereby an organization's plans for a given period are translated into financial terms. The usefulness of budgeting extends beyond the financial arena. Budgeting compels management to plan and gives organizations the capacity to anticipate and adapt to change. It also improves coordination of operations and provides a standard against which performance can be measured and evaluated.

Managers should involve their staff in budget formulation and management activities, discussing organizational goals, eliciting and using ideas, providing feedback on actual performance, and working on strategies for corrective action when needed.

Each organization has its own process for developing an operating budget. Major steps include long-range planning, development of the budget format and guidelines, distribution of the approved budget package, communication, forecasting of volume, preparation of preliminary budgets, holding of hearings, preparation of a tentative operating budget, approval of the budget, and distribution and implementation of the approved budget with regular feedback.

An organization's budgeting philosophy influences its budgeting process. Most organizations use an approach that draws on one or more of four philosophies: program budgeting, which casts a budget in terms of its major programs; incremental budgeting, which bases a budget on the previous year's costs plus an inflation factor; zero-base budgeting, which rank-orders current and new activities and funds only those that are most beneficial to the organization; and management by objectives, which involves budgeting resources based on a commitment to achieve measurable objectives to improve departmental performance within the budget period.

References

1. Berman HJ, Weeks LE: *The Financial Management of Hospitals*, 5th edition. Ann Arbor, MI: Health Administration Press, 1982
2. Longest BB Jr: *Management Practices for the Health Professional*, 3rd edition. Reston, VA: Reston Publishing Co Inc, 1984
3. Beck DF: *Principles of Reimbursement in Health Care*. Rockville, MD: Aspen Systems Corp, 1984
4. Alternative delivery arena evokes melange of approaches. *Business and Health* 1(3):29–34, 1984
5. Johnson AN, Aquilina D: The cost shifting issue. *Health Affairs* 1(4):101–106, 1982
6. Meyer JA, Johnson WR, Sullivan S: *Passing the Health Care Buck: Who Pays the Hidden Cost?* Washington, DC: American Enterprise Institute for Public Policy Research, 1983
7. American Hospital Association: *Managing Under Medicare Prospective Pricing*. Chicago: American Hospital Association, 1983
8. Mistarz JE: Hospitals redefine their business: Competitive hospitals manage network of relationships, not just buildings, with alternative delivery systems. *Hospitals* 58(3):71–72, 74, 1984
9. Sloan FA, Vraciu RA: Investor-owned and not-for-profit hospitals: Addressing some issues. *Health Affairs* 2(1):25–37, 1983

10. Kahn L: Departmental contract management up as much as 162 percent. *Hospitals* 58(3):62, 64, 1984
11. Beck DF: *Basic Hospital Financial Management*. Rockville, MD: Aspen Systems Corp, 1980
12. American Hospital Association: *Chart of Accounts for Hospitals*. Chicago: American Hospital Association, 1976
13. Young DW: *Financial Control in Health Care: A Managerial Perspective*. Homewood, IL: Dow Jones-Irwin, 1984
14. Bolandis JL: *Hospital Finance: A Comprehensive Case Approach*. Rockville, MD: Aspen Systems Corp, 1982
15. American Hospital Association: *Managerial Cost Accounting for Hospitals*. Chicago: American Hospital Association, 1980
16. Spiro HT: *Finance for the . . . Nonfinancial Manager*, 2nd edition. New York: John Wiley & Sons Inc, 1982
17. Gordon MJ, Shillinglaw G: *Accounting: A Management Approach,* 5th edition. Homewood, IL: Richard D. Irwin, 1974
18. Cleverley WO: *Essentials of Hospital Finance*. Germantown, MD: Aspen Systems Corp, 1978
19. Suver JD, Neumann BR: *Management Accounting for Health Care Organizations*. Oak Brook, IL: Hospital Financial Management Association, 1981
20. Horngren CT: *Cost Accounting: A Managerial Emphasis*, 5th edition. Englewood Cliffs, NJ: Prentice-Hall Inc, 1982
21. American Hospital Association: *Cost Finding and Rate Setting for Hospitals*. Chicago: American Hospital Association, 1968
22. Budd GB: Case mix product costing using relative cost factors. In *Cost Accounting Strategies Under PPS,* Hospital Financial Management Association, First Illinois Chapter, Audit and Reimbursement Committee, Editor. Conference Proceedings, April 11, 1984
23. Mansfield M: Micro-costing analysis: A measure of accountability. *Am J Occup Ther* 37:239–246, 1983
24. Esmond TH Jr: *Budgeting Procedures for Hospitals: 1982 Edition*. Chicago: American Hospital Association, 1982

Chapter 6

Marketing

Tina S. Olson, OTR, FAOTA
Carol Urban, BSN, RN

Marketing has become as commonplace as strategic planning, community (or public) relations, and financial management in health care organizations. To compete in the American health care system of this decade and the next, occupational therapy personnel must be familiar with concepts of marketing and their successful application. This chapter reviews marketing concepts and applications within the context of occupational therapy services.

Marketing as a function is accepted in the health care organization, but its place in the structure and its relationship to other, similar functions is not consistent across organizations of similar size and scope. Many individuals in the health care setting confuse marketing with strategic planning or community relations, because the outcomes of these functions seem to be the same as the outcomes of marketing. This confusion is not unlike that which occurs between occupational therapy and physical therapy, or occupational therapy and social work. The outcomes of therapy and counseling seem to be the same in terms of increased function of the patient/client, but the process that is applied through the disciplines is different.

Tina S. Olson serves as vice-president of the Shared Services Division of S-V Enterprises, Inc., a proprietary health services management company affiliated with Stormont-Vail Regional Medical Center in Topeka, Kansas. In this position she directs a large shared services program for a regional medical center and a multihospital system in northeast Kansas.

Carol Urban serves as the marketing director for shared service arrangements between Stormont-Vail Regional Medical Center in Topeka, Kansas, and rural hospitals in the northeast section of the state.

Just as occupational therapy can be described as a system of knowledge and skills applied within the framework of theory, marketing is a system for operational planning from an information base. This information is gathered and analyzed through a disciplined study of the needs of the patient/client (the customer), the physician (the referral source), the administrator (the source of departmental funding), and the reimburser (the source of facility funding). These four groups are referred to as the target market. Of all the individuals who could be influenced, the target market is the portion, or segment, that the marketer wishes to influence.

A DEFINITION OF MARKETING

The definition of marketing offered by Kotler (1, p 5) describes the basic components of a marketing system:

> Marketing is the analysis, planning, implementation and control of carefully formulated programs designed to bring about voluntary exchanges of values with target markets for the purpose of achieving organizational objectives. It relies heavily on designing the organization's offering in terms of the target market's needs and desires, and on using effective pricing, communication, and distribution to inform, motivate and service the markets.

From that definition marketing can be seen as a function that results in the development of a product or program designed to appeal to particular customers or groups of customers with the same or similar needs. Traditionally, health care and other nonprofit or charitable organizations developed their products or services based on what they thought the customer ought to want relative to their own plans for the organization. With increasing competition in the health care system, it is now necessary to organize products or services in terms of what will be most appealing to the customer.

ESSENTIAL CONCEPTS OF MARKETING

Traditionally, marketing theory is based on several key concepts, classically called the four P's of market plan development: product, price, place, and promotion. In addition, the concept of position is essential to theory application and implementation. An understanding of these basic concepts provides a base on which to build a specific market plan.

Product

The concept of product underlies the entire marketing effort. A product is defined as "any complex of tangible and intangible attributes that might be offered to a market to satisfy a want or need . . . " (1, p 174). In health care a product is most commonly a service that can be provided to a patient/client directly, or indirectly through other organizations. The patient/client is often thought to be the target market, but more frequently the target market may be the physician or the organization to which the patient/client looks for care and therapy decisions.

The concept of product line development provides for the grouping of products with like attributes, often around a core attribute such as a body system, a disease entity, or a disability type. Currently, products are being organized around the Diagnosis-Related Group (DRG), which many payment systems use to classify patients/clients by the amount of health care resources consumed during an illness.

As an idea for a product is developed, several questions should be answered:

1. What is the product to be marketed?
2. What attributes of this product will the patient/client desire?
3. What benefits will be derived by the provider for developing and marketing the product?
4. What will be the basis for the exchange?

An example of a product is pediatric developmental assessment. The attribute sought by the patient/client is an assessment outcome and information or recommendations for therapeutic intervention. The benefits to be derived by the provider are referrals for therapy and an increase in the number of referrals for assessment relative to the total done in the area (that is, an increase in the organization's market share). The basis for the exchange is that the parties trade something of value: The patient/client gives cooperation and payment for services; the therapist offers expertise and advice.

Price

Generally speaking, price is accepted as the monetary exchange that occurs when a product is purchased. It *may* be that simple. However, other factors should be considered. MacStravic (2, p 11) defines price as "the financial, physical, and psychological costs to people of doing business with you." Often forgotten in determining pricing strategies is the idea of psychological costs. For example, it may be difficult for a parent to seek out developmental assessment services if he or she is not psychologically ready to accept the possibility of an abnormal finding.

Pricing strategies should take into consideration not only financial, physical, and psychological aspects of the product or the service, but also its competition and its fair market value. Decisions to price a service under its actual cost may be valid if the low price can be expected to attract consumers who will also buy other products of the organization. Such a product is called a loss leader. For example, pediatric developmental assessment might be priced below its actual cost if the organization judged that the revenue from treatment of children found to have abnormalities would offset any shortfall in the revenue from assessment and increase the likelihood that the family would seek other services from the organization. Other pricing considerations include third-party payment practices and rates, current charges for similar services offered by the department or program, and the desired profit margin.

Place

The concept of place is more easily understood as a matter of distribution or access—that is, how a product will be distributed to a market or how the market can get access to the product. The following questions related to place might be asked during development of the pediatric developmental assessment service:

1. How will the service be offered (e.g., in the hospital, in an outpatient clinic, or in a school)?
2. When will the service be provided (i.e., what days of the week and what hours of the day)?
3. How will the patient/client gain access to the service (e.g., by referral from a physician, a nurse, a counselor, a social worker, a parent, or by self-referral)?
4. Who will be eligible for the service?
5. How long will an assessment take?
6. On what basis will testing be done (i.e., inpatient or outpatient)?
7. If the service will be available to both inpatients and outpatients, how will the way in which it is delivered differ?
8. Are there physical or psychological obstacles that will impede access to the service (e.g., inadequate parking space, an inconvenient location, or long waiting periods)?

Answering questions like these will assist the provider in developing a product that can be easily accessed by the target market.

Promotion

This is the concept most commonly thought of in developing marketing efforts. Promotion is just one aspect of marketing. It includes all attempts to make the product visible and desirable to a target market or a segment of that market. It may include, but is not limited to, the following:

1. Advertising through newspapers and other print media, radio, television, billboards, and brochures
2. Personal contact by a representative of the organization or the person providing the service, through health fairs, shopping center displays, and presentations at parent-teacher-organization meetings and in other settings frequented by the target market.
3. Atmospherics, a method used to affect the environment so as to produce a specific emotional response in the target market (3)—for example, showing a film on developmental disabilities at a parent-teacher-organization meeting
4. Bonuses, incentives, discounts, and the development of some tangible reward system to encourage use of the product.

Promotional campaigns are often unsuccessful if conducted on a one-time basis and thus they should be repeated at appropriate intervals. Promotion makes the product more visible to the market.

Position

The final concept, position, refers to the relative place a product holds among similar products in the marketplace. A product changes position as it takes on unique attributes, which set it apart from other products. The design of a product and in some ways the promotion of it should be based on these qualities.

For example, perhaps the pediatric developmental assessment being developed and promoted is unique to the community because it is the

FIGURE 6–1
The Planning Cycle of a Traditional Human Service Organization

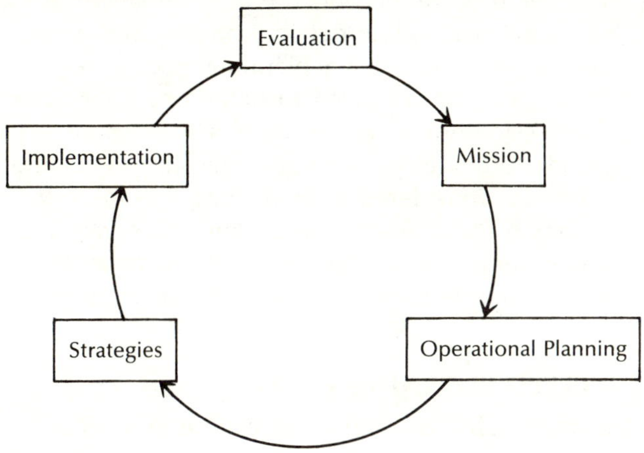

only such service currently available. Or perhaps it is different from others in that the parent is allowed to participate in testing procedures.

A TRADITIONAL PLANNING CYCLE

The impact that marketing orientation has on an organization can be realized by comparing the planning cycles in Figures 1 and 2. These illustrations are based on the works of Berkowitz and Flexner (4) and Stuehler (5).

FIGURE 6–2
The Planning Cycle of a Market-Based Organization

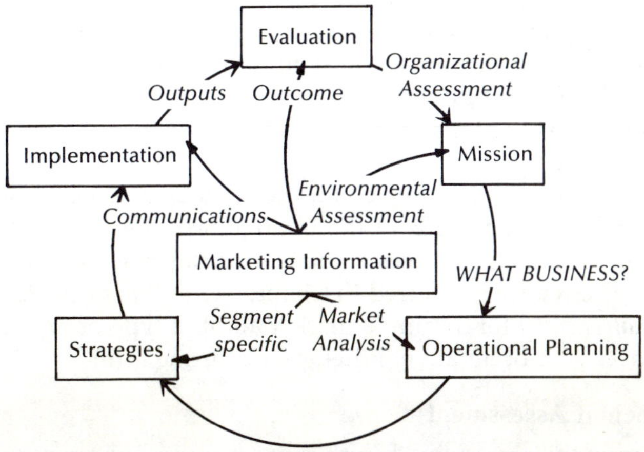

In a traditional planning cycle, illustrated in Figure 1, the *mission* or the purpose of an organization is considered before the actual *operational planning*, or goal setting, occurs. Once the organization's goals for a given period (usually one to three years) are adopted, specific *strategies* or objectives are developed that become the basis for *implementation* of services, new programs, and actual delivery of care to the patient/client. In the *evaluation* phase of a traditional planning model, the organization's programs and services are reviewed to determine their success at implementing the mission of the organization. This is an important point, because this model provides no assurance that the wants and needs of the patient/client are considered in evaluating the work of the organization. The mission statements of most human service organizations express a commitment to serve the needs of the patient/client. These can be overlooked if the organization's programs are not designed around them.

A MARKET-BASED PLANNING CYCLE

In Figure 2 marketing information is the central process that drives the cycle. The components of marketing information are organizational assessment, environmental assessment, market analysis, and communications. These components create an information flow that interacts with and enriches the traditional model.

In market planning, it is essential to understand (a) what was, (b) what is, and (c) what could be. To provide a base for product development, the organizational and environmental assessments conducted at the beginning of a planning cycle should address these three points.

Organizational Assessment

Many organizations are rethinking their missions in light of rapidly changing systems of payment for services and the increase in competition from both health care organizations and non-health-care organizations entering the health care business. Hospitals in particular are becoming "health service corporations" or "human service organizations" to broaden the scope of services they provide and position themselves more effectively. This reevaluation, called organizational assessment, looks at the effectiveness of the hospital relative to the patient/client population, the community, and the health care system itself. Hospital effectiveness in the decade ahead will be determined by the quality of patient/client care as well as the quality of management of the complex systems needed to provide that care.

Much of the information needed for the organizational assessment can be obtained from the records of the occupational therapy organization. A variety of other data sources available for this research are outlined in Table 1. The reader is referred to Chapter 42 of *Willard and Spackman's Occupational Therapy* for a sample market audit (a type of organizational assessment) by an occupational therapy department (6).

Environmental Assessment

In considering their missions, health care organizations are asking themselves the question, What business are we in? Answering the question

TABLE 6–1
Common Sources of Market Data for an Organizational Assessment

Medical records
Occupational therapy department's or program's records
Other departments' records—nursing, physical therapy, etc.
Patient origin studies, conducted annually by the state hospital association
Organization's organizational assessment
Organization's environmental assessment
American Occupational Therapy Association

usually results in a reexamination of the patient/client population to be served and the mode and location of service delivery. This involves a systematic environmental assessment. At this point the disciplines of marketing and strategic planning merge. The role of strategic planning is to affirm and challenge the mission of the organization, to identify future directions, and to establish a context for future development. Chapter 2 discusses this function in greater depth.

Environmental assessment includes a review of the characteristics (demographics) of the organization's current patients/clients and those of other providers. Such characteristics as age, sex, diagnosis, location of treatment (inpatient versus outpatient), referring physician, length of hospital stays, and cost of care are evaluated. The evaluation includes a history of change that may have occurred for groups of patients/clients with similar characteristics, and projections of what may happen with certain patient/client groups based on population changes or new technology.

Physician characteristics such as type of specialty, number, age, and productivity are studied, as are referral patterns. Both a historical and a prospective view are considered in determining whether recruitment of a certain type of physician is indicated. Another important variable that is considered is the physician's use of resources, for example, how extensively he or she draws on ancillary services such as occupational therapy and how long his or her patients tend to be hospitalized.

Environmental assessment gives the organization a sense of what the market is like for its products or services. The assessment also begins to define how the organization can position itself through operational planning, or goal setting, to be most effective in its environment. Table 2 lists some common sources of data for an environmental assessment.

Market Analysis

Market analysis uses information identified in the organizational and environmental assessments to define the market and determine if the organization's perception of the wants and the needs of the market is valid. This is generally done through some form of survey conducted by the organization or by contract with a market research firm. In the survey process the organization asks randomly selected members of the

TABLE 6–2
Common Sources of Market Data for an Environmental Assessment

Physicians' office records
Hospital association reports other than patient origin studies
Reports of the local health systems agency (HSA), where one exists, or the state department of health, where HSAs no longer operate
Professional association publications
Reports from the U.S. Census Bureau
Purchased data base reports and files
Local and state medical societies
Information shared by other health care organizations or private practitioners
Commission on Professional and Hospital Activities (CPHA) reports from the American Hospital Association
Private demographic firms that develop market research data on a regional, state, and local basis in some communities
American Occupational Therapy Association

target market about their wants and needs and their preferences in seeking satisfaction of those needs.

Through market analysis the organization defines (a) whom it will serve, (b) how it will organize its services, (c) how it can group potential consumers with similar needs, and (d) what is unique about its services or products. The decision of who will be served is based on the mission of the organization and on information obtained in the environmental assessment.

How those people will be served depends on how their needs are clustered with similar needs of others. The clustering of people with similar needs is called segmentation of the market. The marketer looks for what people have in common, to which he or she can appeal with a particular product or service. Traditionally, occupational therapy personnel have clustered their patients/clients in categories like Pediatrics, Physical Disabilities, Cardiac, and Learning Disabilities. These categories describe needs around which treatment programs are designed. In categorizing patients/clients this way, by their needs as presumed from their clinical disability, occupational therapy personnel are segmenting a market. The market in this example is all the individuals in need of occupational therapy services. A segment of that overall market is cardiac patients/clients.

The next step in market analysis is categorizing services to meet the needs of a segmented market, or developing a product line. The changing reimbursement system and other economic forces are making it increasingly difficult for human service organizations to offer "all things to all people." If there is not sufficient demand for specialized services, many of them will be abandoned or obtained by contract from another organization. By evaluating its product lines, or the array of services it provides, and comparing this with the potential for services, the organization positions itself in the marketplace.

Occupational therapy managers should be aware of the type of planning cycle that is used in their organization and the personnel who are involved in organizational and environmental assessment and market analysis. In most organizations an occupational therapy manager is unlikely to participate at this level of planning. However, for the occupational therapy department or program to serve the patients/clients it has identified as a target market, the occupational therapy manager must ensure that information about that target market is included in the planning process. Thus, information should flow upward to the organization's decision makers and planners.

Decision makers and planners should, in turn, make information available to the occupational therapy department or program, to aid it in developing effective market plans and promotional activities specific to its segments of the market. It is through department- or program-level planning that implementation strategies are conceived and implemented. At this stage the manager and the staff design new programs, evaluate programs with poor performance records, and make changes in program operation to improve financial effectiveness.

From the marketing information assembled in the organizational and environmental assessments and the market analysis, an organization develops a market plan by applying the four P's with a view to the position it wants to achieve. Figure 3 describes the information flow resulting in a data base for a market plan.

Marketing Communications

Marketing communications are generated between strategy (or objective) development and implementation. Marketing communications include advertising, promotions (unpaid placement of information in the media), and education of those who can assist the organization in marketing its product.

At this stage, marketing overlaps with community relations. The role of community relations is to communicate the values of the organization to the community it serves. A detailed discussion of this aspect of marketing appears in Chapter 16.

The outputs, or the results, of implementing the market plan are measured in terms of the number of members of key segments who are served and the positive or negative financial impact of the programs and the services that are offered. These components are included in the evaluation of the organization's offerings and in the measure of the quality of its services. They serve as the basis for organizational assessment, which begins the planning cycle once again.

THE ROLE OF MARKETING

Throughout the planning cycle the role of marketing is to validate the mission of the organization in relation to the people and organizations to be served. Basic to that role is the organization's understanding and balancing its own wants and needs with those of the target market. This is the voluntary exchange referred to in Kotler's definition of marketing. It involves offering something of value (a service) for consideration by a target market (a desired customer), who will offer something of value (cooperation, payment, support) in return.

FIGURE 6–3
The Flow of Information to Create a Data Base

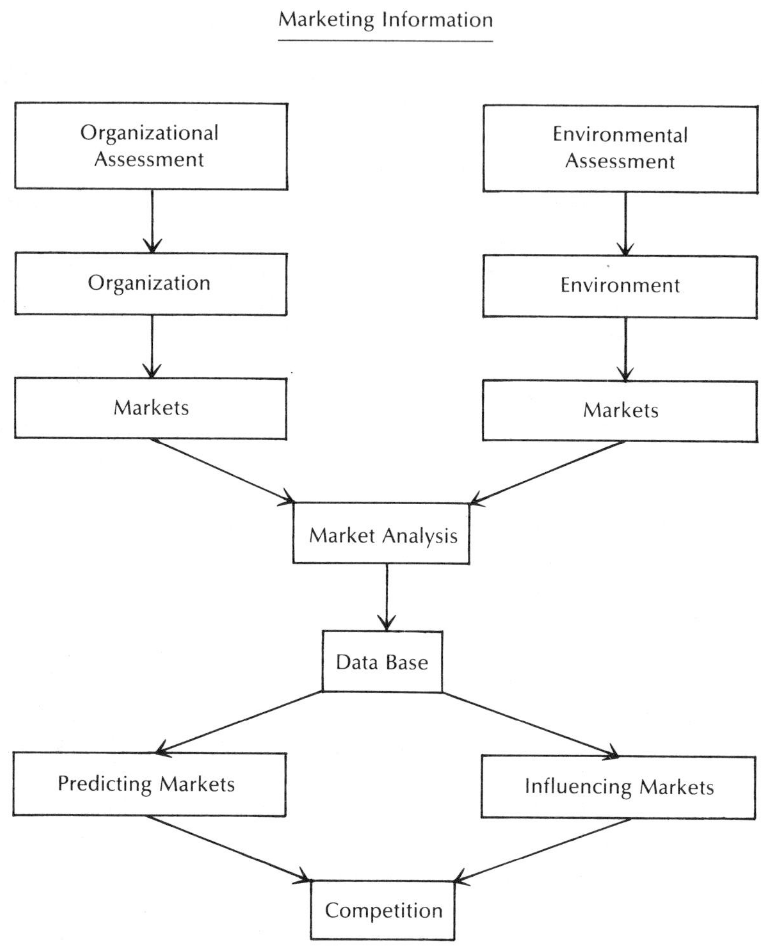

APPLICATION OF THEORY

The example of pediatric developmental assessment provides a vehicle for illustrating the application of marketing concepts. An occupational therapy organization has chosen to market such an assessment, having identified children at risk for developmental delay as a target of its pediatric market.

Organizational Assessment

To develop a plan to attract this population, the organization first undertakes an organizational assessment, seeking information to help it understand its past relationship with the pediatric population—what was. It examines data on previous programs it has provided for children and the response of patients/clients, parents, and referral sources. With these former consumers it attempts to identify wants and needs, psychographic information (e.g., perceptions and feelings about the programs), and demographic data (age, sex, zip code, etc.).

Environmental Assessment

Next, the organization begins an environmental assessment, an investigation of what is and what could be. It explores the market for the service among the portion of the pediatric population it has not served before. Working with population data for its locale, it estimates the number of children at risk. It also investigates the target market being seen for developmental assessment by the competition—nurses, physical therapists, and other occupational therapy organizations.

The organization also assesses government regulations that will affect the assessment program, the program's social impact, and its impact on other providers. Further, the organization studies the competition—available services that are similar, their design, and their position in the marketplace.

Market Analysis

By surveying a randomly selected portion of a potential target market, the organization seeks feedback from potential patients/clients, from physicians, and from others who might refer patients/clients for an assessment. Separate surveys are designed for parents of children at risk, physicians (in family practice, pediatrics, neurology, and internal medicine), and other potential referrers, such as social workers. By separating the surveys the organization learns the following:

From the parents

- Their perceptions of the organization—why they would or would not obtain services from the assessment program and whether they felt they could afford the services
- Their knowledge of the program
- Convenience issues—what time of day they would want the assessment, in what setting, and so forth.

From physicians and others

- Their knowledge of the assessment program
- Their perceptions of occupational therapy as an acceptable intervention for developmental delay
- Their willingness or inclination to refer patients/clients
- The information they would want from an assessment.

The occupational therapy organization uses the survey information to design the program and a communications plan to support it.

The organization is now ready to position itself in the market. First the organization asks itself whether it is unique in the community in providing the pediatric developmental assessment, or whether the assessment has unique attributes that should attract the target market. Finding neither characteristic to be the case, the organization attempts to influence the behavior of the market by enhancing its product through price, place, and promotion.

CONCLUSION

Marketing is a process of applying information based on assumptions about the behavior of the organization doing the marketing, the consumer of products, and the environment in which marketing exchanges take place. This chapter has identified concepts and terminology used in marketing health care services. The concepts are fairly straightforward, but their application is complex. Skills in applying marketing theory and concepts are gained through experience based on the ability to analyze available data and make decisions. The occupational therapy manager must understand the importance of the data base on which marketing decisions are made. Advanced study of business theory, finance, statistics, and organizational design is recommended before occupational therapy managers independently apply marketing theory without the consultation of a marketing professional.

SUMMARY

Marketing is a system for operational planning from an information base. This information is gathered and analyzed through a disciplined study of the needs of patients/clients, physicians, organization administrators (as the source of an occupational therapy department or program's funding), and reimbursers (as the source of the organization's funding). These four groups are target markets—a portion, of a larger population, that the marketer wants to influence.

A market plan is based on five key concepts: product, that which is offered to a target market to satisfy a want or a need; price, the exchange that occurs when a product is obtained; place, the method of distributing a product to a target market, or the means of giving the target market access to a product; promotion, all the attempts to make the product visible and desirable to a target market; and position, a product's relative place among similar products in the marketplace.

For years, health care organizations have followed a traditional planning cycle oriented to their mission and goals. In a market-based cycle an organization's mission and goals are constantly reexamined in light of available information about the organization's target market. The role of marketing is to validate the organization's mission in terms of the wants and the needs of consumers. An organization first engages in an organizational assessment, in which it studies its effectiveness relative to its patient/client population. The organization then performs an environmental assessment, in which it asks, What business are we in? and reexamines its patient/client population, its mode of delivery, and the location of delivery in terms of the characteristics of its target market. In both activities the organization is seeking to determine (a) the need for its product, (b) the market environment for its product, and (c) the competition its product will face—all in terms of the consumer's wants and needs. Marketing data can be drawn from many sources—any that help the organization understand (a) what was, (b) what is, and (c) what could be.

A market analysis follows. Through it an organization defines (a) whom it will serve, (b) how it will organize its services, (c) how it can group potential consumers with similar needs, and (d) what is unique about its services or products.

Communications, the fourth component of marketing information, includes advertising, promotions, and education. Marketing and community relations overlap here.

Marketing concepts are fairly straightforward, but their application is complex. Advanced study of related fields such as business theory, finance, statistics, and organizational design is recommended to help the occupational therapy manager apply marketing theory.

References

1. Kotler P: *Marketing for Non Profit Organizations*. Englewood Cliffs, NJ: Prentice-Hall Inc, 1975
2. MacStravic RES: *Marketing by Objectives*. Rockville, MD: Aspen Systems Corp, 1980
3. Lauback PB, Rand R: *Marketing Management for Health Care Executives*, seminar of the American College of Hospital Administrators. Wichita, KS, May 19–21, 1980
4. Berkowitz EN, Flexner WA: The marketing audit: A tool for health service organizations. *Health Care Manage Rev*, Fall 1978, pp 52–53
5. Stuehler G Jr: How hospital marketing and planning relate. *Hospitals*, May 1, 1980, pp 96–99
6. Olson TS: Health care marketing. In *Willard and Spackman's Occupational Therapy*, 6th edition, HL Hopkins, HD Smith, Editors. Philadelphia: JB Lippincott Co, 1983, pp 848–854

Additional Resource

Levitt T: *The Marketing Imagination*. New York: Free Press, 1983

Section III

Organizing

Three chapters constitute Section III, which focuses on the manager's role as an organizer. The role encompasses activities aimed at creating and maintaining a formal structure for accomplishing tasks. Chapter 7, "Management: Styles, Structures, and Roles," discusses traditional and contemporary theories of management and the effect of organizational climate on employees' motivation. The powerful influence of a manager's style and the important effects of organizational structure are stressed. Because of its effectiveness, participative management and its attendant skill of consensus building receive special attention.

A systems approach to management is the subject of Chapter 8. Systems thinking is explained as a way of relating the activities of an organizational unit to the larger organization, a way of focusing a manager's attention on goals and objectives, and the unit's success in meeting them. Many concrete examples are provided to help the occupational therapy manager understand the relevance of a systems approach to organizing the work of an occupational therapy department or program.

Chapter 9, "Managing Change," focuses on the dynamic aspect of organizing, on the fact that change is inevitable, even desirable, but also manageable. Change in five contexts is explained: problem solving, personal growth, interpersonal interaction, organizational development, and social evolution. The extensive discussion of theory is well balanced with guidelines and techniques for managing change and examples of its implementation.

Chapter 7

Management: Styles, Structures, and Roles

Ruth Ann Watkins, MBA, OTR, FAOTA

The ultimate responsibility of a manager is to get work done through other people. The theories that have influenced the way in which people manage have changed over the years, as have the roles of the manager. Also, the worker and the meaning of work have changed.

THEORIES OF ORGANIZATION

Historically the classical school of organization was the first formalized approach to management. It is authoritarian in nature and "emphasizes the need for well-established lines of authority equal to responsibility" (1, p 61). Principles of management that have evolved from this school include the scientific approach, which emphasizes "economic incentives and specialization of work," and the administrative approach, "which concentrates on departmentalization and forecasting" (2, p 2). Remnants of the classical school are still in existence in some settings. The current emphasis on efficiency, productivity, and cost reductions, and the trend

---

In 23 years as a professional, Ruth Ann Watkins has held a succession of management positions, from supervisor to vice-president. Currently she is the vice-president of allied health at the Rehabilitation Institute of Chicago, supervising ten department heads and administering a budget of $11 million.

toward specialization are conducive to a resurgence of an authoritarian approach.

Such a resurgence, however, would not be congruent with today's worker and the modern meaning of work, which reflect an opposite approach most commonly referred to as participative management. It is democratic in nature and incorporates human relations principles stressing the psychological and social factors that underlie individual and group performance (2). Workers' involvement in decision making is considered desirable and essential to high motivation. Balancing workers' needs and desires to be involved in decisions that affect their work environment with the needs and the goals of the organization requires great skill on the part of today's manager.

In these turbulent times of revolutionary changes in health care, a manager must also be able to determine how the parts of the system in which he or she works are interrelated and influenced by external systems. A helpful approach in this regard, of fairly recent origin, is systems theory. This approach analyzes "the relationship between various parts of the organization or system, and the role importance of each to overall performance. [It] also looks at external systems" affecting the organization (2, p 2). Chapter 8 discusses systems theory in detail.

THEORIES OF MOTIVATION

Underlying the different management approaches have been various theories of motivation, from Maslow's ideas about the hierarchy of needs (3) to Herzberg's motivation-hygiene model (4). McGregor (5) developed Theory X and Theory Y, which describe the assumptions about human motivation that are the basis for the concepts of authoritarian and participative management. Theory X assumes that people dislike work; must be directed, controlled, and coerced; and are primarily motivated by money. Theory Y assumes that people have an intrinsic interest in their work, that they desire to be self-directing and to seek responsibility, and that motivators include participation in establishing goals and solving problems that affect the organization.

Morse and Lorsch (1, p 61) have proposed the contingency theory, which contends that "the proper 'fit' among task, organization, and people seems to develop strong 'competence motivation' in individuals regardless of organizational style." Sense of competence is a continuing motivator, and when one competence goal is achieved, a new, higher one is set.

THE EFFECT OF ORGANIZATIONAL CLIMATE ON MOTIVATION

In recent years increased attention has been given to the environment of the organization and its influence on the motivation and the self-esteem of workers. Organizational environment is also referred to as organizational climate or organizational culture. Hamner and Organ (6, p 278) define *climate* as "a set of properties of the work environment that is assumed to be a major force in influencing the behavior of employees on the job. These properties include the size, structure, leadership patterns, interpersonal relationships, systems complexity, goal direction and communication patterns of the organization." The type and the characteristics of an organization influence the roles, the responsibilities, and the behaviors of the employees.

Formal Characteristics

Morse and Lorsch (1, p 63) group organizational characteristics into two sets of factors: formal and climate. Formal characteristics include the "pattern of formal relationships and duties as signified by organizational charts and job manuals, patterns of formal rules, procedures, control and measurement systems, time dimensions incorporated in formal practices and goal dimensions incorporated in formal practices." The goals of an organization reflect what it is trying to achieve and become. The policies indicate how the goals are to be attained and how employees are to behave in order to contribute to the achievement of the goals. Staff should be informed of the goals and should have a working knowledge of the policies and the procedures of the organization for which they work.

Climate Characteristics

Climate characteristics are the subjective perceptions and orientations that individuals have developed about their organizational setting. These include the character of superior-subordinate and colleague relationships, top executives' management style, structural orientation, distribution of influence, and time and goal orientation (1).

Organizations have traditionally been hierarchical in nature, but they are changing and so are workers. The characteristics of a health care organization that used to make it unique in comparison with a business organization are rapidly blurring. Health care organizations are becoming more businesslike, and some are even becoming for-profit businesses. Performance used to mean something quite different to people who provided services and people who received them than it does today or will tomorrow.

Hamner and Organ (6, p 279) conclude that the "traditional hierarchical system of organization breeds a climate of fear and mistrust, which reduces management effectiveness." To build an organizational climate that encourages achievement, management must focus on "an approach that offers warmth and support to each individual, communicating organizational goals and standards but not attempting to control the means of reaching those goals and standards."

In *The Art of Japanese Management* Pascale and Athos (7) report on a study in which they compared Japanese and American management practices. Much insight can be gained by reading the book. The authors conclude that the "best firms linked their purposes and ways of realizing them to human values as well as economic measures like profit and efficiency" (p 332). Pascal and Athos refer to seven "levers": superordinate goals, strategy, structure, systems, staff, style, and skills. The successful managers were able to integrate these significant levers into the fabric of the organization.

A manager must develop an atmosphere that motivates employees to work toward the achievement of the organization's goals and at the same time to satisfy their own needs for a sense of accomplishment, competence, recognition, appreciation, and "winning." Toffler and others have pointed out that the new worker seeks meaning in his or her work, along with financial rewards. Individuals vary in the values, the needs, and the skills that they bring to the workplace, and they differ in their manner of responding to identical organizational environments.

MANAGEMENT STYLE

The type of climate a manager creates for staff and the way in which he or she organizes work and motivates employees are influenced by the organization and the workers. They are also a function of a manager's own needs, goals, motives, abilities, values, and biases. All these contribute to a manager's style. "Style is what other people say it is" (7, p 277). Metzger (8) and others have pointed out that the manager's leadership style has the single greatest effect on a group's productivity and growth.

Collaborative Versus Competitive Styles

Many managers underestimate the powerful influence their behavior has on employees. A manager's behavior is a strong form of symbolic communication. Employees look to the manager for cues about what behavior is expected, how to perform it, and what the consequences of it will be. For example, if a manager works closely with his or her peers in other areas of the organization, seeks their counsel, treats them as respected colleagues, and deals with conflict openly, his or her management style could be categorized as collaborative. The message this behavior gives to the manager's staff is that collaborative relationships are expected.

A collaborative style facilitates working relationships among staff. An organization that values team work and promotes it in direct care invites a collaborative style. If a manager worked in such a setting but rarely met with peers except in meetings called by a superior, and if that manager planned programs in a hands-off manner and referred to other departments in demeaning ways, he or she would be conveying the message that competition rather than collaboration was to be the flavor of working relationships. Such a style does not fit a setting in which teamwork is expected. It creates an atmosphere of conflict for employees, who are torn between the behavior their manager expects of them and the behavior their team members expect. Conversely, a manager whose style was collaborative would not fit in an organization where competitive behavior was valued and rewarded.

Situation Management

The range of problems facing a manager is so great that one habitual set of responses or alternatives is inadequate (9). A manager must be able to perceive differences—between situations, people, circumstances, motives, assumptions, and physical and technological realities(9)—and tailor his or her style of action to fit the situation. In order for employees to trust a manager, however, they must feel comfortable in predicting how the manager will behave in various situations. The key to effective situation management is understanding how to define the situation for others. Once a manager has defined a situation in a certain way, people will continue to see it that way (10). The manager must be able to look beyond the day-to-day details of the job, develop an ability to understand what motivates individual employees, communicate in terms they comprehend, master techniques of introducing change in the face of resistance, and analyze situations using facts and logic while controlling subjectivity (8).

ORGANIZATIONAL STRUCTURE

The formal structure a manager creates is an important ingredient in influencing the behavior of employees on the job and accomplishing the goals of the organization. The formal structure provides a framework for dividing work, developing specific job functions, and making task assignments. It also establishes lines of authority, working relationships among staff, and systems of communication. Whether a manager is dealing with a newly created program or department or a well-established, perhaps entrenched one, he or she is working within the structure of the organization.

The size of work groups, the tasks to be done, the roles staff have taken, the resources available, and the expectations of the leadership of the organization influence the structure the manager develops. Frequently managers find themselves in the middle, between their employees and the administration, the administration and the physicians, or the administration and the governing board. This is particularly true if a manager is working in a hospital.

Work and Role Demands

As mentioned earlier, the tasks to be performed by a group must be taken into consideration in creating or changing a structure. If a manager is responsible for several groups of occupational therapy personnel who provide services to different areas of the organization, he or she must consider the commonalities as well as the differences in work and role demands placed on the staff. The manager has to decide whether to be centralized or decentralized in relation to authority, responsibility, and staff assignment. For example, more authority may need to be delegated to a work group that is physically located in another building, such as an outpatient clinic or an extended care facility.

The transformations in health care and society, higher expectations from employees, and a more educated work group call for a structure that accommodates rapid change and is characterized by involvement, participation, and commitment of the employee. In addition, the structure must allow the manager to maintain a balance between the ideals of health care and the financial resources of the organization. Systems that enhance efficiency, effectiveness, productivity, and accountability must be built.

Participative Management and Consensus Building

Studies have shown that successful managers use participative management. This approach is complex but effective. It emphasizes joint problem solving and decision making by some or all persons who are relevant to the problem (8). The skill of building consensus is needed under this form of management. Staff must come to a consensus on what the real problem is in a specific situation and how they will solve it. The manager's role is to be an active listener, paying close attention to reservations and doubts, encouraging expression of different views, and dealing with conflicts openly and candidly. The manager must be willing to accept a solution that is different than the one he or she favors.

The manager must define the framework within which a consensus decision can be made. For example, if the board of a hospital decides that the facility will provide services seven days a week, a manager should bring staff together and build consensus on how the decision is to be implemented, not whether it will be. In such a situation the manager will most likely have to spend time providing information so that staff understand the reason for the decision and its relationship to organizational goals. The manager will also have to deal with staff feelings, because such a change will affect their work and personal lives. These feelings should be acknowledged and discussed on an individual as well as a group basis. Providing staff with an opportunity to express their feelings and participate in decision making will help establish group ownership of the implementation plan.

According to Metzger (8), tasks that are performed through cooperation rather than competition are more efficiently accomplished. Ad hoc committees, focus groups, peer reviews, and recognition for individual and group efforts are methods a manager can use to facilitate participative management. The astute manager will surround himself or herself with competent people and let them do their jobs. Staff should be involved in setting performance standards that deal with quality and productivity, and they should participate in developing departmental or program procedures. Job descriptions should reflect tasks and responsibilities, including participation in identifying problems and helping to find solutions. Kanter (11, p 102) has found that "companies that produced the most entrepreneurs have cultures that encourage collaboration and teamwork." They also have complex structures that link people in multiple ways and help them go beyond the confines of their defined jobs to do "what needs to be done."

Communication

An effective communication system is basic to successful management. The communication process is complicated because so many different messages are being conveyed and each individual interprets them differently. The amount and the type of experience an individual therapist or therapy assistant has affects how messages are interpreted. Communication is covered in detail in Chapter 15.

ROLES AND RESPONSIBILITIES

As stated at the beginning of this chapter, the roles of managers have changed over the years. Continual change is the environment in which managers will function. To Toffler (12, p 281), managers of the future must be "trained for instant adaptation and they must feel comfortable in a wider repertoire of available organizational structures and roles, . . . [ranging from the] hierarchical mode to the open-door, free-flow style."

Roles

The manager has many roles, as well as explicit and implicit responsibilities. These change from situation to situation and task to task. Whether a manager is a director, a supervisor, or an administrator, an important role he or she plays is that of liaison between his or her staff and other centers of authority in the organization. The manager also represents the administration to the employees as the interpreter of the organization's policies and the implementer of its programs. A manager's real power is achieved through a network of satisfactory relationships (8) built on personal contact, negotiation, support, shared goals and values, and trust. Well-developed interpersonal skills are necessary to develop such relationships.

The occupational therapy manager also fills the roles of professional, leader, counselor, coach, decision maker, trainer, supervisor, supervisee, facilitator, mediator, group member, visionary, planner, and change agent. In today's climate he or she must be a risk taker as well. A more complete discussion of roles is contained in Chapter 11.

Role modeling is a powerful tool. With it, the manager can encourage self-rewarding behaviors among staff and achievement of competence goals. The manager who conveys the message that employees are an organization's most important asset will be effective at motivating staff and engendering trust.

Explicit Responsibilities

Explicit responsibilities that accompany these roles include making decisions, providing feedback, motivating employees, securing resources, managing conflict, and collaborating. Some of these responsibilities are examined in Chapters 10 and 15.

A reality of management is that managers and the people they manage sometimes do not see eye to eye on what workers want most (8). However, managers do make assumptions about how their actions influence the performance and the satisfaction of their subordinates. The validity of their perceptions is based on their previous experience, their value systems, the information they receive, and the method by which it is processed.

Implicit Responsibilities

The implicit responsibilities of the managerial role include being trustworthy and possessing and fostering integrity. Also implied is a subordination of the manager's and staff's interests to organizational goals. This can create a conflict for the manager, and great skill is required to maintain a climate that balances the needs and the interests of the staff with the values and the goals of the organization.

SUMMARY

The theories that have influenced the way in which people manage have changed over the years, as have the roles of the manager. Also, the worker and the meaning of work have changed. The classical school of organization, authoritarian in nature, was the first formalized approach to management. Both the scientific and the administrative approach have evolved from it. Today's worker and the modern meaning of work reflect an opposite approach, participative management. These turbulent times also call for an understanding of systems theory.

Underlying the different management approaches have been various theories of motivation—for example, Maslow's hierarchy of needs, Herzberg's motivation-hygiene model, McGregor's Theory X and Theory Y, and Morse and Lorsch's contingency theory. In recent years increased attention has been given to organizational climate and its influence on the motivation and the self-esteem of workers. An organization's climate is characterized by the subjective perceptions and orientations that individuals have developed about the setting.

Organizations have traditionally been hierarchical in nature, but they are changing and so are workers. The "traditional hierarchical system . . . breeds a climate of fear and mistrust" (6, p 279). Management must focus on "an approach that offers warmth and support to each individual" (6, p 279).

Many managers underestimate the powerful influence their behavior has on employees. For example, through his or her actions a manager can communicate that collaborative relationships are expected.

The range of problems facing a manager is so great that one habitual set of responses is inadequate. The key to effective situation management is understanding how to define the situation for others.

The formal structure a manager creates is an important ingredient in influencing employees' behavior and accomplishing organizational goals. The size of work groups, their tasks, staff members' roles, available resources, and top management's expectations influence the structure the manager develops. The transformations in health care and society, higher expectations from employees, and a more educated work group call for a structure that accommodates rapid change and is characterized by involvement, participation, and commitment. Also, systems that enhance efficiency, effectiveness, productivity, and accountability must be built.

Successful managers use participative management, which emphasizes joint problem solving and decision making. Tasks that are performed through cooperation rather than competition are more efficiently accomplished.

The manager has many roles, among them, liaison between his or her staff and other centers of authority in the organization. A manager's real power is achieved through a network of satisfactory relationships.

Explicit responsibilities of the manager are making decisions, providing feedback, motivating employees, securing resources, managing conflict, and collaborating. Implicit responsibilities include being trustworthy, possessing and fostering integrity, and subordinating staff's interests, and his or her own, to organizational goals.

References

1. Morse JJ, Lorsch JW: Beyond Theory Y. *Harvard Business Review*, May–June 1970, pp 61–68
2. American Occupational Therapy Association: *Manual on Administration*. Rockville, MD: American Occupational Therapy Association, 1978
3. Maslow A: *Motivation and Personality*. New York: Harper & Row Publishers Inc, 1954
4. Herzberg F: *Work and the Nature of Man*. New York: Thomas Y Crowell Co, 1966
5. McGregor D: *The Human Side of Enterprise*. New York: McGraw-Hill Book Co, 1960
6. Hamner W, Organ DW: *Organizational Behavior: An Applied Psychological Approach*. Plano, TX: Business Publications Inc, 1978
7. Pascale R, Athos A: *The Art of Japanese Management*. New York: Warner Books Inc, 1982, p 125
8. Metzger N: *The Health Care Supervisor's Handbook*, 2nd edition. Rockville, MD: Aspen Systems Corp, 1982, pp 3, 162
9. Skinner W, Sasser EW: Managers with impact: Versatile and inconsistent. *Harvard Business Review*, November–December 1977, pp 140–148
10. Ritti RR, Funkhouse GR: *The Ropes to Skip and the Ropes to Know: Studies in Organizational Behavior*. Columbus, OH: Grid Publishing Inc, 1977, p 169
11. Kanter RM: The middle manager as innovator. *Harvard Business Review*, July–August 1982, pp 95–105
12. Toffler A: *The Third Wave*. New York: William Morrow & Co Inc, 1980

Additional Resources

Kennedy MM: Negotiate for cooperation and support. *Hospital Manager* 14(6):1–2, 1984

Klein JA: Why supervisors resist employee involvement. *Harvard Business Review*, September–October 1984, pp 87–95

Knox TA: Hospital manager role demanding more complex skills. *Hospital Manager* 14(4):3–4, 1984

Lawrence PR, Kolodny HF, Davis SM: Human side of the matrix. *Organizational Dynamics*, Summer 1977, pp 43–61

Peters TJ, Waterman RH Jr: *In Search of Excellence: Lessons from America's Best-Run Companies*. New York: Harper & Row Publishers Inc, 1982

Schwartz KB: Balancing objectives of efficient and effective occupational therapy practice. *Am J Occup Ther* 38:198–200, 1984

Tilles S: How to evaluate corporate strategy. *Harvard Business Review*, July–August 1963, pp 111–121

Wysocki B Jr: The chief's personality can have a big impact—for better or worse. *Wall Street Journal*, September 11, 1984, pp 1, 16

Zaleznik A, Moment D: *The Dynamics of Interpersonal Behavior*. New York: John Wiley & Sons Inc, 1964

Chapter 8

A Systems Approach to Management

Winifred E. Scott, PhD, OTR/L

An occupational therapy manager in a university hospital setting might catalog a typical Monday morning as follows:

1. I step off the elevator and unlock the clinic door at 8:30 AM, thirty minutes earlier than usual in order to prepare an agenda for a 9:00 unit meeting and to get the cost of another phone line for the Pediatrics Unit.
2. The phone rings. Dr. Gates needs a splint checked for a patient who is going home at noon today.
3. Two more phone calls come in before 8:55:
   - The university fieldwork supervisor wants to know if the department can take an occupational therapy student next month whose fieldwork site was canceled.
   - Dr. Bahr cannot attend the Occupational Therapy Medical Advisory Committee meeting. I was relying on his moderating voice as a knowledgeable user of occupational therapy services to counter Dr. Rada's attempt to interpret narrowly the Joint Commission

Currently the head of the occupational therapy department at the University of Illinois at the Medical Center, Winifred E. Scott has developed and taught a graduate course in systems theory in the university's College of Allied Health.

on Accreditation of Hospital's (JCAH's) specifications of the purpose of an advisory committee. Perhaps Dr. Rogers can serve this purpose.

4. I prepare a tentative agenda for the 9:00 meeting.
5. In the unit meeting I hear the following news:
   - The roof in the Psychiatry and Outpatient Unit is leaking, and the ceiling tiles are falling. A tile barely missed a wheelchair patient yesterday. I must call Physical Plant about the tiles and then see that someone will be in the unit when Physical Plant's estimators come.
   - The Ortho-Neuro-Rehabilitation Unit needs splinting material—tomorrow. There is not enough money in that unit's budget to buy the materials. I must find the funds in another unit's budget and transfer them.
   - Susan Smith, the staff therapist in the Pediatrics Unit, is resigning. She will be leaving in two weeks and would like her vacation time in pay. (Later I learn that when Susan departs, Tom Brown will be absent from the Psychiatry and Outpatient Unit to take the neurodevelopmental training course, and Laura Bockstiegel will be going on vacation.)

6. At lunch I learn that during the unit meeting a person from the Safety Committee came to the department and reported that we did not have a three-prong adapter on the sewing machine in the Ortho-Neuro-Rehabilitation Unit.

7. In a phone call I am informed that the performance rating for my secretary must be in today.

8. A social worker stops by to be filled in on what happened at the last Geriatric Committee meeting.

9. The chairperson of the Geriatric Committee, Dr. Smith, requests an organizational chart of the occupational therapy department. She also wants to know, by tomorrow, how the new geriatric occupational therapy position (if it is funded) will fit in to the organizational chart.

10. Nancy Beal, the staff therapist in the Medicine and Surgery unit, calls. The new physician does not want the department to see mastectomy patients until they have been discharged from the hospital because treatment may increase sanguineous secretions. He wants to conduct a new study. I wonder why this comes up now. Will the staffing pattern need to be changed?

11. The day's mail arrives:
    - It brings correspondence from students who are due to arrive in two weeks. Responses must be written telling them when and where to meet, and what to wear.
    - I receive the minutes of the semiannual college faculty meeting, at which the faculty voted to establish a nontenure clinical track and maintain the tenure track. The faculty also voted to support the provision that the doctorate be required for promotion to associate professor and for tenure at the university. What implications will these changes have for my staff, who, with one exception, are clinical, not academic, faculty? Will more clinical

occupational therapy staff be required to have master's degrees? Will the demand for research increase?

- Three letters arrive from occupational therapy assistants interested in a position. None come from occupational therapists.

12. I must begin to prepare the inventory report due in two weeks.

13. I must prepare to participate in the inservice sessions on infection control and safety control, in anticipation of the accreditation site visit.

14. My department head calls to schedule two meetings: one with me alone and one with all hospital occupational therapy staff to introduce the new faculty member, who will coordinate clinical research between occupational therapy's hospital staff and academic faculty.

15. Quality assurance meetings now conflict with those of the Occupational Therapy Medical Advisory Committee. I need to delegate a staff member to attend quality assurance meetings and help write a quarterly department report for JCAH.

A manager of an occupational therapy department or program in a large organization needs a way to sort out issues like these that occur daily. How can the whole situation be seen in perspective? How can various actions be put in the context of a manager's broad responsibilities? Often decisions must be made for which an adequate base of information does not seem to exist. Problems are sometimes so interconnected that knowing where to begin is difficult. A manager needs a way to define the nature of the subsystem he or she manages so that decisions get made in a logical way that includes the environment in which the subsystem operates. A manager also needs a way to measure how well the subsystem executes its responsibilities. A systems approach can provide a framework for meeting these needs.

THE LIVES OF MANAGERS

Some aspects of the lives of managers bear elaboration. According to Mintzberg (1), a manager is not "like an orchestra leader, controlling the various parts of his organization with ease and precision" (p 32). They are rarely reflective workers with routinized jobs, who are advised by information systems. Although they may say that they plan, organize, control, and motivate, managers "play a complex, intertwined combination of interpersonal, informational, and decisional roles" (1, p 32). Mintzberg (1) has found that certain facts appear consistently in the lives of managers:

- They "work at an unrelenting pace . . . their activities are characterized by brevity, variety, and discontinuity, they are strongly oriented to action and dislike reflective activities" (p 32). From the time they arrive at their place of work until the time they leave, they meet a steady stream of callers. "They jump from issue to issue . . . responding to the needs of the moment" (p 33).
- They perform a number of regular duties in addition to handling exceptions, "including ritual and ceremony, negotiations, and processing of soft information that links the organization with its environment" (p 33). Often they substitute for absent personnel.

• They favor oral media and word-of-mouth communication—for example, telephone calls and meetings.

• They find mail processing a burden because mail does not provide much live, current information.

• They cherish gossip, hearsay, and speculation because of its timeliness. "Today's gossip may be tomorrow's fact" (p 33). This means that much of the important data regarding the organization is stored in the manager's head rather than in a file cabinet or a computer, rendering the transmittal of the information, and hence delegation of responsibility, difficult.

"The manager is overburdened with obligations; yet he cannot easily delegate tasks . . . he is driven to overwork and is forced to do many tasks superficially" (p 34). Pressures are becoming worse because in addition to their having to respond to superordinates, subordinates with democratic expectations constantly reduce the manager's freedom to give unexplained orders, and a growing number of people with influence and vested interests expect the manager's attention.

In Mintzberg's (1) words, "the manager is challenged to deal consciously with the pressures of superficiality by giving serious attention to the issues that require it, by stepping back from his tangible bits of information in order to see a broad picture, and by making use of analytical inputs" (p 66). How can systems thinking help? It may be a waste of time for managers to list all of the problems that trouble them, all of the things that they have to do, and then begin doing them without logically thinking about the function being served. Managers need objectives to measure the performance of their system and to judge how well it is doing. How do managers do this? How do they get on top of the situation and see the whole system so that their objectives can be accomplished with minimum delay? Some answers to these questions can be found in the systems approach.

THE ORIGIN OF SYSTEMS THINKING

Systems theory was developed by Ludwig von Bertalanffy (2) in the 1920s and 1930s. Early in his career as a biologist, von Bertalanffy noted that his field, which dealt with living matter, analyzed biological phenomena by using the methods of physics and chemistry. Examinations were conducted reductionistically, by breaking phenomena into their component parts: protons, neutrons, atoms, molecules, cells, reflexes, behavior. How these parts were organized to maintain the whole organism was not considered important, nor was the maintenance of the whole organism well explained.

The critical difference, von Bertalanffy (2) observed, was that biological (and social) structures were open systems. Open systems must have a continuing relationship with their environment in order to maintain life. If input from the environment ceases, death or disorganization results.

Closed systems are not connected to their environments. In chemistry one studies chemical reactions, their rates, and the chemical equilibrium that is established—for example, in a closed bottle when a number of reagents are brought together. No input from the environment is needed for the reaction to occur.

Input, Throughput, and Output

In open systems, inputs from the environment—energy in some form—pass through an organism in a process called throughput, and a resulting output is discharged back into the environment. In an organization the available energy is transformed into new products, refined materials, trained people, or services, which are exported into the environment. For example, occupational therapy students enter a university, and through their efforts and those of the faculty (input), they learn and develop entry-level skills (throughput). They then graduate, pass the certification examination, and enter the work force as products (output) of the occupational therapy school.

Feedback

Some input is transformed into a product. Other input—feedback—provides information to a system on how it is doing. In the preceding example the students' passing the certification examination provides feedback to them on their performance in learning entry-level skills and to the occupational therapy school on its performance in choosing and educating students. Negative feedback allows the system to correct deviations from its desired course. The evaluations occupational therapy students receive midway through their fieldwork enable them to improve their performance in key areas before the end of the experience.

SOCIAL ORGANIZATIONS AS SYSTEMS

Systems have been defined in many ways. One way to look at any system is as "a set of parts coordinated to accomplish a set of goals" (3, p 29). A system's goals or objectives are generally its motivating force. Although a systems perspective lends itself to examination of a variety of systems—physiological, technological, etc.—in this chapter, discussion is confined to social systems, specifically social organizations.

Social organizations, like other open systems, receive replenishing supplies of energy from the physical environment, institutions, and people. Social structures are not self-sufficient or self-contained.

Katz and Kahn (4) state, "In using an open systems approach, our objective is to understand human organizations, to describe the essential elements of their form and function, to explain cycles of growth and decline, to predict the effects and effectiveness, and to introduce purposeful change into the organization" (p 18).

Systems as Cycles of Events

The structure of a system can easily be seen when the system has physical boundaries and the component parts are located within them. For example, a human body has limbs that are bounded by skin. Unlike biological systems, social systems are not physically bounded. Parts can be, and are, shed and replaced. Yet these systems have a basic continuity, which can be explained by viewing a system's structure as a cycle of events. The component activities are events that are structured to form a pattern, a repetitious cycle in which energy is exchanged. All social organizations are patterned activities of many people. The patterned activities in which people engage are dependent on one another and complementary in relation to a shared goal. The cycle lasts over time and is enacted more than once. The system is stable, based on the recurrent events (4).

For example, a university's publications office annually prepares a catalog that contains the requirements for entry into the occupational therapy program, among others. From September to February of each year the admissions office accepts the applications of potential students. The occupational therapy faculty, who depend on those two offices to recruit appropriate students each year, interview acceptable applicants. An admissions committee, consisting of representatives of the admissions office, the student affairs office, the occupational therapy department, and the department's parent college of allied health, meets to determine that the objective of admitting fifty students per year has been fulfilled and that the university's norms for admission (e.g., completed application forms, an adequate grade point average, and preadmission experience) have been satisfied. This cycle of events or set of coordinated parts is necessary to the life of the occupational therapy department and the university.

Another example of a social system is evident when an occupational therapist sees patients/clients in a hand rehabilitation clinic. Each week three or four patients/clients are referred to the clinic. They are treated and eventually discharged. To sustain this pattern, the therapist must continue to provide energy by staffing the clinic (an event in the cycle). From his or her energy expenditure emerge patients/clients whose hand functions are improved. The therapist's continued presence in the clinic yields additional referrals and a reputation for occupational therapy as a contributor to successful treatment. These events become a source of continuing referrals.

Katz and Kahn (4, p 21) use two basic criteria for identifying social systems and determining their functions: "(1) tracing the pattern of energy exchange or activity of people as it results in some output and (2) ascertaining how the output is translated into energy that reactivates the pattern."

Control

Preservation of physical and biological structures is not as difficult as preservation of social structures. Limbs do not drift away from the body. People, however, do wander away from social systems. For example, dissatisfied employees resign when they find other jobs, and unmotivated employees take sick leave on Monday to extend the weekend. For their preservation, social organizations depend on both production inputs, energy transformed to yield a product or outcome, and maintenance inputs, energy that sustains a system. People must be motivated to stay in an organization and produce work, because social systems require that people be physically present and carry out particular behavior patterns (work roles). The behavior of individuals must be predictable rather than spontaneous. Katz and Kahn (4, p 41) observe, ". . . the core problem of any social system is reducing the variability and instability of human actions to uniform and dependable patterns."

Thelan (as reported in 4) proposes three types of pressures or forces that control the variance of human action in organizations:

1. Environmental pressures: external forces or demands that induce a coordinated group effort. Environmental pressures may be seen as a prime motivation in the opening example, when, to comply with hospital and JCAH standards (outside pressures), the occupational therapy manager decides to delegate to a staff member the responsibility of attending Quality Assurance meetings and helping write the department's Quality Assurance report.

2. Shared values: common goals and mutual expectations that people have about how they should behave to achieve their shared objectives. In that first illustration the occupational therapy manager and the university fieldwork supervisor value education of occupational therapy students. When the fieldwork supervisor calls, the manager readily agrees to accept the student who needs a fieldwork site on short notice.

3. Rule enforcement: the use of sanctions. The violation of rules calls for some form of penalty. Again with reference to the opening scenario, safety regulations require a three-pronged adapter on all electrical devices. Failure of the occupational therapy department to comply with the directive to change the sewing machine plug will result in a warning notice or a citation.

System Integration

To enforce control, social organizations rely on formal prescriptions of acceptable and unacceptable behavior. Formal patterns of organizational behavior are achieved through roles, norms, and values, which Katz and Kahn (4) describe as furnishing three interrelated bases for social integration in organizations:

1. *Roles* describes specific behavior expectations associated with given positions. "People are tied together because of the functional interdependence of the roles they play . . ." (p 44). Therapist, patient/client, physician, social worker, must perform in accordance with a particular sequence and time schedule. Because the requirements of different roles are interrelated, people who perform them are bound together, and as a result, the organization achieves a degree of integration. In the opening example, Dr. Bahr has agreed to serve on the Occupational Therapy Medical Advisory Committee. He is expected to attend the meetings or to notify the occupational therapy manager when he cannot. The social worker who could not attend the last Geriatric Committee meeting asks to be informed about what she missed, that is, what she needs to know in order to play her role on that committee.

2. Norms are general expectations of all people who occupy a given role. "The normative requirements for roles add an additional cohesive element [to people's behavior]" (p 44). To return to the scenario that opens this chapter, the request from Dr. Gates that an occupational therapist check a patient's splint reflects a norm that patients be treated quickly (before discharge) and as successfully as possible (with the best possible splint for their condition).

3. "Values are the more generalized ideological justification for roles and norms, and express aspirations [that tell why an activity is required]" (p 44). The value of improving the human condition is probably shared by all the people who play parts in the opening example.

A FRAMEWORK FOR EXAMINING A SYSTEM

Readers may be convinced now that systems exist and that some knowledge of their own system may be helpful in their everyday working experience. How then does one keep a finger on the pulse of a system? To do this, according to Churchman (3), it is desirable to delineate the system, to identify the parts that are coordinated to accomplish a set of goals. Churchman (3, p 29) suggests examining a system in terms of five considerations: objectives, environment, resources, component activities, and management.

Objectives

As noted earlier, the goals or the objectives of a system are generally its motivating force, what its efforts are intended to attain or accomplish. The objectives should be expressed in specific terms so that measures of performance can be applied to them. Churchman (3) sees the measure of performance of a system as a score that tells how well the system is doing. One of the objectives of the occupational therapy manager in the opening example may be to run a cost-effective department with a certain number of patients seen by each therapist every day and a certain volume of quality treatments per unit. The maintenance of a full staff despite a turnover of therapists is a critical factor in maintaining the number and the volume. One of the manager's measures of performance of this objective might be that for no more than three weeks per year will any unit be without its full complement of staff. To ensure that this measure of performance is met, the manager could develop strategies—for example, periodic advertisements, a resume file, and cross listings with other occupational therapy managers.

To develop specific measures of performance, an organization must make choices about the kinds of products it will and will not consider and the kinds of markets it will and will not serve (5). In the university hospital scenario the occupational therapy manager and the unit heads may have decided to provide a range of services to fill the current and emerging needs of patients, physicians, and third-party payers in the hospital and its community operations (a teaching nursing home, an ambulatory care facility, and a home health program). They search constantly for new ways of satisfying their present markets, and they are alert to new needs in their medical center. (For a lengthier discussion of products and markets, see Chapter 6.)

Inhabitants of a system, especially managers, often talk about its objectives. Their statements have a number of purposes that are independent of how the system performs. For example, the medical director of a hospital may state that the purpose of the organization is to cure disease and prevent illness in the community. This statement may be an attempt to increase the hospital's credibility. It may be called into question when patients are turned away from the emergency room because they are unable to pay for treatment. In examining a system, therefore, the real objectives must be differentiated from the publically affirmed ones. Churchman (3, p 31) suggests that "the test of the objective of a system is the determination of whether the system will knowingly sacrifice other goals in order to attain the objective."

Environment

The environment of a system is that which lies outside it, over which it has little control—for example, tenured faculty and a facility's location. Although the environment lies outside the system's control, it determines in part how the system performs. To determine whether a particular phenomenon is a part of the environment, one asks, Do my objectives depend on it? and Can I control it? If the answer is yes to the first question but no to the second, "it" is a part of the environment. In the opening example Susan Smith's resignation fits into a pattern; on the average, two to three occupational therapists leave the staff of that program each year. Therapist turnover is a part of the program's environment.

The environment also makes demands on the system. It has a "requirement schedule" (3, p 36). For example, to maintain a viable department or program, there must be a certain ratio of therapists to patients/clients. A certain number of patients/clients must been seen by each therapist every day if the department or the program is to be cost-effective. If Susan Smith, the staff therapist in the example, is not replaced immediately, some adjustments will have to be made to maintain the treatment schedule without her.

Not all energy exchanges occur only between the organization and its environment. Emery and Trist (6) discuss how environments can become increasingly turbulent. Processes occur outside a system whereby elements of the environment become related to one another and become the determining condition for the system's exchanges (input, throughput, and output). The environment then controls its system's objectives. The initiation of Diagnosis Related Groups (DRGs) provides an example. A clustering of environmental forces—that is, increasing hospital and Medicare costs, the wide range of costs at different hospitals, and the inadequacy of per diem rates to measure hospital services—led to a federal decision to separate revenues and costs (at least for the largest hospital payer, Medicare). The traditional hospital governance groups (trustees, administration, and medical staff) were no longer able to set their own (often fragmented) goals in their respective spheres of responsibility. Hospital managers were charged to see that performance throughout the organization met cost-effectiveness objectives. Many hospitals had to redefine their identity, reexamine their basic objectives, and in some cases refashion themselves.

Resources

Resources are the instruments that a system uses to do its work, the things a system can employ or change to its advantage. Resources are people, capital or endowments, the willingness of employees to work, the prime location of a facility. They are the pool from which component activities take shape.

According to Churchman (3), it is difficult to think adequately about real resources. Usually an organization creates a list of resources, a balance sheet. The problem with this approach is that it leaves many resources out—the educational background of personnel, their personal capabilities, goodwill, and so forth.

Important questions to ask regarding resources are, How can they best be used? and How can they be increased? In examining resources, their current use should be monitored, and so should the opportunities that are lost because resources are employed somewhere else. Churchman (3) recommends the development of a management information system to monitor resources. Such a system for an occupational therapy department or program might cover the following types of information:

1. The resources (e.g., treatment activities, volume, procedures) that occupational therapy supplies to the larger system and the usefulness of those activities to the system
2. The reliability of treatments for given conditions
3. The needs and the resources of occupational therapy users, both patients/clients and physicians (to be able to point out options the users have and to generate new programs to respond to existing and developing needs)
4. Potential problem areas in patient/client treatment, or changes in other aspects of the environment.

In regard to the second category, an information system about patient/client conditions could have alerted the occupational therapy manager in the opening scenario to the possibility of an increase in sanguineous fluids in mastectomy patients. Such forewarning might have enabled the manager to forecast the best time for treatment. The Occupational Therapy Medical Advisory Committee on which that manager sits functions as a monitor of the fourth category of information listed.

Component Activities

The objectives of a system are accomplished by the specific activities of its parts or subsystems. Although an organization chart divides people into groups, offices, departments, and divisions, these groupings are not the true components of a system. To look at the true components, the "missions," traditional lines of authority or divisions of people must be ignored. The missions cut across the usual department or program lines. To return to a previous example, the mission of admitting occupational therapy students to a university is carried out by several offices located in different divisions: The publications office prepares the catalog of entry requirements, a recruitment group in the college of allied health attends high school career days, the admissions office sends out and receives applications, occupational therapy faculty interview students, and so on.

Analyzing missions enables a manager to estimate the worth of an activity to the total system. According to Churchman (3, p 43), "the ultimate aim of component thinking is to discover the components (the mission) whose measure of performance is truly related to the measure of performance of the overall system." An occupational therapy department or program might determine that its activities in a hand rehabilitation clinic facilitate patients'/clients' return to work and thus serve the mission of the larger system. In this instance the measure of performance of the occupational therapy component increases the measure of performance of the total system. Otherwise the component is not truly contributing to the system's performance.

Management

Management is defined by Hersey and Blanchard (7) as working with and through individuals and groups to accomplish organizational goals. Four functions are generally considered vital to the role of manager: planning, organizing, controlling, and motivating. Managers generate plans for a system. In so doing they consider the system's goals and objectives, environment, use of resources, and component activities.

In carrying out their organizing function, managers set goals for the components of a system and organize activities by bringing together a systems' resources—people, capital, equipment, etc.—in such a way that the goals are most effectively accomplished.

Managers see that plans they have generated are carried out. If the plans are not carried out, managers determine why. This function is called control. It implies an evaluation of plans based on feedback of results and a comparison of outcomes with the original plan. Also implied are adjustments, in cases when outcomes have deviated from expectations and a consequent change of plans is needed.

Motivation may be management's most important function. For an organization to be effective, managers must stimulate people to participate and do the work required. They must also set expectations for behavior in relation to the organization's goals and provide some form of feedback.

USING A SYSTEMS APPROACH IN MANAGEMENT

An application of systems thinking to the situations faced by the manager of the hospital occupational therapy program in the opening scenario may help the reader to understand the preceding discussion of systems. The program in which that manager operates can be viewed as a cycle of events, a set of patterned activities that are complementary and interdependent, that return on one another to complete the cycle, and that serve to achieve an objective.

With this perspective the manager examines the program using Churchman's five considerations (3). First, the objectives of the program are identified:

1. To deliver cost-effective treatment to patients who are referred to the program; specifically to see appropriately referred inpatients or outpatients in treatment units of fifteen minutes
2. To develop treatment strategies for patient populations of the hospital, where appropriate; specifically to explore new treatment possibilities as the patient mix changes

3. To monitor continually the objectives, environment, resources, component activities and management of each unit through weekly unit meetings and monthly reports.
4. To maintain continuing communication with other members of the system, especially in relation to patient treatment, quality control, safety, and other hospital policies
5. To provide a quality educational experience for four to five occupational therapy students every three months, in the areas of physical disabilities, psychiatry, medicine and surgery, and pediatrics.
6. To keep abreast of changes within and outside the organization that affect the delivery of the occupational therapy program; specifically, to involve staff members in monitoring university and hospital publications, policies, meetings, and reports.

Next, the manager delineates the environment of the program, the phenomena that are largely beyond control but that make demands on resources:

1. The requirement schedule of patient treatment
2. The turnover of occupational therapy staff
3. The lack of an adequate data base on the efficacy of treatment
4. Budgetary constraints
5. The number of meetings that require attendance to sustain involvement in the service program of the hospital and the educational program of the university
6. The demand schedule of student training.

The resources of the program are then listed:

1. Adequate space and support services
2. High-level, well-motivated staff who like their work, enjoy working together, and with only a few exceptions are interested in acquiring more information on treatment in their areas
3. Fieldwork students, who are often an excellent source of new staff.

Turning to the subject of component activities, the manager notes that the hospital program is located within an occupational therapy department, which is a part of a college within a university. The department is made up of an undergraduate program, a graduate program, and the hospital program. Occupational therapy is one of several departments in the college that have service programs, although the university's primary missions are teaching and research. Historically the teaching and service missions of the occupational therapy department were united. An outgrowth of this former union is that the college pays about two-thirds of the hospital program's salaries. The hospital program itself comprises five units: Medicine and Surgery, Ortho-Neuro-Rehabilitation, Pediatrics, Psychiatry, and Outpatient.

In terms of management, the hospital program manager directs a staff of eight full-time and one half-time occupational therapists and three occupational therapy assistants, who are assigned to the various units. The hospital program is located in a different building from the department, and in part because of this, the manager has broad responsibility for running it. The manager reports to the occupational therapy department director, who also supervises the academic faculty and who reports to the dean of the college.

Having considered these five broad aspects of the program, the manager decides to focus the immediate analysis on the relationship between two environmental issues: the demand schedule of patient treatment and staff turnover. The manager notes first that patient scheduling is embedded in a larger system of hospital discharge procedures; the patient's financial resources; the value the patient places on treatment, which may be related to what he or she sees as its outcome; and transportation. Staff coverage too is rooted in larger systems: the female dominance of the occupational therapy profession (one result of which is that therapists generally leave their positions at least for a few years to raise a family), the time staff spend in educational pursuits (condoned by the university, which offers tuition reimbursement), the time staff spend teaching occupational therapy students, and the time staff spend attending meetings.

The manager decides to expand the resources of the program by developing a management information system with the help of staff. The system will be used to gather data on some of the issues that have been identified and their relationship to one another.

From the patient information office the manager learns that although the patient population's economic status has been relatively stable over time, its racial and ethnic makeup are changing. Patients have characteristically been poor, but there are fewer whites now and more blacks and Hispanics.

Other information that the manager wants is not readily available, but it is itemized for further study: the predominant means of transportation used by patients in coming to the facility; the average number of treatments per particular disability; the number of treatments associated with successful outcomes; treatment procedures, goals, and outcomes in each unit; sources of referrals for outpatient occupational therapy; patients' and their families' familiarity with the program; and patients' conceptualizations of the goals of occupational therapy.

In the area of staff coverage the manager also develops a list of information needed: the most likely candidates to leave, their average length of employment, their level of education, their unit assignment, their reasons for leaving, and the educational opportunities they pursued while they were in the university hospital setting.

The program's meeting schedule comes under the manager's scrutiny next. Many of the meetings that staff attend relate to activities in the teaching component. Fives types of meetings seem to require staff's presence: hospital—patient treatment; hospital—governance; occupational therapy department—teaching and research missions; occupational therapy department—governance; and college—governance.

There is also the general pressure for staff to acquire advanced degrees because of the teaching and research missions of the university. Further, because more salaries of the hospital program staff are paid from the college budget than from the hospital budget, it is expected that hospital staff will teach occupational therapy students laboratory skills and supervise their fieldwork.

The manager looks at all these issues and determines which can be controlled or turned into resources and which cannot. In a meeting with the staff, the manager reviews hospital discharge policies. A new orientation plan is developed for patients who will be treated only after discharge (in this case, mastectomy patients). The plan includes setting a limited number of outpatient sessions, with the possibility of negotiating more if they are needed; introducing the patients to a prosthesis and to the clinic; viewing a videotape with patients that explains the need for treatment; stating and reiterating the specific goals of treatment; discussing patients' financial resources with them; and sending a postcard to notify patients of their first appointment visit.

This plan can be carried out relatively easily with a full complement of staff, the manager notes. When staff coverage is interrupted, however, patient follow-up is not as vigorous, and patients are more likely to miss scheduled appointments. Staff turnover is a part of the environment. Often when staff leave, they move out of town, but for some women who remain in the local area and become mothers, the possibility of part-time employment exists. The manager makes a mental note to include a part-time position in the next budget request. A part-time person might provide treatment when staff attend meetings. Perhaps one position could be allocated to two part-time therapists. Benefits would also accrue to the field, because these therapists' treatment skills would remain up-to-date.

The management information system the manager and the staff are developing will provide an important data base with regard to patient treatment. Eventually, the manager thinks, patients may be offered options of which they are not now aware. Moreover, the information gathered on staff who leave may prove helpful in reducing turnover. The manager's counterparts in other organizations might be interested in participating in this aspect of the management information system because many therapists move laterally rather than vertically.

Membership in the university community could be a great resource, the manager notes, and this should be developed. A certain type of clinician might be attracted who could, in time, contribute significantly to the teaching and research missions of the university as well as the service program of the hospital.

SUMMARY

Managers are rarely reflective workers with routinized jobs, who are advised by information systems. They play a complex, intertwined combination of interpersonal, informational, and decisional roles. They are overburdened with obligations, yet they cannot easily delegate tasks. To deal with the pressure of superficiality, the manager must give serious attention to the issues that require it, keep his or her view focused on the broad picture, and make use of analytical inputs. Systems thinking can help the manager do this.

Systems thinking was developed to explain the interaction of some types of systems with their environment. Biological and social systems are open systems, which must have a continuing relationship with their environment in order to maintain life. Closed systems, such as chemical reactions, are not connected to their environments.

In open systems, inputs from the environment—energy in some form—pass through an organization in a process called throughput, and a resulting output is discharged back into the environment. Some input provides feedback to a system on how it is doing.

Both closed and open systems have boundaries. These can easily be seen in closed systems. Social systems are not physically bounded, but they have a basic continuity, which derives from the patterned activities in which people engage. These activities are dependent on one another and complementary in relation to a shared goal.

For their preservation, social organizations depend on both production inputs, energy that is transformed to yield a product or an outcome, and maintenance inputs, energy that sustains a system. People must be motivated to stay in an organization and produce work. Their behavior must be predictable rather than spontaneous. Three types of pressures or forces control the variance of human action in organizations: environmental pressures, shared values, and rule enforcement. Roles, norms, and values help to integrate a system, tying people together in functional interdependence.

To keep a finger on the pulse of a system, it is helpful to delineate the parts of a system. A system can be examined in terms of five considerations: its objectives, or its motivating force, which should be expressed in specific terms so that they can be measured; its environment, or external and largely uncontrollable forces, which determine in part how the system performs, and make demands on it; resources, or the things that a system can employ or change to its advantage; component activities, or missions, whose measure of performance is related to the measure of performance of the system; and management, or working with and through individuals and groups to accomplish organizational goals.

References

1. Mintzberg H: Folklore and fact. *Harvard Business Review*, January 1977, pp 32–35, 66
2. von Bertalanffy L: *General Systems Theory: Foundations, Development, Application*. New York: George Braziller Inc, 1968
3. Churchman CW: *The Systems Approach*. New York: Dell Publishing Co Inc, 1979
4. Katz D, Kahn RL: *The Social Psychology of Organizations*, 2nd edition. New York: John Wiley & Sons Inc, 1978
5. Tregoe BB, Zimmerman JW: *Top Management Strategy: What It Is and How to Make It Work*. New York: Simon & Schuster, 1980
6. Emery FE, Trist EL: The causal texture of organizational environments. In *Systems Thinking*, FE Emery, Editor. New York: Penguin Books Ltd, 1978, pp 241–257
7. Hersey P, Blanchard KH: *Management of Organizational Behavior: Utilizing Human Resources*. Englewood Cliffs, NJ: Prentice-Hall Inc, 1982

Chapter 9

Managing Change

Sylvia Harlock, PhD, OTR

People cannot prevent change. The question is, Can they manage it in ways that are satisfactory, in both process and outcome, to themselves and to other people and organizations about which they care? Professional personnel as individuals are constantly changing. As they master certain professional tasks, they may want to acquire and practice new skills. They may have the opportunity to do so without changing the position they hold or the organization for which they work. After a time they may wish to vary the priority of their professional activities relative to other aspects of their lives. At the same time that professional personnel are experiencing change, those around them at work may in turn be changing, and influencing them. Similarly, developments within the larger organization, their community, and society may affect them.

The more that a manager understands himself or herself, the environment, and the changes that are occurring in it, the more able the manager is to influence change to his or her satisfaction. To enhance the ability to influence change, a manager may need to acquire new skills and resources. However, the effective design and selection of strategies and action plans depend first on obtaining a clear and accurate picture of what is happening.

The literature on change is vast if change is conceptualized as (a) a problem-solving process, (b) a personal growth process, (c) an interper-

---

In her various career positions, Sylvia Harlock has been responsible for managing change at the individual, organizational, and community levels. She has worked as a psychiatric occupational therapist, an occupational therapy department director, an academic instructor, and a health planner. She is now the assistant administrator for Rehabilitation Services at St. Joseph Hospital and Health Care Center in Tacoma, Washington.

sonal interaction process, (d) an organizational development or adaptation process, and (e) a sociological evolutionary process. The factors that may be involved and the strategies and skills that may be needed to effect change in personal, small group, organizational, interorganizational, and societal realms vary. In a given instance, it is important to turn to the literature in that area for help in understanding and developing strategies to influence events.

This chapter presents only an introduction to understanding and managing change. The first section covers change as a problem-solving process. The second focuses on personal change, the third on small group change, and the fourth on change within an organization. In each section some key concepts of change are highlighted and examples provided.

CHANGE AS A PROBLEM-SOLVING PROCESS

Two important concepts in the literature on problem solving are particularly applicable to understanding the management of change. One is that sequential phases are involved in solving a problem. The second addresses the development of creative or new solutions to problems in contrast to the application of known solutions.

Phases in Problem Solving

The general phases in problem solving are as follows (1–6):

1. Recognition that there may be a problem.
2. Clear identification of the nature of the problem.
3. Generation of possible strategies to solve the problem.
4. Selection of a particular strategy.
5. Implementation of the strategy.
6. Evaluation of the effectiveness of the strategy in conjunction with a reassessment of the continued presence of the problem.
7. Corrective action as needed.

An illustration of the first two phases is provided by the following sequence of events. An occupational therapist appears in a patient's/client's room to provide a scheduled self-care treatment session and finds the patient/client absent. This is the recognition phase. There may be an immediate, real problem for the therapist at that moment, but it is actually only a clue to the possibility that there is a general problem of adherence across disciplines to the system of scheduling treatments.

To verify whether there was a general problem, the therapist would have to communicate the experience to other occupational therapists, find out that they had had similar experiences, determine that the number of missed treatments exceeded an acceptable standard, and discover the cause(s) of the missed appointments. If the general incidence was unacceptably high and the cause was the lack of timely return of the patient/client from another discipline's treatment session, such as physical therapy, one could say that the existence of a problem had been verified.

However, the nature of the problem would still not have been clearly identified. For instance, were patients/clients not returning to their rooms on time because of too few distribution personnel to transport them or too tight a scheduling between occupational and physical therapy to accommodate transport time? Or perhaps the physical therapists were running behind schedule in providing treatment because of overscheduling, understaffing, lack of sufficient treatment space or equipment, or a particularly slow physical therapist. Maybe the physical therapists simply lacked consideration of other therapies. Each of these possible definitions of the problem suggests different constellations of people who would need to be involved in the problem-solving process and different solutions to the problem.

Common shortcomings in the use of the problem-solving process are several. One is inadequate attention to the recognition phase. A problem may then reach crisis proportions before problem solvers deal with it. A second is superficial exploration of the nature of the problem—the implementation of a solution, but for the wrong problem. Insufficient exploration of the impacts of possible solutions on related aspects of functioning is another shortcoming. It results in unwitting creation of additional problems. A fourth pitfall is lack of systematic evaluation of progress toward solving the problem and failure to assess the general impact of the changes being instituted. This is a form of inadequate attention to the recognition phase.

The following types of activities enhance management of the recognition phase:

- Greater attention to the changes one is experiencing in carrying out one's daily activities on the job.
- Communication of those changes to others to verify whether others are experiencing similar changes.
- Development and maintenance of a network with people in other disciplines and in other management positions in the organization and with people working in similar organizations in the community.
- Breadth of exposure to literature and other media that communicate changes occurring in one's field, related fields, one's community, and society.
- Generation of ideas about the possible impact of changes on oneself, one's organization, field, and environment.

Creative Problem Solving

Special mention should be made of the literature dealing with creative problem solving because survival in the face of major changes frequently necessitates the generation of new solutions rather than the application of familiar or known solutions (2, 5). Creativity involves seeing things in different ways, discerning new patterns in old information. DeBono stresses the importance of learning skills of creative thinking so that a person can manage change before changes become so all encompassing that they manage the person. In his book, *Lateral Thinking for Management*, he offers a number of techniques for acquiring skills in creative thinking or for restructuring patterns of information (2). Following is a sample of them:

1. Develop an attitude that encourages new ideas, change, exploration.

2. Develop tools for escaping from familiar ways or patterns of viewing events.

a. Don't let yourself focus for a moment on the familiar pattern.

b. Rotate attention to various aspects of the problem.

c. Change the point of attention in the sequence of events that led up to the current situation.

d. Divide the problem into subproblems.

e. Work backward from the outcome one wants to the current situation.

f. Withhold judgment in determining whether a possible view of the problem or situation matches reality.

3. Develop tools for provoking new ways of viewing events.

a. Look for commonalities in things that seem to have no relation to each other.

b. Put things together that have no reason to be put together.

c. Distort and exaggerate.

d. Consider things that are irrelevant and try to make connections between them.

e. Try to solve the problem through an analogy, then go back and try the solution on the original problem.

Managing change means solving problems in creative ways. However, people do the managing, and people have motives, interests, capabilities, and limitations. In the next section concepts relative to understanding and influencing personal change are presented.

PERSONAL CHANGE

The literature on personal growth and change is vast. Rather than attempting to summarize all the concepts on personal change, selected concepts are highlighted. A convenient way to address these concepts is to associate them with the phase of the stimulus-response-outcome-stimulus cycle on which they focus.

Stimulus Concepts

Understanding what motivates one's own behavior or that of another is key to trying to shape or change behavior (7–14). Sometimes what stimulates an individual to act in a particular way is obvious. At other times the reasons may not be clear. People spend thousands of dollars annually on such aids as psychoanalysis, therapy, and self-help books to try to understand themselves more clearly and direct the forces that shape their behavior.

Therapeutic approaches vary in what they consider to be likely origins of current problems and helpful sources of information in analyzing the nature of a current problem. For example, psychoanalysis (10), rational emotive therapy (11), and focusing (12) differ greatly in this regard. Psychoanalysis places a strong emphasis on the influence of early, repetitive, and symbolic experiences. The recall of early events and relationships, and the analysis of dreams and other symbolic representations of feelings and thoughts are viewed as helpful in understanding a person's present feelings and reactions. Rational emotive therapy focuses on the analysis of a person's current belief structures as the method for identifying points of difficulty and opportunities for change. Focusing stresses that a person's own body sensations provide a primary source of clues to when the person is and is not functioning in an integrated way. Increasing one's awareness of one's body sensations (tight, slowed down, speeded up, etc.) and the linkage between those sensations and recent events is helpful in identifying the source of problems and in generating solutions.

The organizational management and conflict management literatures, along with the therapy literature, offer many techniques to better understand what is motivating an employee's actions (15–17). Managers and supervisors can use these methods to help elicit information from employees. Below are some examples:

1. Ask the employee to state how he or she perceives things.
2. Nonjudgmentally accept what is said (although not necessarily agreeing with it).
3. Reflect back to let the employee know he or she was heard and to make sure that one has heard correctly.
4. Use a combination of conceptual statements and concrete examples.

Expectations of a particular outcome can exert a powerful influence on one's behavior (7–9, 13). For example, if an employee expects—and wants—daily personal positive interaction with his or her supervisor to result in the supervisor's paying closer attention to the employee's ideas and opinions, he or she is likely to use that strategy. Much of the literature on the power of positive thinking is based on the assumption that what a person "expects" is what will come to pass because the person's expectations influence his or her responses and those responses influence the responses of others. Also because of the power of expectations, effective change agents always strive to get those who will be affected by a change to "buy into" it (or at least agree not to resist it) in the very beginning.

As an illustration, the manager of an occupational therapy department has decided that it must change from a strictly individual treatment mode to some treatment with two to three patients in a group. When the idea is first presented, some therapists resist it, believing that the quality of care will decrease. At some point in the problem-solving process the manager feels that discussion and clarification must cease and the change must be implemented. It is now important for the manager to get a commitment from the "disbelievers" to suspend judgment temporarily and put their energies into making the idea work, with the agreement that the process will be reassessed in, say, six months.

Response Concepts

So far, concepts that focus on understanding or structuring the stimulus have been presented. The next type is concepts that focus on the response. To evoke a particular response from a person, one first has to be sure the person has the capability, the skills, and the knowledge to perform in that way.

Today's increased emphasis on marketing provides an example. What skills does one need to market one's "product" effectively? How well can occupational therapy personnel describe their product to nurses, patients/clients, families, and various types of physicians, in terms of who can benefit from occupational therapy? How comfortable are they initiating contact with people in these various audiences? How effectively can they describe the benefits of occupational therapy in the language and value systems of the people in these different audiences? At the next level of complexity, how well can occupational therapy personnel participate in conducting market research activities to identify the need for occupational therapy services and develop and implement promotional plans to increase their use?

Occupational therapy literature offers a wealth of information on analyzing activities in terms of the cognitive, perceptual-motor, social-emotional, and interpersonal skills involved (18). Drawing on this literature, managers and employees can assess the skill requirements of the "new" marketing tasks being asked of them.

Assuming that a person has the basic skills to perform in a new way, clarification that the new performance is desired and expected may also be important to making it happen. That expectation may be communicated explicitly, by identifying how, when, and where the behaviors are to occur, or implicitly, by modeling (19) and rewarding the performance desired (9).

Outcome Concepts

The actual outcomes form the third focus in understanding personal change. If valued outcomes happen and a person associates his or her responses with them, the responses are likely to be repeated (9, 20). So one way for a manager to change behavior is to reward the behavior he or she wants, whether it is his or her own or someone else's. That sounds simple. If things are not happening as expected, however, there may be problems in three areas:

1. Are the outcomes that are valued occurring with the frequency and strength desired or expected?
2. What behaviors is the person associating with those outcomes?
3. Does the person feel the outcomes are worth the time and energy required to make the response, or worth the inadvertent consequences?

In the first problem area, salary and salary increases are often expected to be reinforcers. At a person's annual performance appraisal, overall expectations may be reviewed and a raise may be communicated. Is a raise once a year frequent enough to serve as a strong reinforcer? Probably not. These days, raises tend to have two components, an inflation component and an actual raise or merit increase. In today's economy the raise is likely to have a 90 percent inflation component, if it even keeps up with inflation. A five-cents-an-hour merit raise is not a very strong reinforcer.

If a discipline's salary scale is better than other disciplines' salary scales, that in itself, or a reminder of it, can be a positive reinforcer. Salary scales are difficult to change once they have been set in an organization or a field, however. Thus reinforcers other than money, such as recognition, praise, job security, and opportunities for participation in job tasks that are particularly valued by the individual, tend to be more frequently used to shape behavior.

In the second problem area, the behaviors a person associates with valued outcomes can be difficult to sort out because so much is going on all the time. A change agent does not have time to address everything. It is extremely important that he or she keep people focused on the key behaviors and the key outcomes.

For example, in today's shrinking hospital market, the management of a particular facility might reason that each employee could contribute to the survival and success of the hospital, and thus to the continuation of his or her job, by being positive about the hospital in interactions with friends and acquaintances in the community. The employees' positiveness and confidence might make people want to come to that hospital. In this example, management would be identifying a behavior it desired (positive attitude and communication about job and hospital) and clearly linking that behavior to an outcome desired by the employee (job security).

The third possible problem area, whether the outcome is worth the time, energy, and other consequences resulting from the response, again acknowledges the complexity and interconnectedness of events. For example, a therapist may have an interest in developing a new program, but may also feel that he or she just does not have the personal time and energy to do so.

In a different example, a therapist may gain a lot of attention and stimulation from always opposing the ideas of others. He or she may view supporting and facilitating others' ideas and contributions as unrewarding and dull. The manager might use disciplinary action and job security to effect change—keeping one's job may be worth the boredom. The therapist's peer group may effect change by rewarding supportive and facilitative participation and reducing the degree of attention paid to oppositional behaviors.

In summary, to effect personal change, the change agent must identify and build on what will motivate (or at least not be resisted by) the individual. He or she must work with the individual to identify a desired change and to develop skills and procedures to implement it. Once the changes occur, the change agent must reinforce them.

SMALL GROUP CHANGE

Working in the context of a small group adds additional dimensions that must be taken into account in effecting change. When an individual is trying to make a change, the conceptual process, the execution of the behaviors, and the evaluative process all take place within the same person. Although the experience and representation of that experience in a concept or a thought are not exactly the same, they are certainly more alike within an individual than between two or more people.

Change in Groups of Two People

Changes that depend on coordinated actions and communication between two individuals are more complex. In communicating with another person the sender must translate his or her experience into a concept, which in turn is translated into symbols (words and gestures). These are sent to the receiver through a medium (air, paper, a relationship, an environment), and received. The receiver then reacts conceptually and experientially to the symbols. At each of these points in the communication process, the original experience of the sender is modified somewhat (21). It is a wonder that people understand one another as well as they do. Change that involves a division of labor, as in the case of a supervisor guiding a supervisee's change, introduces another element, a difference in the experiences of the two people.

Change in Groups of Three or More People

Changes that depend on coordinated actions and communication among a small group of people are even more complex, both in the variety of differences in the division of labor or roles to be taken and in the opportunity for imperfect understanding and lack of coordination. Various researchers who have studied small groups in action have developed schemes for categorizing the roles or types of behaviors that occur as a group solves a problem (22–23). Some of the roles involve actions that facilitate the resolution of the problem. Other roles contribute actions that help maintain an energized, constructive social-emotional environment in the group.

Bales's role scheme is shown in Figure 1. It indicates the types of problems that occur when there is a breakdown in the execution of the different roles (22). The types are explained below:

- Problems of communication: The availability, sharing, and understanding of factual information is vital to the development of an accurate picture of the problem and generation of solutions.
- Problems of evaluation: The giving of and asking for opinions about the factual information and suggestions provide the group with needed evaluative comments.
- Problems of control: Suggestions offered and sought by group members may relate both to potential strategies for resolving the problem and to the group's process of working together.
- Problems of decision: Agreeing and disagreeing may be explicit or implicit. In either case effective change depends on all affected members of the group reaching a decision and agreeing to act in accordance with the decision.
- Problems of tension reduction: The degree of tension inherent in groups varies by the group's dynamics and by the nature of the problem or change with which it is dealing. If there is high tension, methods for expressing and reducing tension by positiveness, humor, dramatization, or whatever, are needed.
- Problems of reintegration: Change that depends on the interaction of two or more people is facilitated by a positive relationship between the individuals involved and hampered by negative relationships.

Benne and Sheats have developed a more comprehensive set of roles (23). As Figure 2 shows, they divide the roles into group task roles, group building and maintenance roles, and individual dysfunctional roles

FIGURE 9–1
Bales's Small Group Interaction Role Scheme

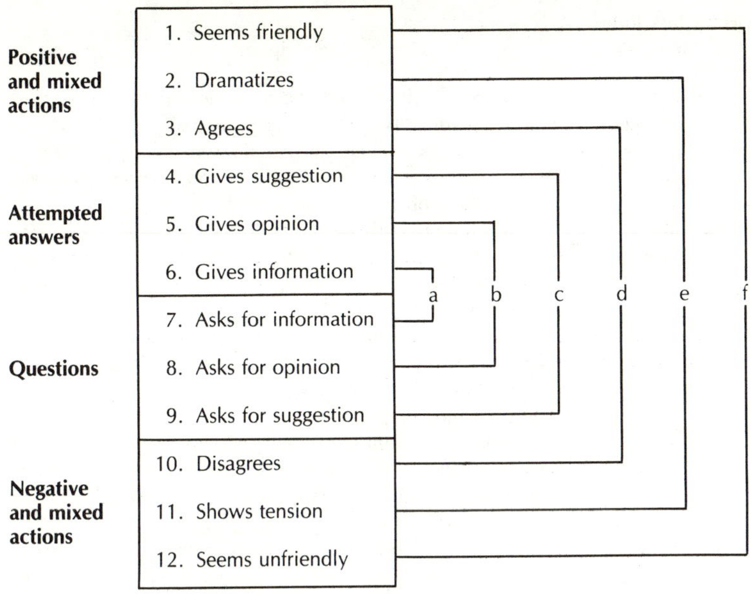

a — Problems of communication
b — Problems of evaluation
c — Problems of control
d — Problems of decision
e — Problems of tension reduction
f — Problems of reintegration

Note: Reprinted with permission from RF Bales, *Interaction Process Analysis: A Method for the Study of Small Groups*, Cambridge, MA: Addison-Wesley Publishing Co, 1950, p 59.

that often block the progress of a group when performed excessively. Their delineation of roles helps one appreciate the complexity of group interaction. Many behaviors must happen correctly and at the right time for a given change to occur constructively and successfully.

The greater the number of people involved, the longer the time period needed for change to occur. More complex change requires clear specification and written documentation of the anticipated process, decision points, plan of implementation, actual implementation, and reevaluation activities (21). Such documentation reduces the dependence on individual interpretation and memories, and also provides a basis for evaluating the change process itself.

Insufficient use of documentation as a procedural tool for clarifying, validating, and coordinating views, decisions, and actions is a common problem in managing change in a small group. Problems relating to roles include lack of clarity about them, competition over them (particularly leadership roles), gaps within them, and use of dysfunctional ones. Inappropriate sequencing or rate of movement through the phases of problem solving is another frequent difficulty, as is inconsistent participation

FIGURE 9–2
Benne and Sheats's Group Member Roles

Group Task Roles

Role	Description
(a) initiator-contributor	. . . suggests or proposes to the group new ideas or a changed way of regarding the group problem or goal.
(b) information seeker	. . . asks for clarification of suggestions made in terms of their factual adequacy, for authoritative information and facts pertinent to the problem being discussed.
(c) opinion seeker	. . . asks not primarily for the facts of the case but for a clarification of the values pertinent to what the group is undertaking or of values involved in a suggestion made or in alternative suggestions.
(d) information giver	. . . offers facts or generalizations which are "authoritative" or relates his own experience pertinently to the group problem.
(e) opinion giver	. . . states his belief or opinion pertinently to a suggestion made or to alternative suggestions.
(f) elaborator	. . . spells out suggestions in terms of examples or developed meanings, offers a rationale for suggestions previously made and tries to deduce how an idea or suggestion would work out if adopted by the group.
(g) coordinator	. . . shows or clarifies the relationships among various ideas and suggestions, tries to pull ideas and suggestions together or tries to coordinate the activities of various members of subgroups.
(h) orienter	. . . defines the position of the group with respect to its goals by summarizing what has occurred, points to departures from agreed upon directions or goals, or raises questions about the direction which the group discussion is taking.
(i) evaluator-critic	. . . subjects the accomplishment of the group to some standard or set of standards of group functioning in the context of the group task.
(j) energizer	. . . prods the group to action or decision, attempts to stimulate or arouse the group, to "greater" or "higher quality" activity.
(k) procedural technician	. . . expedites group movement by doing things for the group—performing routine tasks, e.g., distributing materials, or manipulating objects for the group, e.g., rearranging the seating or running the recording machine.
(l) recorder	. . . writes down suggestions, makes a record of group decisions, or writes down the product of discussion.

Group Building and Maintenance Roles

Role	Description
(a) encourager	. . . praises, agrees with and accepts the contribution of others.
(b) harmonizer	. . . mediates the differences between other members, attempts to reconcile disagreements, relieves tension in conflict situations through jesting or pouring oil on the troubled water, etc.
(c) compromiser	. . . operates from within a conflict in which his ideas or position is involved.
(d) gatekeeper/expediter	. . . attempts to keep communication channels open by encouraging or facilitating the participation of others . . . or by proposing regulation of the flow of communication.
(e) standard setter	. . . expresses standards for the group to attempt to achieve in its functioning or applies standards in evaluating the quality of group processes.

(f) group-observer	. . . keeps records of various aspects of group process and feeds such data with proposed interpretations into the group's evaluation of its own procedures.
(g) follower	. . . goes along with the movement of the group, more or less passively accepting the ideas of others, serving as an audience in group discussion and decision.

Dysfunctional Roles

Role	Description
(a) aggressor	. . . may work in many ways—deflating the status of others, expressing disapproval of the values, acts or feelings of others, attacking the group or the problem it is working on, joking aggressively, showing envy toward another's contribution by trying to take credit for it, etc.
(b) blocker	. . . tends to be negativistic and stubbornly resistant, disagreeing and opposing without or beyond reason and attempting to maintain or bring back an issue after the group has rejected it.
(c) recognition seeker	. . . works in various ways to call attention to himself, whether through boasting, reporting on personal achievements, acting in unusual ways, struggling to prevent his being placed in an "inferior" position, etc.
(d) self-confessor	. . . uses the audience opportunity which the group setting provides to express personal, nongroup-oriented "feeling," "insight," "ideology," etc.
(e) playboy	. . . makes a display of his lack of involvement in the group's processes.
(f) dominator	. . . tries to assert authority or superiority in manipulating the group or certain members of the group.
(g) help-seeker	. . . attempts to call forth "sympathy" response from other group members or from the whole group.
(h) special interest pleader	. . . speaks for the "small business man," "the grass roots" community, the "housewife," "labor," etc., usually cloaking his own prejudices or biases in the stereotype which best fits his individual need.

Note: Reprinted with permission from K Benne, P Sheats, Functional roles of group members, *J Soc Issues* 4(2):43–46; 1948.

of the members of the group, particularly if the process goes on over a long period.

Small group change may seem complicated. However, all of the participants are usually present throughout the whole process. Such commonality of experience among them helps minimize the opportunity for imperfect understanding and lack of coordination. In the next section organizational change, with its added complexity, is explored.

CHANGE WITHIN THE ORGANIZATION

Inherent in an organization is a true division of labor, with a specified set of roles and responsibilities for each position and an organizational structure that identifies the lines of interaction, authority, and responsibility. In addition, sets of formal policies and procedures identify the rules by which decisions and problems will be addressed and who should be involved in addressing them. There are also sets of informal networks of individuals in the organization and informal ways of dealing with problems. A given individual in the organization may at various times be an instigator of change, an implementer of it, and a participant in it. Figure 3 illustrates the complexity of effectively managing change in an organization. The elements involved are listed below, along with pertinent references in the literature.

1. Problem identification skills (1–3, 5–6, 16, 24, 27).
2. Problem-solving skills (1–3, 5–6, 16, 24, 27).
3. Implementation skills (1, 3, 6, 16, 18, 22, 25, 27).
4. Access to information relevant to problem identification and problem solving (1, 3, 5, 17, 24–25, 28).

FIGURE 9–3
Effective Management of Change

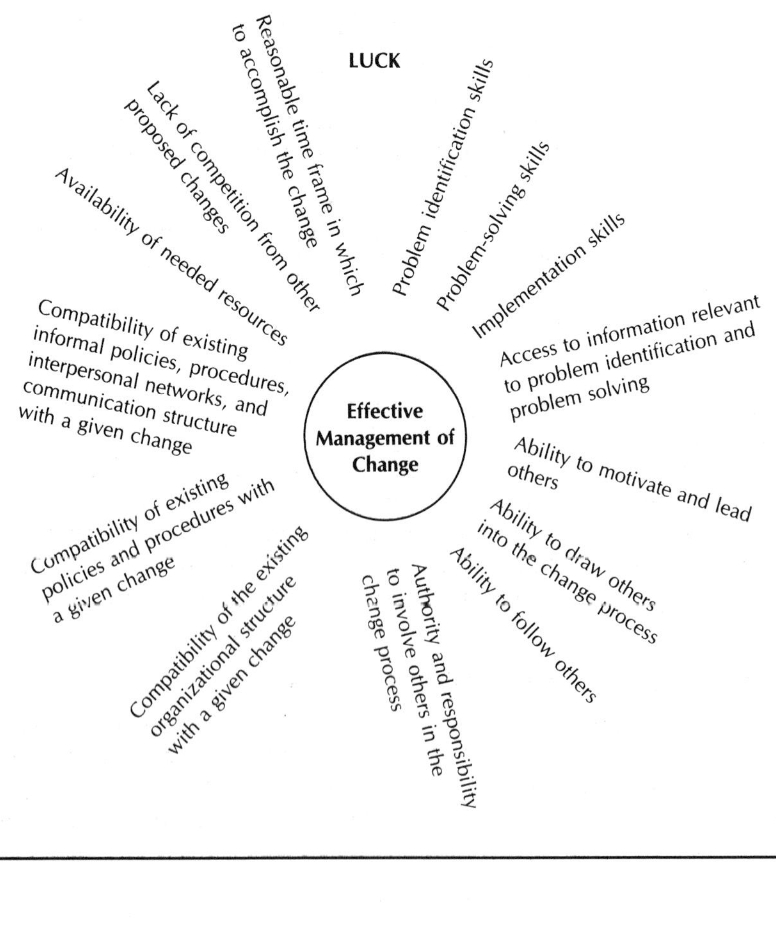

5. Ability to motivate and lead others (1–3, 6, 14–17, 20, 22, 24, 27, 29).
6. Ability to draw others into the change process (1, 3, 6, 14–16, 22, 24, 27, 29).
7. Ability to follow others (3, 16, 22, 24).
8. Authority and responsibility to involve others in the change process (1, 3, 6, 14, 16–17, 22, 24).
9. Compatibility of the existing organizational structure with a given change (1, 3, 15–17, 24, 26, 29).
10. Compatibility of existing policies and procedures with a given change (1, 3, 15–17, 24, 27, 29).
11. Compatibility of existing informal policies, procedures, interpersonal networks, and communication structure with a given change (1, 3, 14–16, 24–26, 28–30).
12. Availability of needed resources (1, 3, 17, 24–25, 28).
13. Lack of competition from other proposed changes (1, 3, 24, 28).
14. A reasonable time frame in which to accomplish the change (1, 16, 24, 26, 29).
15. Luck.

When one considers all the aspects that might go wrong, it is easy to see why people are likely to resist change. Some common reasons for resistance are economic threat; the threat of inconvenience; uncertainty about what others will do, how events will unfold, how one will respond; and the threat of change in social relationships or social status because of new skills required or changes in interpersonal networks. Also causing resistance are competing interests; inaccurate perceptions of the intended change; personal disagreement with the change; a perceived decrease in freedom to engage in alternative behaviors, that is, a narrowing of options; a low tolerance for change; insufficient consideration given to problems that are likely to occur as a result of the change and ways of dealing with them; fear of failure; and overload (14, 16, 29).

A number of authors have identified points to keep in mind in managing a change in an organization (1, 5, 14, 16, 24, 27):

1. Clearly communicate the objectives the anticipated change is to accomplish.
2. State the specific changes that are required.
3. Ask for employee reaction.
4. Clear up misunderstandings and fill in information gaps.
5. Ask employees to support the change, even if they disagree; seek prior commitment.
6. Don't move too fast.
7. Involve the people affected.
8. Focus on the options available.
9. Share responsibility and credit.
10. Anticipate an occasional rebuff.
11. Plan for all contingencies; think and plan ahead.

An example is provided by the proposed adoption of the American Occupational Therapy Association's Product Output Reporting System (31) by the occupational therapy department in a large hospital. The department would use the system as a data collection tool for documenting productivity and billing patients/clients and third-party payers for services. The department is currently using a simple, non-time-based system to bill for five services: individual evaluation, group evaluation, individual treatment, group treatment, and splinting.

The occupational therapy manager needs to deal with several components of the organization to accomplish this change effectively: (a) staff of the department; (b) his or her supervisor; (c) the medical directors of hospital programs affected by the change (e.g., physical medicine and rehabilitation and mental health); (d) financial components (e.g., the vice-president for finance, the comptroller, the billing department, the budget director, and the data department); and (e) the medical records department.

First, the occupational therapy manager has to identify clearly the benefits of the change in the value systems of each set of people affected. The benefits might include greater descriptive clarity of the treatment goals or outcomes and increased accuracy and detail of information on which to base staffing decisions, program planning, and budget planning. This information, in turn, could be used to educate hospital personnel and third-party payers about the benefits of occupational therapy services to the patient/client, the productivity of the occupational therapy staff, and the comparative use of hospital resources.

The occupational therapy manager also has to think through the potential impact of the change on the various components of the organization and be ready to make suggestions regarding methods of implementation. The manager must have the full backing of his or her supervisor and the affected medical directors. This support must be reviewed and renewed periodically throughout the process of managing the change. The impact on the supervisor will vary at different stages of the change process. Review of the commitment will allow the supervisor to become aware of the impacts and provide an opportunity for both the manager and the supervisor to deal with them.

A possible reason for resistance by the supervisor is the threat of changes in social relationships. For example, the supervisor might have to relate to the comptroller in new ways, or the supervisor might have to oppose another employee and not want to do so at that point. Other possible sources of resistance are the threat of inconvenience during the transition, a perception of little or no benefit to be gained from the new system, and a low tolerance for change in general.

Assuming the supervisor offers no objections, the manager is ready to guide the occupational therapy staff in an exploration of the change. In eliciting the staff's reactions, concerns, and suggestions, the manager may uncover resistance on several fronts. For one, staff may disagree with the categorization of services, or the relative values assigned to services, under the new system. They may perceive that the assignments do not accurately reflect what occupational therapy personnel do in this hospital or what the relative worth of the different services is. Another source of resistance may be that they see little value in the change. Also, they may fear that they will not be able to learn the new system and, further, that it may overload them with work. The unknown "productivity measures" may threaten them economically, and with all the detail in the system, they may perceive a decrease in their freedom. Finally, their general tolerance for change may be low, and they may anticipate great disruption of routine during the changeover.

The manager and the staff design strategies to deal with these concerns. Among them is a three-month pilot project in which "double books" are kept. This allows the manager and the staff to gather information about the problems that they will face if the system is actually implemented and to gather data about the occupational therapy services to use in presenting the proposal to the financial component of the organization. Throughout the pilot project the manager and his or her supervisor plant seeds regarding the benefits of the system and the possible implications for change in other departments, such as the budget and billing offices.

At the end of the three months the manager and his or her staff review and deal with their concerns regarding implementation of the change. The manager then makes a formal proposal to appropriate personnel in the financial components of the organization. The earlier informal communication has alerted him or her to possible concerns of the various financial officers so that they can be effectively addressed in the presentation.

Some of the possible sources of resistance from these people are the same as those the manager encountered earlier: the threat of inconvenience, a perception of little or no benefit from the change, the threat of a transformation in social relationships, a perceived decrease in freedom, and a low tolerance for change. Moreover, they may fear failure, in this case because their personnel may not know enough about occupational therapy to design the data collection and billing systems and justify bills to patients/clients and insurers. These people may also have competing interests, preferring to use their time and data system space for other information-tracking activities in the hospital.

In preparing to address these potential concerns, the occupational therapy manager familiarizes himself or herself with the job tasks and stresses of these personnel, in order to relate potential benefits and problem-solving strategies in terms they will understand. Through informal relationships with personnel in these departments, the manager gathers information and establishes support.

Implementation of the change is approved. Time is made available to everyone who is affected to work through the problems that arise. The manager checks frequently to determine how well things are proceeding. Attention is paid to departments or components that are affected but not sufficiently *impacted* to have been a major part of the decision making. For example, the new system requires the development of new forms, which must be approved by the medical records department before they can be used. When the change is successfully accomplished, the manager organizes a celebration, during which he or she makes a point of thanking everyone for their cooperation and support.

In the implementation of a major change, it is easy to overlook "details" such as working with the medical records department and organizing a celebration. They may be very important to the success of the change, however, and to the development of a base of credibility and support for future changes.

INTERORGANIZATIONAL AND SOCIETAL CHANGE

The principles of managing change in an interorganizational or societal environment are similar to those in a large organization (32). There must be a clear identification of the change desired, whether that identification is embodied in an individual leader or in written documents. Usually a small core of individuals directs or manages the change process, and a larger following of people lends support and carries out the myriad actions needed to implement the change. A coalition of organizations may be necessary to accomplish the change at this level. The passage and implementation of a state occupational therapy licensure bill is a good example of an interorganizational or societal change in the political arena.

SUMMARY

Change may be conceptualized as (a) a problem-solving process, (b) a personal growth process, (c) an interpersonal interaction process, (e) an organizational development or adaptation process, and (d) a sociological evolutionary process. The literature in each of these fields offers a wealth of information applicable to the issue of managing change.

Two important concepts in the literature on problem solving are the sequential phases involved and the development of creative, new solutions. The phases of problem solving are recognition that there may be a problem, clear identification of it, generation of possible strategies to solve it, selection of one strategy, implementation of the strategy, evaluation of the strategy, and corrective action as needed. Creative problem solving involves seeing things in different ways and discerning new patterns in old information. The literature suggests many techniques for restructuring information.

Personal change can be studied in terms of groups of concepts related to the stimulus-response-outcome-stimulus cycle. Some examples of stimulus concepts are the theories various kinds of therapists have about the origins of personal problems and helpful sources of information in understanding them. Response concepts focus on the capabilities, skills, and knowledge that people need to respond in the particular ways that a change requires. Outcome concepts relate to such issues as identifying the behavior that a person associates with a valued outcome, so that the behavior can be rewarded and structuring various reward or reinforcement systems.

Change at the level of the small group is more complex because it depends on coordinated action and effective communication among two or more people. In small groups people play different roles. Two prominent theorists characterize these as task roles (e.g., initiator-contributor, information giver, and evaluator-critic), group building and maintenance roles (e.g., harmonizer and follower), and dysfunctional roles (e.g., aggressor and dominator).

Managing change in an organization is extremely complex because of the extensive division of labor, the formal policies and procedures for decision making and problem solving, and the informal networks of employees. The literature identifies several categories of likely resistance to change and identifies strategies and techniques for uncovering and addressing them.

Change at the interorganizational or society level can be managed using principles similar to those that apply to an organization. Sometimes a coalition of organizations is necessary to effect a desired outcome.

Solving problems, growing and adapting, and resolving conflicts are all integral aspects of managing change. Knowledge of the normal functioning and the growth and adaptation processes of the system in which a change is taking place—an individual, a small group, an organization, or society—is important to the effective management of the change.

References

1. Beyers M: Getting on top of organizational change. Part 1, Process and development. *J Nurs Administration* 44(Oct):32–39, 1984
2. DeBono E: *Lateral Thinking for Management: A Handbook*. New York: Penguin Books Inc, 1971
3. Kaluzny AD, Hernandez SR: Managing change in health care organizations. *Med Care Rev* 40(3):161–203, 1983
4. Miller GA, Galanter E, Pribram H: *Plans and the Structure of Behavior*. New York: Holt Rinehart & Winston Inc, 1960
5. Spradley BW: Managing change creatively. *J Nurs Administration* 40(May):32–37, 1980
6. Welch LB: Planned change in nursing: The theory. In *The Nursing Clinics of North America*, B Worthington, LB Welch, Editors. Philadelphia: WB Saunders Co, 1979. 14(2):307–321
7. Bandler R, Grinder J: *Frogs into Princes: Neuro-Linguistic Programming*. Moab, UT: Real People Press, 1979
8. Bandler R, Grinder J: *Reframing: Neuro-Linguistic Programming and the Transformation of Meaning*. Moab, UT: Real People Press, 1982
9. Binder V, Binder A, Rimland B, Editors: *Modern Therapies*. Englewood Cliffs, NJ: Prentice-Hall Inc, 1976
10. Freedman AM, Kaplan HL, Editors: *Comprehensive Textbook of Psychiatry*. Baltimore: Williams & Wilkins Co, 1967
11. Ellis A: *Humanistic Psychotherapy: The Rational-Emotive Approach*. New York: Julian Press and McGraw-Hill Paperbacks, 1974
12. Gendlin ET: *Focusing*. New York: Everest House Publications, 1978
13. Kelly GA: *A Theory of Personality: The Psychology of Personal Constructs*. New York: WW Norton & Co Inc, 1963
14. Olson EM: Strategies and techniques for the nurse change agent. In *The Nursing Clinics of North America*, B Worthington, LB Welch, Editors. Philadelphia: WB Saunders Co, 1979. 14(2):323–336.
15. Deal TE, Kennedy AA: *Corporate Cultures*. Reading, MA: Addison-Wesley Publishing Co, 1982
16. Labovitz GH: *Motivational Dynamics*. Minneapolis: Control Data Education Co, 1975 (Address: P.O. Box O, Minneapolis, MN 55440)
17. Liebler JG, Levine RE, Dervitz HL: *Management Principles for Health Professionals*. Rockville, MD: Aspen Systems Corp, 1984
18. Hopkins HL, Smith HS, Editors: *Willard and Spackman's Occupational Therapy*, 5th edition. Philadelphia: JB Lippincott Co, 1978
19. Bandura A: *Social Learning Theory*. Englewood Cliffs, NJ: Prentice-Hall Inc, 1977
20. Weisinger H, Lobsenz NM: *Nobody's Perfect: How to Give Criticism and Get Results*. Los Angeles: Stanford Press, 1981
21. Littlejohn SW: *Theories of Human Communication*. Columbus, OH: Charles E Merrill Publishing Co, 1978
22. Bales RF: *Interaction Process Analysis: A Method for the Study of Small Groups*. Cambridge, MA: Addison-Wesley Publishing Co, 1950
23. Benne K, Sheats P: Functional roles of group members. *J Soc Issues* 4(2):41–49, 1948
24. Carner DC: Managing change: Carner's codes. *Hosp Forum* 26(6):59–62, 1982
25. Carr EM: Networking: A resource for change. *Nurse Practitioner* 7(April):32–34, 1982
26. King ES: Coping with organizational change. *Topics in Clin Nurs* 4(July):66–73, 1982
27. Levenstein A: Effective change requires change agent. *J Nurs Administration* 9(June):12–15, 1979
28. Naisbitt J: *Megatrends: Ten New Directions Transforming Our Lives*. New York: Warner Books Inc, 1984
29. New JR, Coullard NA: Guidelines for introducing change. *J Nurs Administration* 11(March):17–21, 1981

30. Rheiner NW: Role theory: Framework for change. *Nurs Manage* 13(3):20–22, 1982
31. American Occupational Therapy Association: Uniform terminology for reporting occupational therapy services and occupational therapy product output reporting system. In *Reference Manual of the Official Documents of the American Occupational Therapy Association*. Rockville, MD: American Occupational Therapy Association, 1983
32. Kahn S: *Organizing: A Guide for Grassroots Leaders*. New York: McGraw-Hill Book Co, 1982

Section IV

Directing

In the directing role the manager is concerned with motivating and stimulating staff and promoting morale and job satisfaction. Chapter 10, the sole component of this section, discusses major theories and principles of managing. Its five main topics are leadership, decision making, supervision, delegation, and conflict resolution. Various styles of accomplishing these responsibilities are described, and the appropriateness of the styles in different situations is pointed out. Numerous references are included as resource material for the manager, and an appendix offers advice on conducting successful meetings.

Chapter 10

Directing

Susan Haiman, MPS, OTR/L

This chapter explores the concepts that occupational therapists in administrative positions must understand to turn the tasks of management into the process of management. The assumption of management roles in hospitals, schools, clinics, and other settings requires more than a passing familiarity with skills in leadership, decision making, supervision, delegation, and management of conflict. Following is an overview of these topics, intended to provide a basic framework around which growth in managerial and administrative competence can begin.

LEADERSHIP

Leadership occurs informally or formally any time one attempts to influence the behavior of an individual or group. The informal leader influences others through strength of personality, whereas the formal leader has legitimate authority over them. Managers, then, must not only have charisma but also the ability to synthesize leadership into the administrative structure of their organization (1, 2, 3). To accomplish this, professional education, training, and clinical experience are not enough. Occupational therapists must begin to think not only in terms of patient/client relationships, but in terms of big business, for that is what health care delivery systems have become. In this context, patients/clients are "inputs," or raw material that is processed through treatment systems and returned to the environment as products with enhanced

Susan Haiman is the assistant director of the department of therapeutic activities at Payne Whitney Clinic, which is affiliated with Cornell University Medical College. Her master's degree is in health services administration, and she has five years of experience as a manager.

capacity to function in daily life (4). Unempathic as this observation may sound, it emphasizes the harsh reality of today's disappearing health care dollars and the need to develop both cost-effective and efficient treatment approaches. Thus, an occupational therapy service must be seen as a unit that delivers direct care and as an organization or a part of an organization concerned with remaining in the business of caring for people.

The manager must function as the link between an organization's policy makers and those on the front lines of service delivery. He or she must operate in two highly differentiated spheres, identifying with both the upper levels of administration and the professional group he or she represents, to facilitate meeting their common goals and objectives. The manager who is able to negotiate between these spheres is in a better position to use his or her discretion in interpreting and implementing directives from above and can influence superiors to formulate policies and procedures that are in keeping with the competencies of his or her staff (5, 6). He or she can also help those in primary service roles not lose sight of or misunderstand the inseparable relationship between direct care and the organization's mission.

Another consideration is the manager's need for relationships with his or her counterparts in other departments or services. Informally, managers must rely on friendship or exchange of favors to ensure collaboration with other services that affect their programs (7). This approach might be taken with such an issue as whether occupational therapy intervention takes priority over other treatment modalities when multiple services are being delivered (5, 8).

Historical Perspectives on Leadership

The study of leadership began with the belief that natural leaders were born, not trained. The notion was that leaders could be defined in terms of a certain constellation of personality traits that were observable and measurable. Efforts to support this premise through research, however, met with failure (1).

The next step in leadership research was attention to observed behaviors. The first notable contributions of the leadership behaviorists emerged from the work of Fredrick Winslow Taylor and the School of Scientific Management (9). This group posited that what was important in leadership was behavior that demonstrated *orientation only toward the task*, toward efficiency and production. People (employees) were of little concern; they were viewed as merely an aspect of the technology of production. With the emergence of the behavioral sciences and their application to better understanding of employees' values, goals, and motivations, this view of management became obsolete.

The human relations movement grew out of these increased efforts to understand human psychology. The strength of any organization was believed to rest in the interpersonal relationships within and between work groups. Thus, leadership was explored in terms of behavior that facilitated cooperation among employees and demonstrated concern for individual growth and development. Research was intended to prove that people-oriented behavior and task-oriented behavior were mutually exclusive styles of leadership (1). Instead, the findings demonstrated that these two distinct styles of leadership existed, but neither was more effective in every situation.

Leadership then began to be viewed as a *dynamic process* in which attention to human resources and to task might vary under different circumstances. Fiedler (10) developed the Contingency Model of Leadership, which was concerned not only with the variables of human resources and task, but also with the power and authority mandated by the leader's position. Others wrote of effective or ineffective leadership as determined not by actual behavior but by the appropriateness of that behavior in a given environment (e.g., an occupational therapy department). A third variable, context or environment, thus emerged as important, reflecting such issues as the number of staff, available space, required technology, variety of services, and organizational structure (1).

Finally, the concept of environment was expanded to include the complexity of conditions outside the leader's span of control. In this view, effective leaders had to be aware of the resources available to other departments or services and be cognizant of the degree to which their department depended on others to meet stated goals. In addition, they had to monitor such variables as political climate within and outside the organization, economic and public policy shifts, and advances in their profession (11).

Given this wide range of considerations, leadership style can be understood as an adaptive capacity. In occupational therapy it calls for more than clinical competence. It requires the ability to use analytic powers, interpersonal skills, excellence in communication, and a high degree of discretion. Once these skills have been developed, the effective leader can juggle the multiple missions of service, research, and education in occupational therapy with the mandates and missions of a given health care setting. Then too, he or she can use leadership styles that, at any moment, may be tight or loose, paternal/maternal or fraternal, authoritarian or egalitarian, or win over–take over (12).

Power and Authority

No clinician can become a manager without dealing with the implications of obtaining power and authority. Stated simply, "Authority is the power that is legitimized by virtue of an individual's formal role in an organization" (13, p 177).

Power is a complex issue. Being powerful means having access to essential resources and information and having the support of both superiors and subordinates. Power brings with it the freedom to take risks without approval from above, and the discretion to be flexible in interpreting organizational policies for one's own department. It also means having essential peer networks and political alliances. Most important, power is the leadership of a department or service that is seen as critical to an organization's mission. An illustration of this point is the relative power of a chief of medicine and a director of housekeeping in a large medical center (3, 8, 11, 14).

The hallmark of power is the *ability to get things done and to influence the internal and external environments*. As this ability is demonstrated, power also becomes a manager's source of credibility with subordinates. In fact, subordinates' perceptions of how much power a manager holds is as important an influence on their behavior and compliance as the manager's real power within the organization (11, 14).

Occupational therapists educated and professionally socialized to provide direct care do not find it easy to make the transition to positions of management and power. Such transitions often evoke feelings of isolation from the professional peer group. There is often marked discomfort with heightened status and increased authority. This is especially true in settings where the strength of the medical model may leave occupational therapy to be viewed as an ancillary service (3, 8, 11). But just as power can be used or abused, it can be depleted through disuse. Occupational therapists in management roles must recognize the scope and strength of their power and not allow themselves to be controlled or ignored by the system.

DECISION MAKING

"The common denominator of all administrative functioning" (15, p 7) is the process of making decisions. One key to successful management is knowing whether decision making in an organization is centralized or decentralized (11). Who in the administrative hierarchy can make decisions? How many and what kinds of decisions can be made at each hierarchical level? *Centralized* decision making occurs at top levels in the management structure. *Decentralized* decision making pushes that process down the line to incorporate full participation by subordinates. The following sections explore the decision-making process in greater detail so that the implications of both approaches are clear (1).

Components of Decision Making

Purists believe that decision making by managers is a certain and predictable process. Reality dictates that like all humans, managers have some cognitive limitations and can act only on the basis of how they perceive and process information in a given situation. Ambiguous problems, too little or too much information, make optimal decisions a dream. The hope instead is to make satisfactory ones (1). Decisions, then, are choices between two or more courses. They are made either rationally, by analysis and consideration of alternatives, or irrationally, by habit and instinct. Under either circumstance one must consider the interplay between *facts* and *values*. Without this interplay decision making could be accomplished by a computer. Yet remarkably it remains in human hands (15, 16, 17).

It is an able manager who can separate facts from values and keep a perspective on both throughout the decision-making process. Only thus can he or she assess whether the values themselves are those of an individual or a group; whether they are related to the means or the ends of the organization; and what effect they have on identifying problems as well as solutions (16).

Steps in Decision Making

Cooper (18) has neatly defined the steps to be followed in decision making. First is defining the problem in terms of its basis rather than its "presenting symptoms." For instance, that patients are chronically late to individual or group sessions held at 1:00 p.m. is a presenting symptom. Its basis might be the unavailability of staff to transport at that hour because of scheduled lunch breaks, or that the patients themselves are not receiving their noon meal from the kitchen until 12:45 p.m. Next, alternative solutions should be developed. One alternative is then selected, and the reasons for that selection (including factual and value-related aspects) are delineated.

Decision making does not stop with these steps. It continues through the implementation of the solution. At this point, managers should recognize that staff are learning new approaches and must work through the resistances that are corollaries to change regardless of the degree of their involvement in the process. Finally, plans for feedback on the success or failure of the decision must be in place, because an outcome depends not on the manager alone but on the communication with all who are involved in implementation. This is of particular importance when feedback or new data make it essential to critically revise the original decision or to make a different one.

Styles of Decision Making

In selecting a decision-making style, an effective manager must make some hard choices about the degree to which his or her staff are to be a part of decision making. In a highly bureaucratic setting, the person in authority makes decisions and communicates them to subordinates as commands. Another approach is for the person in authority to consult with staff for opinions and information, after which he or she reaches a decision. The group or consensus method, in which a manager and staff work together to reach decisions, is the most democratic approach. Its success depends on such factors as effective interpersonal and group interaction, the competence of group members, and the presence of similar goals within the group (11).

As with leadership styles, no single decision-making method should be used at all times. Differentiation must be made between the kinds of decisions that the group has the legitimate power to make and those that must be handled by administrative fiat (19). It has been suggested that autocratic methods are better when decision making is simple and clear-cut, whereas democratic methods are better in complex, ambiguous situations. This distinction does not always apply, however. For example, deciding whether to promote an existing staff member to a senior position or hire someone from outside the organization is a highly complicated, loaded issue. It cannot and should not be settled democratically. After consultation with staff, the manager alone must choose who is best qualified to fill a position, as the manager is responsible for the competence of the professionals in his or her department.

Managers must be sufficiently at ease in their roles to be democratic when they can and autocratic when they must. Supporting and encouraging autonomy and the professional identification of occupational therapy personnel is an important aspect of a manager's role. So is balancing staff growth with the mandates and constraints imposed by the organization.

SUPERVISION AND DELEGATION

AOTA's Position on Supervision

In 1983 the American Occupational Therapy Association (AOTA) published guidelines describing supervision as a mutual undertaking between supervisor and supervisee, intended to promote growth and development while evaluating performance and maintaining standards (20). Supervision must take place within the framework of the organization and be relevant to its legal guidelines and organizational structure (20). Although entry-level occupational therapists can provide services independently, they must be encouraged to pursue educational experiences (13). Too often, new graduates work in settings where supervision by an experienced occupational therapist is not available. On this issue the AOTA states that although registered occupational therapists may be administratively supervised by professionals in other disciplines, clinical practice should be supervised only by members of the profession (20). In addition, state licensure acts may dictate both the amount and type of supervision an occupational therapist or an occupational therapy assistant must receive.

Styles of Supervision

Supervision can range from close daily contact, such as one might have with a new staff member, to less frequent weekly or monthly individual contact, with group meetings, phone calls, and written reports filling the gaps (20). Frequency of supervision can depend on multiple factors, for example, the expertise of the supervisor, the determinations of need by the supervisee, and the organization's style and structure (13).

Occupational therapy managers bear responsibility for the work of other professionals, students, and nonprofessionals. In light of that responsibility supervision cannot always be a collaborative process (21). At times the supervisor must be directive and/or didactic, such as when newly mandated policies and procedures are introduced. The supervisee must accept the limitations that are occasionally imposed on autonomy, such as not unilaterally changing programs or not altering the caseload without permission. Although such limitations seemingly impede growth and development, they can in fact support it, because the supervisee learns more about his or her relationship to a larger system and develops into an effective group/team member (8, 21).

Clinical and Administrative Supervision

There is some debate over whether clinical and administrative supervision should be separated or integrated. Decisions about this depend on the size and complexity of the occupational therapy organization and the number of supervisory-level, registered occupational therapists. When the two types of supervision are combined, supervisors tend to be seen as jacks-of-all-trades, and the weight of the bureaucracy can interfere with clinical functions (21). There is also the possibility that individual clinical issues will not be kept separate from administrative decisions.

On the other hand, when clinical and administrative supervision are split, the administrator's authority is not weakened by the performance of dual roles. Depending on the setting, this can be an advantage or a disadvantage. There is, however, a risk that under such a division of supervisory tasks, communication will be cumbersome and inefficient. Both gathering and disseminating information become increasingly complex processes with much time spent on clarification, individually and in group meetings (21, 22). Finally, the success of split supervision depends very much on the manager's ability to delegate, the next topic covered in this chapter.

Delegation

When clinicians become managers they must expand their focus from a hands-on patient/client orientation to one of responsibility for the programs through which services are delivered. In a sense they must delegate direct care, the first step in that difficult transition to management. But delegation of authority over direct care or even programs does not mean abdicating responsibility (23). Managers, therefore, must call on their clinical competence as well as their capacity to establish effective program structures to ensure the level of excellence for which supervisors hold them accountable. This means creating a climate of mutual trust and professional respect in which staff have confidence in the judgment of managers and managers can rely on staff to fulfill expected roles and functions. Often a willingness to delegate has less to do with trusting people per se than with trusting staff to meet goals and objectives because the tasks themselves are understood (8, 24).

Delegation requires many capacities:

- Patience in helping others develop skills and judgment they may not yet have acquired.
- Clarity about the extent and limitations of the power/authority to be delegated.
- Judiciousness in establishing priorities.

Thus, delegation at times becomes an emotional rather than a procedural issue. Because of this, managers may not do enough of it. Failure to delegate may be attributable to a manager's lack of confidence in staff. The problem may be an inflated self-image, leading a manager to believe that he or she is pivotal to departmental functioning. Such a self-image can contribute to an unwillingness to decrease the power a manager perceives himself or herself as holding by sharing it. Alternatively, lack of self-confidence and fear of taking risks can keep managers tied to routine and familiar tasks. Finally, they may fear competition from subordinates, be concerned about appearing lazy, and mistakenly believe that if they delegate responsibility, they will be left with nothing to do (25).

Managers who cannot delegate are likely to feel overwhelmed and overworked. They are just as likely to be poor managers of time. Without delegation they have little opportunity to develop long-range plans, evaluate programs, and keep abreast of the politics, the technical advances, and the economics of health care delivery systems (8).

It is helpful to think of managers' time as falling into one of two categories. The first is time on which the organization, supervisors, and staff impose realistic constraints. This may be time spent in committee meetings with other department or service heads, on tasks mandated from above, or in regularly scheduled meetings with individual staff members or staff groups. The second category is time that may be called discretionary—the minutes, hours, or days that can be spent however the manager chooses (26).

The key to managing discretionary time is to set limits and to make choices about what truly requires the attention of management. If delegation has been effective, staff should have been encouraged to take initiatives and make independent decisions (26). It is better to review those decisions in supervision sessions than to be faced with frequent interruptions and disruptions of work. Other than in emergencies, problem identification should be kept to scheduled appointments or group meetings. By so doing, managers will find more time than they imagined for creative thinking and planning about how the entire department can expand professional objectives. This is not to recommend isolation from day-to-day issues. Rather, what is needed is to balance "being there" and giving to staff with being a "getter," a proactive leader who has the available time and energy to gather resources and move his or her department ahead (3, 8, 26).

MANAGING CONFLICT

Although not by design, managers spend approximately 20 percent of their time dealing with conflicts (27). That is as much as one full work day per week. So they must learn to manage the time spent in this way. Moreover, they must learn to manage the conflicts. Like leadership ability, supervision, and decision making, conflict resolution depends heavily on effective communication skills (8).

Types of Conflict and Stages of Resolution

Conflicts may be either substantive or emotional; that is, they may be based on disagreements over interpretation of facts or on differences in feelings and values. Sometimes they are a combination of both. At other times conflicts are the result of competition for status, resources, or favors. Conflicts of this nature usually result in a win-lose situation in which one party stands to gain at the expense of the other. Under any of these circumstances, resolution depends on the capacity of the manager, as a neutral third party, to impartially facilitate both ventilation around feelings and communication around facts (11).

Conflicts evolve through a variety of stages before becoming full-blown. Stage one develops as a result of ambiguity about professional roles and functions, communication barriers, competition among staff, or individual differences among staff in perceptions of needs, goals, values, and motivations. The second stage can be identified by the mounting of interpersonal tension among those who perceive these differences. It is only when tension is perceived by all parties that the antecedents to the tension can be analyzed and there is motivation to change. This is the third stage and the point at which conflict resolution can begin (11).

Conflict can be managed in ways ranging from simply ignoring it (which in itself is a decision) to negotiating for resolution. At one end of the spectrum, nonattention can result in destructive solutions or solutions that inhibit individual or departmental growth. Negotiation is the process that occurs at the other end of the spectrum, not unlike the collective bargaining model used in union strike settlements (28, 29). Negotiation or bargaining is characterized by each individual or group presenting a "public" stance that is favorable to its own position. Each side withholds information and slowly makes concessions until an acceptable solution or agreement is reached (28). It is not unusual for managers in unionized organizations to participate in formal collective bargaining. Nor is it unusual for managers to negotiate with others in an organization around such issues as the redistribution of diminished resources, cutbacks in space, and overall reductions in staff. Communication skills, discussed in chapter 15, are essential in negotiation.

More frequently, occupational therapy managers will be faced with resolving conflicts that arise over program and service priorities, and differences among staff about professional values. In these instances creative resolutions can be found if issues are confronted directly. However, direct confrontation is useful only when conflicts are not interpersonal or emotional but involve a higher level of goals (28). Then, there must be a willingness among all parties to immediately share all available information and initiate a collaborative search for alternatives (28).

Interpersonal or emotional conflict can be managed quite differently. The neutrality of the manager is still required, but resolution is reached via individual supervision of both parties, with the expectation that professionals can independently overcome personality conflicts. Time need not be spent fielding complaints about what's wrong with "him" or "her." Rather it should be spent in gentle exploration and, if necessary, confrontation of how the individual at hand contributes to the conflict through his or her own feelings and behavior. This can lead to both personal and professional growth for the supervisee, as well as better understanding of the other person. More important, efforts should be geared toward averting such conflicts through administrative commitment to team building and administrative awareness of group process.

Team Building and Group Process

Unfortunately, much of the knowledge base on group process derives from the body of literature on the theory and practice of group psychotherapy. Application of these theories in a professional setting can lead to the "false expectation that such knowledge automatically enhances administrative practice" (30, p 147). In fact, at times such an approach actually diminishes administrative effectiveness by overdetermined attention to personal issues.

What is useful in understanding group process is some basic knowledge about the nature of work groups, which are the key to organizational change. All work groups share some features that should be recognized by a manager whether he or she is functioning as the leader of his or her own department or as a group member at a higher administrative level (31).

1. These groups function best when made up of people who share similar job responsibilities.
2. Groups should be of reasonable size, allowing for frequent and productive communication.
3. Individuals should have opportunities to become involved not only in routine tasks, but also in concerns that affect them and the larger organization.

A work group has four major components: task, social structure, culture, and social process. The task involves the mode of work, resources, and evaluation of performance. The social structure incorporates divisions of labor and of authority. Within this component, issues of professional roles, identity, autonomy, and loyalty to the organization versus loyalty to professional groups come into play. The group culture comprises "values, assumptions and beliefs that characterize a given situation" (32, p 130). The social process relates to how the team does its work in terms of both tempo and methods used (32–35).

For a team to function well, there must be a clear distinction between "the domains of disciplinary competence or specialization and the sharing of organizational tasks or responsibilities" (36, p 836). The functions to be performed should determine which team or group members are best qualified to perform them (36). The primacy of each task may vary from setting to setting, or even moment to moment, requiring group/team members to have a strong sense of professional identity, to be flexible, and to tolerate some degree of role blurring (21, 33, 34, 37).

Managers should neither fear nor ignore the "social" and "cultural," or sentient, processes of group functioning, the informal aspects on which members depend for emotional support (14). These can be the key to understanding both organizational dynamics and group resistance to change. Addressing resistance to change rarely achieves the desired result. Awareness of that resistance, however, can lead to awareness of the need to engage staff in the change process by establishing working departmental committees that both increase problem solving and improve communication among group members. In this way group process can provide a forum for peer group identification in settings where occupational therapy personnel's time and loyalties are split between the department and the various interdisciplinary teams on which they serve.

An important aspect of team building and group process is effective meetings. Appendix A discusses this topic.

CONCLUSION

The manager's role has been described as bearing a closer resemblance to "that of a benign dictator than to that of an elected official" (12, p 5). This role can be both uncomfortable and unpopular. But managers do not have to be "lonely at the top" if they can expand their sources of gratification to include the sense of pride and mastery that comes from establishing a highly visible, relevant, and fiscally viable occupational therapy organization within a complex health care delivery system. Then, and only then, can occupational therapists offer themselves as prime movers in health care management and as role models, mentors, and educators for students of management.

SUMMARY

Occupational therapists in management positions must balance skills in leadership, decision making, supervision, delegation, and conflict management with the concrete tasks demanded by their roles and functions. They must also strike a balance between competence in direct clinical care delivery and concern with programmatic issues. Finally, they must balance their clinical values, rooted in professional identities as occupational therapists, with the constraints, values, goals, and missions of the organization and its monitoring agencies.

In his or her formal leadership role, the department manager must function as the link between an organization's policy makers and those on the front lines of service delivery. The manager who is able to negotiate between these highly differentiated spheres is in a better position to use his or her discretion in interpreting and implementing directives from above and can influence superiors to formulate policies and procedures in keeping with the competencies of his or her staff. Informally, managers must rely on friendship or exchange of favors to ensure collaboration with other services that affect their programs.

Leadership style can be understood as an adaptive capacity, calling for analytic powers, interpersonal skills, excellence in communication, and a high degree of discretion. Occupational therapists educated and professionally socialized to provide direct care do not find it easy to make the transition to positions of management. They must recognize and use their power, however, or they will be ineffective managers.

Decision making is "the common denominator of all administrative functioning." A key to successful management is knowing how decisions are made in an organization, that is, whether decision making is concentrated at the top or dispersed throughout the organization. Decisions are choices between two or more courses. They should be made with an awareness of the interplay between facts and values. Steps in decision making are (a) defining the problem, (b) developing alternative solutions, (c) selecting one alternative, (d) delineating the reasons for the selection, (e) implementing the choice, and (f) arranging for feedback on it.

In selecting a decision-making style an effective manager must make some hard choices about the degree to which his or her staff are to be a part of decision making. Styles range from autocratic to democratic. No single style should be used at all times. Managers must be sufficiently at ease in their role to be democratic when they can and autocratic when they must.

Supervision is a mutual undertaking between supervisor and supervisee, intended to promote growth and development while evaluating performance and maintaining standards. It can range from close daily interaction to weekly or monthly contact. There is a debate over whether clinical and administrative supervision should be separated or integrated.

Decisions about this depend on the size and complexity of the occupational therapy organization and the number of supervisory-level registered occupational therapists.

Delegation of authority offers managers the opportunity to develop long-range plans, evaluate programs, and keep abreast of the politics, technical advances, and economics of health care delivery systems. At times delegation becomes an emotional rather than a procedural issue, and because of this managers may not delegate enough. It is helpful to think of managers' time as falling into two categories: nondiscretionary (that demanded by the organization and personnel) and discretionary. The key to managing discretionary time is to set limits and to make choices about what truly requires the attention of management. If delegation has been effective, staff should have been encouraged to take initiative and make independent decisions.

Conflict resolution depends heavily on effective communication skills. Conflicts evolve through a variety of stages before becoming full-blown. Stage one develops as a result of ambiguity about roles and functions, communication barriers, competition among staff, or individual differences among staff. The second stage can be identified by the mounting of interpersonal tension among those who perceive their differences. When tension is perceived by all parties, stage three has been reached, and conflict resolution can begin.

There is a range of ways to manage conflict, from simply ignoring it to negotiating a resolution. Frequently, occupational therapists in management will be faced with resolving conflicts that arise over program and service priorities and differences among staff about professional value systems. In these instances creative resolutions can be found if issues are confronted directly. Interpersonal or emotional conflict can be managed quite differently, via individual supervision and the expectation that professionals can independently overcome personality conflicts.

More important than resolving conflicts is averting them through team building and group process. Work groups, which are the key to organizational change, have four major components: task, social structure, culture, and social process. The task involves the mode of work, resources, and evaluation of performance. The social structure incorporates divisions of labor and of authority. The culture comprises "values, assumptions and beliefs that characterize a given situation." The social process relates to how the team does its work in terms of both tempo and methods used.

Work groups function best when made up of people who share similar job responsibilities. They should be of reasonable size, allowing for frequent and productive communication, and individuals should have opportunities to become involved in concerns that affect them and the larger organization.

References

1. Hersey P, Blanchard K: *Management of Organizational Behavior: Utilizing Human Resources*, 4th edition. Englewood Cliffs, NJ: Prentice-Hall Inc, 1982
2. Mark B: A psychoanalytic approach to organizational diagnosis. *Admin Ment Health* 8:113–123, 1980
3. Fine SB: Weighing in: A consideration of leader-

ship and the occupational therapist in multidisciplinary settings. Paper delivered at Special Interest Group Breakfast, American Occupational Therapy Association Conference, Portland, Oregon, April 1983

4. Schulberg HC, McClelland M: Ethical dilemmas in administering mental health services. *Admin Ment Health* 9:20–31, 1981
5. Dolgoff T: The organization, the administrator and the mental health professional. *Admin Ment Health* 2:47–59, 1975
6. Kouzes JM, Mico PR: Domain theory: An introduction to organizational behavior in human service organizations. *J Appl Behav Sci* 15:449–469, 1979
7. Elridge WD: Coping with accountability and evaluation: Some guidelines for supervisors of direct service staff. *Admin Ment Health* 11:195–204, 1984
8. Henning M, Jardin A: *The Managerial Woman*. New York: Pocket Books Inc, 1977
9. Taylor FW: *The Principles of Scientific Management*. New York: Harper & Brothers, 1911
10. Fiedler FE: Validation and extension of the contingency model of leadership effectiveness: A review of empirical findings. *Psychol Bull* 76:128–148, 1971
11. Schermerhorn JF, Hunt JG, Osborn RN: *Managing Organizational Behavior*. New York: John Wiley & Sons Inc, 1982
12. Greenblatt M: Management succession: Some major parameters. *Admin Ment Health* 11:3–10, 1983
13. Minimal occupational therapy classification standards for supervisory administrative level personnel. In *Reference Manual of the Official Documents of the American Occupational Therapy Association*. Rockville, MD: American Occupational Therapy Association, 1983, pp 151–153
14. Kanter RM: Power failure in management circuits. *Harvard Bus Rev* 57:65–75, 1979
15. Foley AR, Brodie HKH: The administrative process as an instrument of change. *Hosp Community Psychiatry* 20:1–8, 1969
16. Simon HA: *Administrative Behavior*. New York: MacMillan Publishing Co Inc, 1945
17. Kraft S, Kraft S: Leadership strategies and values in times of scarcity. *Admin Ment Health* 9:177–183, 1982
18. Cooper JW: Six steps in problem solving for work supervisors. *Stout Vocational Rehabilitation Institute National Reporter*, Fall–Winter 1979–1980
19. Vroom VH: A new look in managerial decision-making. *Organizational Dynamics*. Spring:66–80, 1973
20. Guide for supervision of occupational therapy personnel. In *Reference Manual of the Official Documents of the American Occupational Therapy Association*. Rockville, MD: American Occupational Therapy Association, 1983, pp 141–142
21. Benarroch CC, Astrachan BM: Interprofessional role relationships. In *Psychiatric Administration: A Comprehensive Text for the Clinician-Executive*, JA Talbott, SR Kaplan, Editors. New York: Grune & Stratton, 1983, pp 223–236
22. Barton WE: Leadership development. *Admin Ment Health* 8:34–39, 1981
23. Allison MA, Allison E: Picking the right management style. *Working Woman*, October 1984, pp 31–38
24. Johnson AC, Forrest CR: Evaluating the effects of organizational variables on task performance of administrators. *Admin Ment Health* 11:92–105, 1983
25. Ransepp E: Why supervisors don't delegate. Newsletter of Princeton Creative Research Inc, undated.
26. Oncken W, Wass D: Management time: Who's got the monkey? *Harvard Bus Rev* 52:75–80, 1974
27. Thomas KW, Schmidt WH: A survey of managerial interests with respect to conflict. *Acad Manage J* 19:315–318, 1976
28. Lawrence PR, Lorsch JW: *Organization and the Environment*. Homewood, IL: Richard D Irwin Inc, 1969
29. Association policy: Stance on collective bargaining. *Am J Occup Ther* 37:816, 1983
30. Spiro HR: Psychodynamic theories in psychiatric administration. In *Psychiatric Administration: A Comprehensive Text for the Clinician-Executive*, JA Talbott, SR Kaplan, Editors. New York: Grune & Stratton, 1983, pp 147–166
31. Webster RS, Talbott SW, Loutsch E: Administrative development. In *Psychiatric Administration: A Comprehensive Text for the Clinician-Executive*, JA Talbott, SR Kaplan, Editors. New York: Grune & Stratton, 1983, pp 237–256
32. Newton P, Levinson DJ: The work group within the organization. *Psychiatry* 36:115–141, 1973
33. Astrachan BM, Flynn HR, Geller JD, et al: Systems approach to day hospitalization. *Arch Gen Psychiatry* 22:550–559, 1970
34. Feldman S: The middle management muddle. *Admin Ment Health* 8:3–11, 1980
35. Westbrod M: Why organizational development hasn't worked (so far) in medical centers. *Health Care Manage Rev* 1:17–28, 1975
36. Stone N: Effecting interdisciplinary coordination in clinical services to the mentally retarded. *Am J Orthopsychiatry* 4:835–839, 1970
37. Lewis JM: The organizational structure of the therapeutic team. *Soc Work Health Care* 20:206–208, 1969

Section V

Controlling

Section V takes up the managerial role of controlling, which is defined in this text as influencing the accomplishment of goals through formalized means such as organizational charts, policies and procedures, and job descriptions. "Organizational Roles and Relationships," Chapter 11, addresses controlling in terms of roles, stressing their interactive nature and the ways in which they can be used to influence an organization. Particular attention is given to the different roles occupational therapy personnel play—clinicians, educators, supervisors, managers, researchers, consultants, etc.—both longitudinally, over the span of a career, and simultaneously, as their own interests and their organizations' needs dictate. The chapter also deals with policies and procedures as ways of controlling what happens in an occupational therapy organization.

Chapter 12, "Personnel Management" describes this important managerial function in terms of a theoretical model that places it at the interface between the organization's resources, values, and goals, and the individual's values, goals, and skills. It takes the reader step by step through all aspects of personnel management, from projecting staffing needs to terminating an employee. Appended materials include sample job descriptions, an interview form, a performance appraisal form, and a summary of major legislation affecting employment.

Chapter 11

Organizational Roles and Relationships

Wendy Colman, PhD, OTR

This chapter concerns the particularly human side of management, which is seen when individuals interact with one another. That interaction represents individuals in roles, focused within a framework of influence or control. Webster's dictionary defines *control* as "application of policies and procedures for directing, regulating, and coordinating production, administration, and other business activities in a way to achieve the objectives of the enterprise" (1, p 496). In order to consider control in this context, it is important to examine the relationship of control to authority and power. The kind of power and authority occupational therapy managers exercise influences the settings in which they practice. Whether the setting is clinical, academic, or consultative, the goal of influencing it is ultimately to increase the quality of patient/client services.

The number of arenas that can be influenced varies according to the particular role of the occupational therapist—staff therapist, instructor,

---

Wendy Colman did her doctoral dissertation on the interactions of different ideological groups in AOTA relative to attaining and maintaining control. Her career pattern includes clinical experience as a supervisor and a program director, and academic experience as an instructor and a director of graduate education. She is on the faculty at Temple University in Philadelphia.

manager, or consultant, supervisor or supervisee, and so on. To exert the greatest amount of influence in their setting, that is, to attain the greatest amount of power and authority, occupational therapy personnel need to decide how best to (a) organize their work, (b) define their roles, (c) determine their behavior, and (d) set their boundaries and goals for performance. In this way they begin to assume control in their workplace.

ROLES

The term *role* is a metaphor derived from acting. One imagines favorite screen, stage, or television stars in given roles. Actors play various parts and are applauded when they appear to be most natural. Roles, then, relate to specific actions that clearly demonstrate a known character. Roles may also be identified with different members of a family or a society. Individual roles exemplify a set of predictable actions that are useful to special groups or society in general. Each role is bounded by a set of responsibilities and privileges. The dimensions of any role are determined collectively by the person inhabiting the role and by the group or the society in which the role exists (2–4).

The central point in considering the nature of roles is that they are *interactive*. Individuals in particular roles see themselves in relation to others who also have roles (5). Therefore, roles emerge from human social organizations (6). Groups of actions that exemplify particular task mastery (7) are classified into discrete roles and labeled. Thus, roles are those determinable actions that individuals expect and are expected to perform in social group formations. Roles lend order to a social group, promote the work or the task of a group, and facilitate group members' interactions. Because each member of a group or system, assumes or is assigned a particular role, and because each role encompasses certain expected behaviors, the nature of individuals' interactions in different roles becomes the hallmark of the system's ability to function.

Professions, as special kinds of groups, have their own role definitions, both within the profession and in relation to society. Professionals sustain certain role functions that are valued in the major cultural tradition of the society in which the profession exists (8). Professionals who engage in patient/client treatment are expected to (a) apply their skills, knowledge, and technique within the value orientation of their organization, and (b) work toward realizing the organization's goals (9). Within professions as well, then, the importance of role as an interactive function is stressed.

Perspectives on Roles

Various perspectives on roles that are described in the literature often convey a similar message: An individual should understand the role he or she occupies within a system and use it strategically to meet his or her professional needs. Approaches for identifying and describing roles can be divided into three categories: (a) generic role descriptions identified through particular theoretical frameworks, (b) the notion of professional responsibilities, and (c) the particulars of a job function.

Generic role descriptions. The word *role* pervades the everyday language of the society and has thus taken on a variety of meanings depending on the user's particular experience and intent. In the study of roles, experience and intent are structured within particular disciplinary or theoretical frameworks. For instance, to sociologists, roles describe the behaviors of individuals in specific group settings. The business literature discusses role in terms of workers and their place in an organizational structure or hierarchy. In health care, role is most often identified in terms of an individual's particular responsibilities in delivering health care.

Specifically, discussions of role identification in the workplace have been linked to issues of job status and job satisfaction. These concerns center on the quality of interactions among people in various work roles. Some business theorists have extended the ideas of job status and satisfaction to include achievement potential, advancement possibilities, and increased responsibilities (10–11). These concerns also revolve around role interaction.

Professional responsibilities. The second category of discussions about roles centers on professional responsibilities. For occupational therapy personnel, responsibilities have been identified in such areas as health planning, development of contracts with third-party payers, government legislation, the social situation within the health care system, and interaction between clinical and academic education (12–15). Most recently, the role of occupational therapy personnel in reimbursement has gained national attention (16).

A review of the literature on clinical and academic roles supports the concept of their interactive nature within the framework of professional responsibility. Maintaining relationships between clinical and academic settings is a major arena of professional responsibility according to Snow and Mitchell (15). These authors stress roles as a concept primarily concerned with human interaction. They note that different occupational therapy roles interact frequently in the relationship between clinical and academic settings, and they also identify potential role conflicts within that interaction. Additionally, Snow and Mitchell cite the problems faced by individual therapists when caught between academic and clinical systems, noting that such roles force therapists to clarify their ideas about professional responsibility in order to remain flexible and thus maintain the intersystem relationship. Flexibility is the mark of a role that is determined by professional responsibilities.

Job functions. Finally, roles have been identified as they specify job functions or tasks. The action involved in a role comes into play in this perspective. Many examples from the literature describe the occupational therapist's role as a member of the health care team. This theme appears to be central in the profession's concept of role delineation. It is discussed in terms of both classic and new definitions, relative to both specialty and generic occupational therapy concerns (9, 17–26).

Occupational therapy roles and job functions that extend beyond the scope of direct care have developed primarily within the last decade. The image of occupational therapists functioning effectively and necessarily in other than the practitioner role is now taking hold strongly in the field. What is emerging is a description of the profession of occupational therapy in a multifaceted milieu.

Career Development: New Role Options

Hertzberg, Mausner, and Synderman discuss the need for career development as a means of maintaining job satisfaction (11). As occupational therapy has expanded its scope academically and clinically, a number of new roles have emerged, broadening career possibilities for individual occupational therapy personnel. The choices available now include not only a diversity of specialty roles for the practitioner, but additional career opportunities in management, administration, teaching, research, scholarship, and consultation. Each of these roles is identified by particular job functions and specific skills necessary for success.

Campbell has categorized the work of the clinical occupational therapy practitioner into direct patient care and supervisory/administrative responsibilities. Her taxonomy of clinical roles identifies emerging managerial concerns for the clinician, noted by these categories: staff therapist, clinical supervisor, assistant chief, and chief therapist. She has also described the management skills necessary for an occupational therapist to acquire in order to fulfill the requirements of these clinical roles, among them, skills in developing and directing policy, and in managing personnel, supplies, time, and competence. Campbell has underscored the importance of occupational therapists' involvement in policy making within the health care system, using their emerging roles to effect changes that meet their professional needs.

Others have continued development of Campbell's taxonomy. Miller has suggested that the position of consultant is becoming one of the major roles in occupational therapy (21). A committee of the American Occupational Therapy Association (AOTA) formed to review administrative issues in the field has described the work of some occupational therapists as solely administrative, thus delineating another career possibility (28–29).

However, as these new roles have emerged, problems have arisen with them. They have put a strain on the educational system in occupational therapy in terms of the training available to meet the skills these roles demand. Additionally therapists have been challenged and taxed to develop an understanding of these new career choices and the expanding notions of role. As discussed earlier, the most critical concern in the study of roles is their interactive character, which demands communication skills if the therapist is to function effectively. As the roles of occupational therapists change, the roles of others within the systems in which occupational therapists work alter accordingly. These changes require adjustments and adaptations in communication skills. Concurrently occupational therapists' roles are shifting in response to the changing job functions of other professional personnel and in response to skill development and an expanding occupational therapy knowledge base. All of these areas affect the interactive process involved in maintaining the functioning of a system through role delineation. What has become clear in much of the recent literature is the need for occupational therapists to begin deliberately to educate themselves for these new roles (30–31).

Linear career choices. Today the three primary arenas in which occupational therapists work are clinical settings, academic settings, and consultative settings. Clinical settings comprise those programs in which the occupational therapist engages in or is responsible for direct treatment of patients/clients. Such settings include traditional hospitals, nontraditional public health or community centers, the public school system, and other health care organizations. Academic settings encompass programs in which occupational therapists are responsible for the education and training of entry-level and advanced occupational therapy students. Consultative settings may be either clinical or academic, their nature being defined by the involvement of an occupational therapy consultant,

FIGURE 11–1
Occupational Therapist's Roles: Potential Linear Career Choices

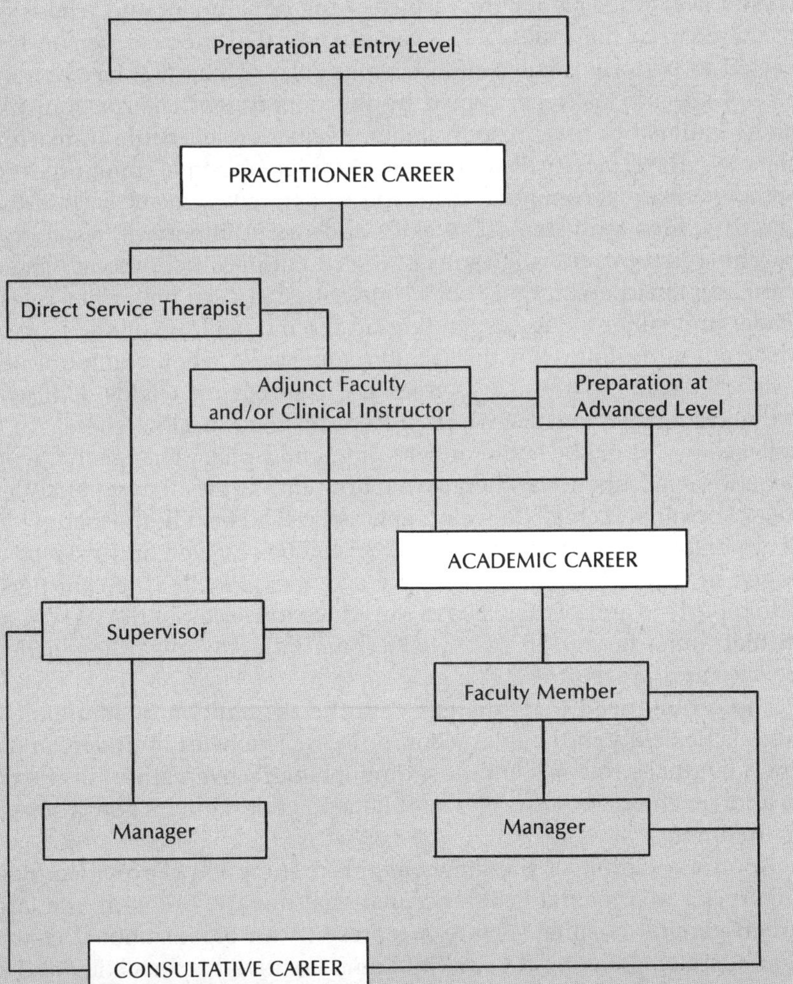

who advises on staff or program development (chapter 17 discusses this role in depth). Within each of these settings occupational therapy personnel may assume one or a number of roles, from direct care through management and administration. The skills necessary to perform the different functions are acquired through experience, mentoring, and continued education. As occupational therapy personnel move from one role to the next, they depend on the skills they mastered in their previous roles. A structure allowing both vertical and horizontal movement between roles emerges, symbolizing career development (see Figure 1). Occupational therapy personnel are afforded a great many options in directing their career and in choosing the type and nature of work for which they are best suited.

Simultaneous roles. Figure 1 only partially describes career development. In some of the career choices available in occupational therapy, a number of roles are in action simultaneously. For example, as illustrated in Figure 2, an occupational therapy department chairperson in a university is responsible for the faculty of the department and responsible to the dean of the college. The varied tasks that the chairperson is expected to perform involve simultaneous roles. Miller (32) has identified eleven specific tasks performed by the department chairperson: planning, leadership, fiscal responsibility, evaluation, curriculum, teaching, climate setting, faculty development, extradepartmental communication, intradepartmental communication, and student advisement. Each of these tasks requires a diverse set of skills and, more important, a variety of psychological positions in terms of the communication process. The department chairperson must shift constantly between his or her roles as leader and subordinate, depending on the moment; he or she is supervisor when dealing with the faculty, supervisee when communicating with the dean. In these two roles the chairperson wields a different influence relative to policies and procedures. Specifically, whereas at the college level he or she might only recommend a policy change that would benefit the occupational therapy department, at the departmental level he or she might actually develop new policies to benefit the faculty. The chairperson often has teaching responsibilities as well and may be engaged in research or other scholarly activities. Finally, the chairperson also reports to and participates in the education sector of the AOTA, and in that arena he or she may wield some influence regarding national policies and procedures.

The central need that emerges with the assumption of simultaneous roles is flexibility in the interaction process. The heart of understanding an individual's role is comprehending its interactive nature. In the case of a career choice that involves simultaneous roles, interaction is stressed to the limit.

Another example of simultaneous role assumption is provided by the supervisor of a mental health occupational therapy program in a large, urban general hospital. Figure 3 represents an organizational chart of that hospital, showing the lines of administrative responsibility and detailing the position of the occupational therapy department. Obviously the supervisor of the mental health program must function through various lines of communication. The supervisor in this case is a woman

FIGURE 11–2
An Occupational Therapy Department in a University

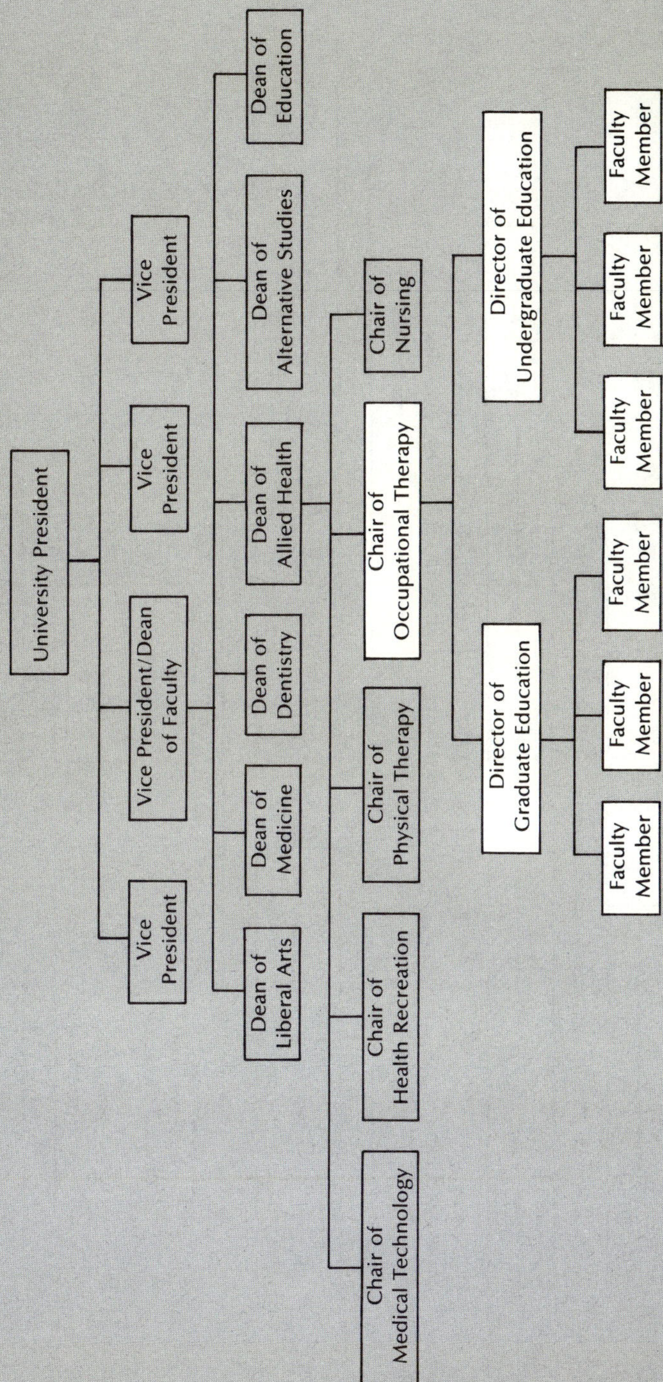

FIGURE 11–3
An Occupational Therapy Department in a Hospital

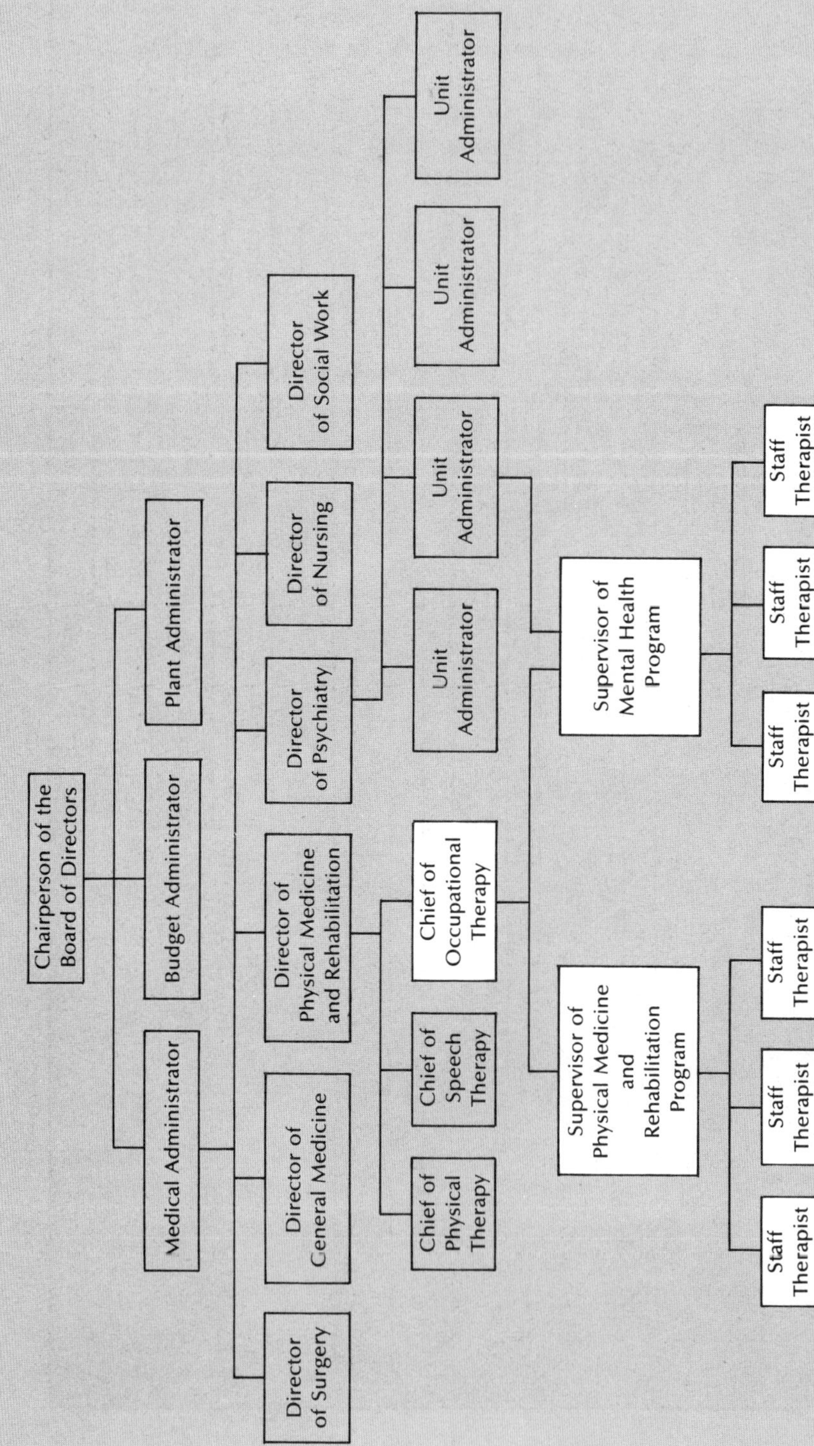

in her mid-twenties who has moved through a linear career pattern, choosing a clinical specialty (mental health) and advancing vertically to the position of supervisor. She brings with her a variety of advanced clinical skills and some emerging administrative ones. Figure 3 indicates that as supervisor of a mental health occupational therapy program, she is responsible for three staff therapists and responsible to both the chief occupational therapist and a psychiatric unit administrator.

The tasks of her position as outlined in Figure 4 indicate that she wears many hats. She is not only supervisor of the occupational therapy mental health program but also the director of fieldwork for the entire department. Each of those roles has required task and communication competencies. As a supervisor, she is responsible for continuing program development, implementation, and evaluation; staff supervision; student supervision; and direct patient care. She may also participate in the occupational therapy department's financial planning and research. As the director of fieldwork, she is responsible for placement, planning, and supervision of all staff therapists who are supervising students.

Finally, as a member of the mental health treatment team, she has program evaluation and patient care responsibilities to her unit and to the hospital department of psychiatry. In this capacity she may also be instrumental in affecting policies and procedures and in controlling the nature and the quality of occupational therapy services.

Communication skills. The critical concern in this discussion is the fact that each career move longitudinally (over time) encompasses an increasing simultaneity of role responsibilities. As occupational therapy personnel make career choices and advances, many of the tasks and the skills that they developed along the way are incorporated into a larger scheme, including a new set of tasks requiring new skill development.

FIGURE 11–4

Clinical Occupational Therapy Department: Organizational Chart

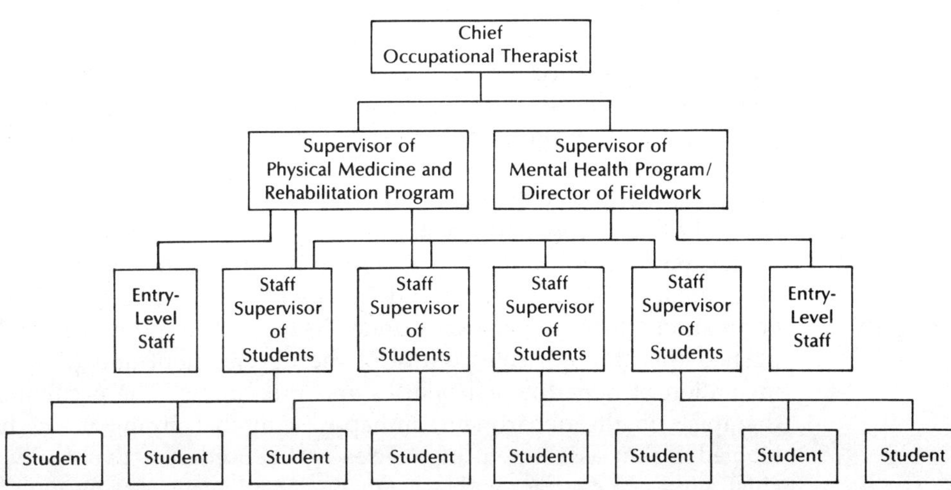

Central to this is the continuous improvement of communication skills. Again, the notion of roles as interactive stresses the need for excellence in a variety of communication processes. Each of the roles and job functions just discussed demands different kinds of communication skills. As developing occupational therapy personnel don new hats with each role change, the nature of necessary communication alters. The primary purpose of that communication is to influence the system. Thus, to affect organizational policies and procedures successfully, it becomes critical to hone those skills. An understanding of the aspects of role simultaneity can facilitate effecting control in a particular work setting.

The exercise of control. The exercise of control varies with the different roles assumed by occupational therapy personnel. Because control represents power and authority, managers often equate it with an attitude of restriction. Limiting or confining a subordinate's scope of responsibility is certainly one means of exercising control. However, given a framework of human interaction, it may not always be the best way to ensure control.

An alternative method of exercising control is by maintaining flexibility. In settings that are soundly organized, with clear role delineations and respect for individual integrity, workers experience a greater sense of freedom while being "well controlled." Therefore, a more positive and productive view of control is that (a) it works well when good planning and organization are at the root of a program, and (b) it is best effected when individuals have freedom to make on-the-spot decisions. A manager's task is to create the balance that allows freedom within reasonable boundaries. A way to create those boundaries and effect control is through policies and procedures.

POLICIES AND PROCEDURES

An organization is generally best influenced through its body of written rules and regulations, known as policies and procedures. Policies and procedures express the value system of an organization, outlining specific directions, goals, and expected behaviors for workers. At any one time, policies and procedures are controlled by the individuals or the groups that hold power in an organization. Often, changes in policies and procedures reflect attitudinal and value changes in an organization's membership or leadership. An example of planning and implementing policy and procedural changes to shift the sphere of influence from the existing leadership to a broader, more encompassing and interactive group is provided by the hypothetical occupational therapy department in Figure 4. A history of the department indicates that the chief has been in that position for many years, during which she has controlled departmental decision making and dominated the functioning of all of the occupational therapy personnel under her jurisdiction. She has accomplished this through sole control of the development and the implementation of departmental policies and procedures. The occupational therapists in the department, unhappy with that arrangement, have lobbied for an assessment of policies and procedures. Eventually the chief agrees to contract with an outside consultant to review the organizational structure and functioning of the department.

Through an in-depth study the consultant finds that the department's organization does not promote adequate or equitable decision making, lacks standard operating procedures, and turns most tasks into ineffective, time-consuming exercises. The consultant also identifies the leadership within the department as factious. This has not only alienated the staff, but it has been detrimental to the growth of the group and has sometimes resulted in inadequate patient care.

The consultant has in effect documented the existing value system of the department as expressed in policies and procedures. At its inception the department apparently valued stable leadership, vesting authority and power in one person for a long period. That leadership structured the department within a limited emphasis. As the department has grown, as new therapists with different educational and life experience have been hired and advanced in their practice, a shift has occurred in the values of the majority in the group.

In light of the findings, the consultant generates recommendations for change. To facilitate better decision making, she suggests a reorganization of the department, starting with the development of committees.

The occupational therapy staff review the consultant's findings and recommendations and discuss a series of other options. Because of the balance of the group, the majority promotes a change in the individual occupational therapist's sphere of influence within the department. The staff struggle with the notion of altering the structure and the administration of the department. Eventually, through the institution of new policies, they move the seat of decision making from the chief to a group of elected members. This change increases staff involvement and responsibility in the running of the department. The occupational therapists promoting the new value system have thus implemented a strategy of taking control of the basic structural components of the department to solidify their place within it, and have increased their influence in policy setting.

In this example roles (positions within an organizational structure), control (the ability to influence the system from one's role), and policies and procedures are used together to promote change in an organization and facilitate control. Understanding that process and implementing actions to effect it will create avenues of influence for occupational therapists in their work arenas.

It is also in the area of policies and procedures that individuals have the greatest potential for long-term influence in an organization. Coupled with an effective managerial style of role definition and expression, policies and procedures can become a central tool of control. To return to the example of the supervisor of the mental health program, in that role she is able to direct the professional socialization of the occupational therapy personnel and students in her charge. This is done by explicitly identifying and defining their roles through particular behaviors. Those behaviors may be called performance evaluation criteria, for example, and be used to determine staff promotions and student competencies. Thus, by outlining the specific roles of supervisees through written policies and procedures, the occupational therapy supervisor exerts control and influences the system in which she works. She can also use policies and procedures to effect control by influencing (a) reporting systems, including record keeping, communication standards, and budget, (b) program evaluation, including goals, objectives, and services, and (c) research directions, including data organization and analysis (33).

Critical to the adequate use of policies and procedures as a tool of control is an in-depth understanding of three aspects of the organization:

1. The intact organizational structure
2. Its current procedures
3. The reasons why those procedures are or are not effecting adequate results in the directions determined important by the leadership.

This knowledge can be used to direct action within an organization. Baum equates that kind of action with stellar treatment planning (34). She suggests that if the organization is viewed as a patient, the procedure is to (a) evaluate in order to determine assets and limitations, (b) identify particular problem areas, and (c) develop a plan to intervene in those problem areas in order to effect change. Change on the organizational level, as on the level of patient treatment, reflects a goal of attaining functional abilities, that is, the supporting functions that promote and enhance the work of occupational therapy and individual occupational therapists.

SUMMARY

Control is the "application of policies and procedures for directing, regulating, and coordinating production, administration, and other business activities in a way to achieve the objectives of the enterprise" (1, p 496). The kind of control occupational therapy managers exercise influences the settings in which they practice. The number of arenas that can be influenced varies according to the particular roles of occupational therapy personnel. To exert the greatest amount of control, occupational therapy personnel must decide how best to organize their work, define their roles, determine their behavior, and set their boundaries and goals for performance.

The central point in considering the nature of roles is that they are interactive, emerging from human social organizations. They are those determinable actions that individuals expect and are expected to perform in social group formations. Roles lend order to a social group, promote the work or the task of a group, and facilitate group members' interactions. Professions, representing a set of special groups, have their own role definitions.

The various perspectives on roles in the literature often convey a similar message: An individual should understand the role he or she occupies within a system and use it strategically to meet his or her professional needs. Approaches for identifying and describing roles can be divided into three categories: generic role descriptions, which represent roles in terms of a profession's experience and intent; role characterizations in terms of professional responsibilities, which identify such areas as health planning and the interaction between clinical and academic education;

and role delineations relative to job functions, which define the actions involved in a role.

In the latter category, the role of the occupational therapist as a member of the health care team appears to be central in the profession's concept of role delineation. However, new roles and job functions for occupational therapy personnel have developed in the last decade. The choices available now include not only a diversity of specialty roles for the practitioner, but additional career opportunities in management, administration, teaching, research, scholarship, and consultation. Each role is identified by particular job functions and specific skills necessary for success in it. What has become clear in much of the recent literature is the need for occupational therapy personnel to begin deliberately to educate themselves for these new roles.

Another way of organizing current occupational therapy roles and possible career moves is to identify the work of occupational therapy personnel. The three primary work settings are clinical, academic, and consultative. Within each of these settings the practitioner may assume one or a number of roles, acquiring the skills to perform them through experience, mentoring, and continued education. A structure allowing both vertical and horizontal movement between roles emerges.

In some of the career choices available in occupational therapy, a number of roles are in action simultaneously. For example, the chairperson of an occupational therapy department in a university is the supervisor of a faculty and the supervisee of the dean. He or she also has responsibilities in planning, leadership, fiscal matters, evaluation, curriculum, teaching, climate setting, faculty development, extradepartmental communication, intradepartmental communication, and student advisement. Flexibility is a central need that emerges with the assumption of simultaneous roles. Also, because roles are interactive, a critical skill that is called for is communication. Communication is necessary if one is going to influence the system, that is, exercise control.

The exercise of control varies with the different roles assumed by occupational therapy personnel. Managers often equate control with restriction, but given a framework of human interaction, flexibility may be a better approach. That is, in settings that are soundly organized, with clear role delineations and respect for individual integrity, workers experience a greater sense of freedom while being "well controlled."

A way to create freedom within reasonable boundaries is through policies and procedures. An organization is generally best influenced through its policies and procedures. These express its value system, outlining the specific directions, goals, and expected behaviors. Often, changes in policies and procedures reflect attitudinal and value changes in an organization's membership or leadership. Coupled with an effective managerial style of role definition and expression, policies and procedures can become a central tool of control.

Critical to the adequate use of policies and procedures as a tool of control is an in-depth understanding of the intact organizational structure, its current procedures, and the reasons why those procedures are or are not effecting results in the directions determined important by the leadership.

References

1. Gove PB, Editor: *Webster's Third New International Dictionary of the English Language Unabridged.* Springfield, MA: G and C Merriam Co, 1981
2. Berne E: *Games People Play.* New York: Grove Press Inc, 1964
3. Sarbin TR: Role theory. In *Handbook of Social Psychology*, G Lindzey, Editor. Menlo Park, CA: Addison-Wesley Publishing Co, 1968
4. Shaw ME: *Group Dynamics: The Psychology of Small Group Behavior*, 2nd edition. New York: McGraw-Hill Book Co, 1976
5. Emmet D: *Rules, Roles, and Relations.* Boston: Beacon Press, 1966
6. Erikson EH: *Childhood and Society.* New York: WW Norton and Co Inc, 1963
7. Szasz TS: *The Myth of Mental Illness: Foundations of a Theory of Personal Conduct*, revised edition. New York: Harper & Row Publishers, 1974
8. Parsons T: *Essays in Sociological Theory*, revised edition. Glencoe, IL: Free Press, 1954
9. Fidler GS, Fidler JW: *Occupational Therapy: A Communication Process in Psychiatry.* New York: The Macmillan Co, 1963
10. Linton R: *The Study of Man.* New York: Appleton-Century, 1936
11. Hertzberg F, Mausner B, Synderman B: *The Motivation to Work.* New York: John Wiley & Sons Inc, 1959
12. Wilson SR: Health planning: An opportunity for involvement of occupational therapists. *Am J Occup Ther* 30:214–215, 1976
13. Meredith F: Perspectives on occupational therapy's role in health systems agency activities. *Am J Occup Ther* 31:454–455, 1977
14. Yerxa EJ: Occupational therapy's role in creating a future climate of caring. *Am J Occup Ther* 34:529–534, 1980
15. Snow T, Mitchell MM: Administrative patterns in curriculum-clinic interactions. *Am J Occup Ther* 36:251–256, 1982
16. Davy JD, Editor: Reimbursement. *Am J Occup Ther* (special issue) 38:293–343, 1984
17. Gillette N, Kielhofner G: The impact of specialization on the professionalization and survival of occupational therapy. *Am J Occup Ther* 33:20–28, 1979
18. Davis JC: Team management of Parkinson's disease. *Am J Occup Ther* 31:300–308, 1977
19. Sieg KW: The nursing home: Occupational therapy service in an institution. *Am J Occup Ther* 31:516–524, 1977
20. Frazian BJW: Establishing and administrating a private practice in a hospital setting. *Am J Occup Ther* 32:296–300, 1978
21. Miller DB: Reflections concerning an activity consultant by a nursing home administrator. *Am J Occup Ther* 32:375–380, 1978
22. Sorensen J: Nationally speaking: Occupational therapy in business: A new horizon. *Am J Occup Ther* 32:287–288, 1978
23. Conine TA, Chritie GM, Hammond GK, et al: An assessment of occupational therapists' roles and attitudes toward sexual rehabilitation of the disabled. *Am J Occup Ther* 33:515–519, 1979
24. Gilfoyle EM, Hays C: Occupational therapy roles and functions in the education of the school-based handicapped student. *Am J Occup Ther* 33:565–576, 1979
25. Rosenfeld MS: A model for activity intervention in disaster-stricken communities. *Am J Occup Ther* 36:229–235, 1982
26. Lindsay WP: The role of the occupational therapist in the treatment of alcoholism. *Am J Occup Ther* 37:36–43, 1983
27. Campbell K: Occupational therapist: OTR/Manager. *Am J Occup Ther* 32:291–295, 1978
28. Ad Hoc Committee on Administrative Issues: Nationally speaking: Final report of the Ad Hoc Committee on Administrative Issues, part 1. *Am J Occup Ther* 34:5–9, 1980
29. Ad Hoc Committee on Administrative Issues: Nationally speaking: Final report of the Ad Hoc Committee on Administrative Issues, part 2. *Am J Occup Ther* 34:81–84, 1980
30. Gilfoyle EM: Eleanor Clarke Slagle Lectureship, 1984: Transformation of a profession. *Am J Occup Ther* 38:575–584, 1984
31. Swartz KB: The issue is—balancing objectives of efficient and effective occupational therapy practice. *Am J Occup Ther* 38:198–200, 1984
32. Miller R: Application of role and role conflict theory to administration in occupational therapy education. *Occup Ther J Res* 2:27–38, 1982
33. Guidelines for an occupational therapist providing services as an administrator. In *Manual on Administration.* Rockville, MD: American Occupational Therapy Association, 1978, pp 56–59
34. Baum CM: Management and documentation of occupational therapy services. In *Willard and Spackman's Occupational Therapy*, 5th edition, HL Hopkins, HD Smith, Editors. Philadelphia: JB Lippincott Co, 1978, pp 675–685

Additional Resources

Durbin RL, Springall WH: *Organization and Administration of Health Care: Theory, Practice, Environment*, 2nd edition. St. Louis: CV Mosby Co, 1974

Grant KH: Nationally speaking: A perspective on occupational therapy education. *Am J Occup Ther* 38:643–646, 1984

Huss AJ: Nationally speaking: Whither thou goest? Report of the AOTA task force on OT/PT issues. *Am J Occup Ther* 38:81–86, 1984

Larson MS: *The Rise of Professionalism: A Sociological Analysis*. Berkeley: University of California Press, 1977

Mintzberg J: *The Structuring of Organizations: A Synthesis of the Research*. Englewood Cliffs, NJ: Prentice-Hall Inc, 1979

Mosey AC: *Activities Therapy*. New York: Raven Press Publishers, 1973

Mosey AC: *Occupational Therapy: Configuration of a Profession*. New York: Raven Press Publishers, 1981

Osterman P, Gross R: *The New Professionals*. New York: Simon & Schuster, 1972

Sartain AQ, Baker AW: *The Supervisor and His Job*, 2nd edition. New York: McGraw-Hill Book Co, 1972

Sergiovanni TJ, Starrat RJ: *Supervision: Human Perspectives*, 3rd edition. New York: McGraw-Hill Book Co, 1983

Yerxa EJ: Consultancy and research. In *Willard and Spackman's Occupational Therapy*, 5th edition, HL Hopkins, HD Smith, Editors. Philadelphia: JB Lippincott Co, 1978, pp 689–693

Chapter 12

Personnel Management

Barbara A. Boyt Schell, MS, OTR/L

Management is accomplishment of work through the efforts of others (1). This chapter highlights concepts important to efficient and effective management of personnel resources. A theoretical model of personnel management is presented in the initial section. The rest of the chapter is devoted to discussions of personnel practices and techniques relevant to occupational therapy management. Included are identification of staffing needs, development and use of job descriptions, and staff recruitment, selection, and orientation. Staff development, performance appraisal, rewards, and management of the difficult employee are also addressed. Appendixes include sample forms and a summary of legislation affecting the personnel aspects of management.

A THEORETICAL MODEL OF PERSONNEL MANAGEMENT

A manager serves as the interface between the individuals forming a department or a program and the larger organization. In the particular function of personnel management he or she designs work roles and acquires, develops, and maintains individuals to perform the roles. To

---

A manager with experience in both the public and the private sectors of health care, Barbara A. Boyt Schell now directs a large (40-plus) occupational therapy department at Harmarville Rehabilitation Center in Pittsburgh. Recently she chaired a task force of AOTA's Commission on Practice that revised the classification standards for occupational therapy personnel.

FIGURE 12–1
Personnel Management Model

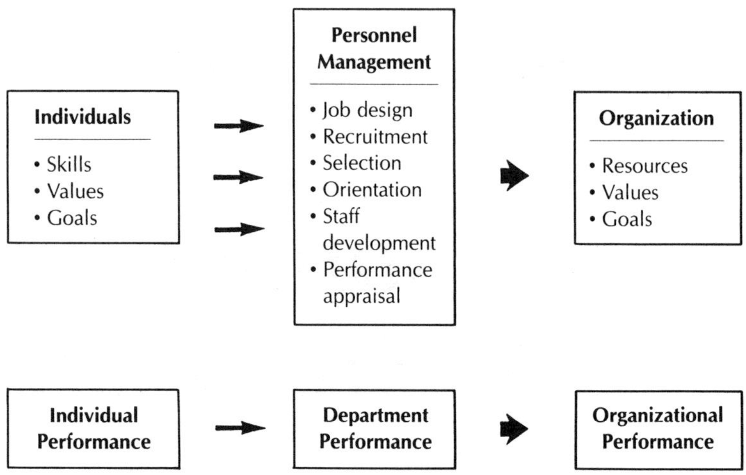

do this effectively, a manager must understand organizational resources, values, and goals. This knowledge provides a context for recruiting, selecting, and developing staff, focusing on identification of individuals with skills, values, and goals consistent with the organizational context. Figure 1 illustrates this pivotal function of personnel management. It also displays the role of personnel management in performance. Individual performance is measured against the desired performance within the department or the program and the larger organization. Performance is enhanced through staff development activities and represents the channeling of individual aspirations and abilities into attainment of department or program and organizational goals. This process of translating individual efforts into an effective work group is one of the most rewarding aspects of management.

QUANTIFICATION OF STAFF NEEDS

One component of personnel management is the ability to quantify and project staffing needs accurately. This process requires that human resources be expressed in quantifiable terms.

Understanding Full-Time Equivalents

Frequently the concept of a full-time equivalent or FTE is used. An FTE is the amount of work time of one full-time staff person. Full-time employment usually represents an 8-hour day and a 5-day week—thus, 260 paid days per year or 2,080 paid hours per year. This measure is helpful for representing the amount of staffing (both full-time and part-time) in a department or a program.

For example, an occupational therapy department in a large teaching hospital employs eleven individuals: one full-time manager, three full-time occupational therapists and one full-time occupational therapy assistant assigned to the rehabilitation unit, one full-time therapist in the burn unit, one full-time therapist and one half-time assistant in psychiatry, and three half-time therapists for outpatient services. The manager could express this staffing as follows:

1	FTE Manager
6.5	FTE Occupational therapists
1.5	FTE Occupational therapy assistants
9.0	FTE Total

The manager could also express allocation of staff by program area:

1	FTE Manager
4	FTE Rehabilitation unit
1	FTE Burn unit
1.5	FTE Psychiatry
1.5	FTE Outpatient services
9.0	FTE Total

Although there are eleven individuals in the department, there are only nine FTEs. This is due to the four half-time employees, who each represent only 0.5 FTE.

Developing Productivity Standards

The quantity of work that a given FTE can be expected to produce is called a productivity standard. Productivity standards vary according to the setting and the population being served. To develop a productivity standard, units of productivity must be determined. The American Occupational Therapy Association (AOTA) has developed a Product Output Reporting System (2) for quantifying aspects of occupational therapy services. This system is designed to be used in conjunction with computer-generated billing systems. When it is used as a productivity measure, data are collected reflecting the number of relative value units (RVU) generated by each individual. RVU are indices of the level of competence at which a category of service is delivered and the sophistication of the equipment and the facilities that are used. A staff member would be expected to generate a predetermined average number of RVU in a given time frame.

Simpler measures of productivity include treatment units and visits. These are less sensitive than RVU because, for example, they do not account for the skill and experience level of the human resources being used. Treatment units represent a given amount of patient/client treatment and are frequently based on therapist time, e.g., fifteen minutes of treatment). Visits usually refer to the number of treatment sessions. Because the definition of these terms may vary from setting to setting, it is important for managers to clarify them in the local context.

Whatever unit of measure is used, it should be meaningful to both staff and administration. Measures of staff's use of time are the basis for determining the need for more staff, different staff composition, and staff reduction.

Once the methods for quantifying work have been identified, productivity standards can be developed. These standards may reflect several parameters of productivity, including the number of patients/clients, RVU, treatment units, and visits per day.

Developing Staffing Plans

To develop staffing plans, managers relate their expectations about productivity to the therapy needs of the patient/client population to be served. Often clinical judgment is required to predict the therapy needs of a given population. Managers must also be sensitive to organizational goals to realistically assess the extent of services to be provided within a given setting. Factors to consider include the ratio of staff to patients/clients and the amount of time needed for indirect patient/client care (such as billing, documentation, and transport). The consistency of demand may also affect productivity. Staff input, time studies, AOTA guidelines, and information gained from continuing education and peer professionals can all be used to assist in the determination of staff needs.

An example may help the reader understand how a manager can weave various factors together into a staffing plan. A manager is responsible for determining occupational therapy staffing needs for a ten-bed inpatient rehabilitation unit that is being planned. The manager has a fairly good understanding of the diagnoses to be admitted. Based on information obtained from a variety of clinical sources, he or she estimates that each patient/client will require a minimum of one hour of individual treatment and one hour of group treatment daily. Maximum group size will be five patients. This unit is expected to be fully occupied throughout the year. In general, the staff can be expected to engage in direct treatment six out of eight hours daily, allowing two hours for indirect service. The following computations would be done to calculate the total number of hours per day that therapists would spend in direct treatment:

Number of individual treatment hours required per day	
10 patients/clients × 1 individual treatment/day = 10 individual hours	
Therapist direct time	10 hours
Number of group treatment hours required per day	
10 patients/clients × 1 group treatment/day = 10 group hours	
Group = 5 patients/clients, lasts 1 hour	
Therapist direct time	2 hours
Total therapist hours required/day	12 hours

Before converting these figures to FTE requirements, it is necessary to identify the average number of days per years that an individual staff member actually works. As noted earlier, there are 260 possible working days a year, assuming a forty-hour work week. This does not reflect the actual days of work per employee, because vacations, holidays, and sick days have not been deducted. Adjustments should be made based on actual experience or estimates that reflect an organization's leave policies. For the example, each staff person is assumed to be absent from work for 33 days (10 holidays, 15 vacation days, 6 sick days, 2 days educational leave).

$$\begin{array}{l} 260 \text{ possible work days/year} \\ -33 \text{ days leave} \\ \hline 227 \text{ productive days/year} \end{array}$$

It has already been determined that the staff have only six hours a day for direct service. The estimated number of hours per year would be as follows:

$$227 \text{ productive days} \times 6 \text{ hours direct care/day} = 1{,}362 \text{ direct hours/year}$$

The earlier computations indicated that twelve hours of direct patient contact would be required for each working day of the year:

$$260 \text{ working days} \times 12 \text{ hours direct care/day} = 3{,}120 \text{ direct hours required/year}$$

The manager now has sufficient data to project staffing needs. By dividing the projected demand (3,120 direct hours) by the actual productivity per FTE (1,362 direct hours), he or she can determine how many staff are needed:

$$\frac{3{,}120 \text{ direct hours}}{1{,}362 \text{ direct hours}} = 2.3 \text{ FTE}$$

A conservative manager would probably recommend two FTEs initially, with contingency plans for allocation of additional part-time staff to the new unit.

If the manager chose to use fifteen minutes of patient/client treatment as the measure of productivity, he or she could set a productivity standard for these employees by converting planning assumptions to treatment units. Assuming that each therapist saw five patients/clients a day individually for an hour, and led one group of five patients, the treatment units (TU) would be calculated as follows:

$1 \text{ hour} = 4 \text{ TU}$
$5 \text{ individual treatments} \times 4 = 20 \text{ individual TU}$
$1 \text{ group} = 5 \text{ patients/clients} \times 1 \text{ hour/ea} \times 4 \text{ TU/hour} = 20 \text{ group TU}$

$$\begin{array}{l} 20 \text{ individual TU} \\ +20 \text{ group TU} \\ \hline 40 \text{ TUs per therapist per day} \end{array}$$

Personnel assigned to this program would then have an understanding of the average volume of patient/client treatment that was expected.

QUALITATIVE ASPECTS OF STAFFING

The kind of personnel hired (occupational therapists, occupational therapy assistants, etc.) and the way in which they are allocated to patient/client programs are referred to as a staffing pattern. A staffing pattern should reflect the amount and the kind of staff necessary to provide acceptable care in the most cost-efficient way. A manager must be familiar with the abilities and limitations of the various levels of occupational therapy personnel. The AOTA has resource information that addresses this subject (3). The information can assist in determining reasonable expectations of entry-level staff as well as of more experienced practitioners.

A manager should also know how to use support personnel in some aspects of department or program functioning. Effectively used clerical staff and aides free treatment staff for patient/client care.

Another consideration is the capabilities of individuals. Some therapists are more effective in developing new programs; others function better in already established programs. Some assistants enjoy working with several therapists; others prefer being teamed with one individual. Successful staffing patterns capitalize on these variances and place individuals in organizational niches where they are most likely to succeed.

JOB DESCRIPTIONS: FORMULAS FOR PERFORMANCE

Developing Personnel Job Descriptions

The job description is a basic tool of management. It is used in employee recruitment, selection, evaluation, and development. It forces the identification of critical aspects of work that are necessary to meet departmental or program demands and patients'/clients' needs. It should reflect organizational expectations and parameters.

In most employment situations job descriptions are developed and modified in conjunction with personnel departments and should be based on a systematic job analysis. There are several approaches to job analysis, many of which were developed in industry (4).

Critical components of job descriptions include a statement of the job's purpose or a summary of the job, a list of the job's duties, an explanation of supervisory relationships, and a delineation of job specifications. The latter indicate education, training, experience, skills, and other special characteristics that are required of individuals filling the position. The occupational therapy manager is usually expected to develop and regularly review the list of a job's duties and the delineation of job specifications. The AOTA has published several documents that can assist in the development of job descriptions: "Entry-level Role Delineation for OTRs and COTAs" (3), "Guide for Supervision of Occupational Therapy Personnel" (5), and "Classification Standards for Occupational Therapy Personnel" (6). Sample job descriptions from the latter document appear in Appendix B.

Developing Functional Job Descriptions

Job descriptions are usually developed to reflect the job roles of a particular group of employees who are doing similar jobs. In most departments or programs there is unlikely to be a job description specifically designed for each employee. At times a more specific description or delineation of duties is desirable—for example, when a manager wishes to delegate a specific function such as student fieldwork coordination to individual staff members. Because these duties may rotate among several people, a personnel job description may not be appropriate, so a functional job description may be developed. Functional job descriptions describe in detail the specific duties associated with a particular delegated responsibility. Also, in organizations in which personnel job descriptions are rather general, functional job descriptions serve to elaborate on them. Functional job descriptions are kept among department or program records and used in conjunction with relevant job descriptions approved by the personnel department.

Writing Performance Standards

Related to job descriptions are performance standards. Performance standards delineate criteria that describe specific expectations related to the performance of job duties. These standards are useful for orienting new employees and form the basis for performance appraisal. Figure 2 is an example of how a performance standard might be written.

RECRUITMENT

The recruitment of occupational therapy personnel is a challenging process in the current climate of shortages. Even with the cost containment strategies being implemented by government and third-party payers, the demand for occupational therapy personnel remains high. Managers must develop strategies to predict turnover and identify potential replacements, often in advance of the actual vacancy. This section addresses approaches to forecasting vacancies and recruiting new staff.

Forecasting Vacancies

Forecasting vacancies requires the ability to identify the variables associated with staff turnover in the department or the program. An understanding of individual staff members' personal and professional goals is helpful. The development of a high level of trust between manager and

FIGURE 12–2
Sample Performance Standard

Responsibility: Responds to referrals for occupational therapy services.
Performance Standard: Performance is satisfactory when therapist consistently does the following:

1. Checks board daily for new referrals
2. Responds to referrals by reviewing medical chart
3. Initiates patient/client assessment within eight working hours
4. Documents initial contact in medical record within same working day
5. Schedules patient/client for routine services within eight working hours of initial contact.

staff facilitates open communications and aids in forecasting. In such an environment staff members may share intentions far enough in advance for the manager to plan for turnover. Staff members who fear negative responses will not change their plans; they will just give less warning. A review of the turnover history of the department or the program, coupled with information obtained from exit interviews, may also increase the accuracy of predictions. Review of existing staff characteristics can assist. For instance, the potential for turnover is highest among employees who have the least longevity (4). In a particular department or program, staff from the local region may tend to stay longer.

All of these approaches help forecast staff turnover. More effective planning for recruitment can occur when a manager can accurately predict vacancies and combine those predictions with knowledge of positions to be added or eliminated.

Recruiting New Staff

Recruitment involves the use of a variety of communication strategies to attract qualified applicants. The AOTA permits paid advertisements in *The American Journal of Occupational Therapy* and *Occupational Therapy News*. Both have early deadlines for acceptance of advertisements (thirty to forty-five days before their issue date); however, they reach a national audience. State and local occupational therapy associations generally accept advertisements and often have job listing services available through placement chairpersons. Classified advertisements in local and regional daily newspapers are being successfully used, particularly in metropolitan areas. Job openings can be posted at conferences and workshops and on bulletin boards in college and university occupational therapy departments. Directors of some occupational therapy curricula will provide a list of recent graduates, which may be used to mail recruitment information.

The selection of one or more of these approaches depends on an assessment of which approaches are most likely to attract qualified candidates who could become effective and stable employees. It is sometimes necessary to experiment to identify consistently successful strategies.

A variety of indirect approaches can be equally effective. Current employees can be encouraged to informally recruit occupational therapy personnel with whom they socialize or have shared educational experiences. Networks can be developed through active participation in professional groups such as local, state, and national associations. These networks can be used for identifying and referring candidates among managers. Professional publications and presentations by staff indirectly advertise the department or the program as a good place for professional growth, thus attracting candidates. The development of student clinical fieldwork experiences often provides an introduction to promising new graduates and may attract candidates interested in an opportunity to supervise students. Finally, the development of reentry opportunities can assist in identifying occupational therapy personnel who may have stopped working for a time and want to reenter the work force gradually. Often volunteer experiences, part-time positions, and temporary-coverage jobs are attractive to this group and may pay off in a full-time candidate at a future date.

SELECTION

The recruitment and selection process should be tailored to identify candidates who will perform well and stay for a desirable length of time. These considerations can be addressed by the development of selection criteria. Selection criteria should reflect characteristics important to successful job performance. The characteristics of current successful employees can be reviewed to determine those apparently related to their success—for example, place of education, interpersonal style, and personal and professional goals. Personal preferences—about the size and nature of the patient/client population, the size of the department, the general work pace, etc.—may have a bearing on job success. Longevity of employment may be linked to the geographic origin of the employees or their history of job tenure. With a sufficient number of employees the prediction value of some characteristics can be statistically determined. Personnel departments can assist in this process, or the reader may refer to personnel literature for methodologies (4). Even without statistical treatment these variables can add an important dimension to the considerations already formulated in the job specifications.

Once criteria are determined, the actual process of staff selection can begin. In organizations with personnel departments the manager and the personnel department will collaborate in staff selection, with the personnel department providing support services. It is desirable to predetermine the division of duties, thus avoiding confusion. The selection process usually involves six stages: screening, ranking, interviewing, checking references, making the final selection, and making a job offer.

Stage 1: Screening

Applicants usually have provided resumés and may have completed application forms provided by the personnel department. Using this written information, the manager should screen applicants against the job specifications. Applicants who lack the necessary qualifications should be informed that they cannot be considered. If it is likely that they may qualify for some future position, their applications can be kept on file. This approach allows for the development of a bank of potential candidates and should be considered for use with any unselected but possibly desirable candidates.

Stage 2: Ranking

Qualified candidates should be ranked according to how well they meet the predetermined criteria. At this stage, and throughout the rest of the selection process, the manager must be sensitive to local, state, and federal employment regulations (see Appendix C for a summary of the latter). The most desirable candidates should then be contacted for an interview. The other candidates are kept on hold, pending the results of interviews.

Stage 3: Interviewing

The interview is a critical stage in the selection process. Not only do managers gain impressions of candidates, but candidates form opinions of both the job and the manager. It is important that the interview be organized to maximize the exchange of information. The candidate should be informed in advance about the interview process, including how long it will take and who will be involved. Adequate time should be allowed for the candidate to tour the facility, obtain an overview of department or program functioning, and be informed of the general conditions of employment.

The interview itself is most effective when the manager structures it, using the predetermined criteria to obtain specific information and impressions from all candidates. One or more people may be involved in the interviews, depending on both the setting and the manager's leadership style. All who are involved should document their impressions on feedback forms that reflect the major selection concerns (see Appendix D for an example). This is best done very soon after the interview to minimize the effects of selective memory and the influence of others. This form can also be used to note (a) specific areas to be explored further during reference checks and (b) preliminary impressions as to whether the candidate should be considered further.

As a result of the interviews, the manager may choose to keep all candidates active, pending reference checks, or may eliminate some candidates. All candidates who are interviewed should be told when a decision is to be made and how they will be notified.

Stage 4: Checking References

At the time of application or during the interview process the candidate should be asked to provide the names of references. These should include individuals who are likely to know information that can help determine the potential success of the applicant in the job. Personnel departments frequently have standard forms that they mail to references. Telephone references may also be taken, with the results documented by the caller or confirmed with a written reference. Telephone references have the advantage of providing timely and sometimes more relevant information.

The manager needs to be sure that any concerns that should be explored have been identified, and that any routine questions related to the selection criteria have been asked. Either the manager or the personnel department should contact the references, depending on the setting. Professional registration and licensure may also be verified at this time.

Stage 5: Making the Final Selection

The final selection of the successful candidate can be the most difficult part of the process. The manager must review carefully all the objective information available, but also be sensitive to subjective reactions to the various candidates. The rankings of candidates should be reexamined, and the acceptable candidates should be listed in order of priority. Candidates who are not ranked first should not be notified until a job offer has been successfully negotiated with the desired candidate.

Stage 6: Making the Job Offer

The final stage of staff selection is the job offer. The desired candidate is usually contacted by telephone and notified of his or her selection. The starting date is identified, and, if necessary, the salary is negotiated. In negotiating salary, the manager must know in advance what is an acceptable range of possibilities. It is advisable to maintain salary equity among employees with similar experience, skills, and responsibilities. Salaries need not be exactly the same, but consideration must be given to existing personnel.

Once the job offer has been made and accepted, a letter of confirmation should be sent. Only after this stage should the remaining candidates be notified, with an indication as to whether they might be considered for additional openings in the future.

ORIENTATION

Any new employee feels insecure during the first days and weeks on a job. This feeling can be minimized by an effective orientation program. Although some aspects of orientation may be handled by the personnel department, much of the specific information of how to perform the new job effectively will need to be provided by the manager or the supervisor. A plan for communicating this information should be developed in advance, and modified in process to suit the learning style of the particular employee. A checklist, handouts, and a manual of information help to ensure that all new employees receive the necessary information about their jobs. Introduction to key coworkers and the identification of one primary resource person facilitate the development of positive peer relations. A tour of the facility and time to learn the location of relevant tools and materials assist the new staff member in beginning to feel at home in the new work site. Chances to observe, assist, and practice are helpful in developing and reinforcing job skills. Regular opportunities to discuss progress and ask questions create a safe environment in which to learn. Every effort should be made to identify organizational and departmental or program values and practices so as to ensure that the employee knows how to succeed (7).

PERFORMANCE EVALUATION

The evaluation of staff performance is probably the most threatening of the various supervisory duties, particularly when the need to give negative feedback arises. Consequently the temptation is to procrastinate or to provide only positive and neutral feedback. Inexperienced supervisors are surprised to learn that employees frequently appreciate tactfully delivered negative feedback, when it is relevant to the job and accompanied by suggestions as to how the employee might alter his or her behavior to be more effective.

Establishing Performance Expectations

The key to effective performance evaluation is the development and articulation of clear performance expectations. If an employee understands how to do a job correctly and receives regular praise and guidance, the performance appraisal itself becomes merely a summary of this information and an opportunity to discuss options for continued growth.

Documenting Performance

Just as in patient/client care, good documentation of employee performance is necessary. Lack of documentation or inadequate documentation can severely hamper the manager's ability to deal effectively with the problem employee. Documentation of positive performance is often necessary to substantiate recommendations for merit increases in salary. Most personnel departments require one or more performance appraisals during the probationary period of employment, with regular evaluations at least annually thereafter. Frequently, standard forms must be completed for the employee's personnel file (see Appendix E for example). A manager may want to develop supplementary forms or procedures that are directed more specifically at the performance standards associated with the job. The performance appraisal should clearly document the employee's strengths and the areas needing improvement. The employee should have a clear picture of how satisfactory his or her current performance is relative to the performance standards and be given examples of when these standards were exceeded or not satisfactorily met.

Discussing the Appraisal

Once the written appraisal is developed, the manager should schedule a meeting with the employee to discuss it. A private and quiet place should be used, with sufficient time allotted to discuss the evaluation and allow the employee to provide feedback on his or her reaction to it. To facilitate interaction, employees may be asked to prepare self-evaluations or to identify performance objectives. Also, employees can prepare feedback for the supervisor on their perceptions of his or her role as a supervisor. This reinforces the importance of two-way communication.

The manager should convey information in a relaxed and matter-of-fact manner, focusing on the documented performance. When sensitive or negative feedback must be provided, it is important to remind the employee that this information is based on observable work-related behavior and is not a reflection of perceived capability. Plans should be made to assist the employee in performing more effectively, and they should be documented as a part of the appraisal. With employees whose work is satisfactory or better, the development of plans or objectives for continued growth and accomplishment is an effective approach to maintaining motivation. In either situation subsequent appraisals should include assessment of whether the objectives were attained. A combination of both approaches can be used with most employees, thus creating a climate of channeled job growth for all staff (7).

DISCIPLINARY ACTION

Special evaluations are required when an employee is demonstrating severe performance problems. For unionized employees the special evaluation procedures and related employee grievance procedures are spelled out in a contract. Even in nonunion situations good personnel practice dictates that clear information be provided to let the employee know that his or her performance is unacceptable. This usually takes the form of written disciplinary actions or warning notices. Information provided to the employee should also refer to the organization's grievance procedures, which delineate the process the employee may use for administrative review of discipline. The importance of clear policies and effective orientation of employees to these policies becomes evident during difficult situations.

In considering disciplinary action, the "red-hot stove" rule can be a useful guide. This rule states that good discipline should be like touching a red-hot stove (8):

1. There is a *warning:* Anyone can see that the stove is red.
2. The consequences are *immediate:* As soon as a person touches the stove, he or she gets burned.
3. The consequences are *impersonal:* Anyone who touches the stove gets burned.
4. The consequences are *consistent:* Touching the stove always results in a burn.

After a series of written notices, accompanied by related counseling sessions, employees may need to be terminated from employment. Although this is not a comfortable situation for either the employee or the manager, it cannot be avoided in the face of inadequate performance. Avoidance of the issue inevitably affects the performance of other employees and creates morale problems. Therefore, effective managers make employee performance problems a priority and deal with them until the employee either sustains a satisfactory performance, resigns, or is terminated.

REWARD SYSTEMS

Rewarding the successful employee is a much more pleasant part of the supervisory process. The obvious rewards for good performance are salary adjustments, such as merit increases. An astute manager soon becomes aware that although money is a nice reward, it is not sufficient to sustain employee motivation. Verbal and written praise and recognition, paid attendance at continuing education seminars, increased responsibility for program development, student supervision, and flexible working hours can all be perceived as rewards. Opportunities for promotion can be powerful motivators.

Each employee has his or her own perception of what is important, and these can change in the course of personal and professional development. Employees also form perceptions of the likelihood of being rewarded in a meaningful way. To use rewards successfully, the manager must identify what is meaningful to the employee, find an organizational context that allows the expression of the meaningful reward, and then relate the reward to good performance (9). The manager must also communicate accurately the range of rewards that are available in a given situation so employees can set realistic expectations. Careful monitoring of staff reward systems and expectations pays off in dedicated and productive personnel.

STAFF DEVELOPMENT

Orientation, performance evaluation, and reward systems are all tools critical to the basic development of staff. In addition, continual upgrading of knowledge and skills is required to support occupational therapy services in the changing health care environment. This is a professional responsibility of individuals and an organizational responsibility of managers.

To upgrade staff performance effectively, areas of concern must first be targeted. Quality assurance activities may identify areas needing improvement. Organizational strategic plans may reveal new areas of service provision for which staff need preparation. Individual staff members can identify areas in which improved competence would enhance patient/client care. Managers who use systematic methods, such as needs assessments (10), are in the best position to justify costly expenditures of time and money.

In many cases educational strategies can be effective methods to enhance existing skills and develop new ones. Most large occupational therapy organizations have regularly scheduled inservice education sessions. Opportunities to attend seminars, professional meetings, and college courses are available to staff in many departments and programs. Follow-up on the outcomes of educational efforts relative to predetermined objectives supports the use of new skills and serves to evaluate the effectiveness of a particular educational intervention.

SUMMARY

A manager serves as the interface between an organization's resources, values, and goals, and the skills, values, and goals of its employees. In personnel management this requires that the manager employ his or her knowledge of the organization in the recruitment, selection, and development of staff. It also calls for the manager to channel individual employees' aspirations and abilities into attainment of the organization's goals.

A fundamental component of personnel management is the ability to quantify and project staffing needs. This involves understanding the concept of full-time equivalents and using it to develop productivity standards and staffing plans. On the qualitative side a manager must be familiar with the abilities and limitations of the various levels of occupational therapy personnel and other types of personnel.

A basic tool of personnel management is the job description. A personnel job description includes a summary of the job or a statement of its purpose, a list of the duties, an explanation of supervisory relationships, and a delineation of job specifications. Job descriptions reflect the roles of a particular group of employees doing similar work. A functional job description may be used to describe in detail certain responsibilities of a particular job.

Performance standards describe specific expectations related to the performance of duties. They are used to orient new employees and to appraise performance.

Staff recruitment involves forecasting vacancies as well as attracting qualified applicants to vacant positions. Forecasting is aided by openness and trust between manager and staff. A variety of strategies for recruiting are possible. Some are direct, such as placing advertisements in professional periodicals and posting job openings. Others are indirect, such as encouraging employees to recruit informally through their social contacts.

The selection process should be tailored to identify candidates who will perform well and stay on the job. This can be aided by the development of selection criteria. The process itself involves six stages: screening, ranking, interviewing, checking references, making the final selection, and making the job offer.

A plan for orienting a new employee should be developed in advance of his or her arrival on the job and should then be modified to suit the employee's learning style. Regular opportunities to discuss progress and ask questions create a safe environment in which to learn.

The key to effective performance evaluation is the development and articulation of clear performance expectations. Good documentation of performance is necessary, both to deal with problem employees and to substantiate recommendations for merit increases. Once an appraisal is written, the manager should discuss it with the employee, allowing sufficient time for feedback. With employees having severe performance problems, special evaluations are needed, such as written disciplinary actions or warning notices. Effective managers make these employees a priority and deal with them until they either sustain a satisfactory performance, resign, or are terminated.

Rewarding the successful employee is also important. An astute manager soon becomes aware that although money is a nice reward, it is not sufficient to sustain employee motivation.

Continual upgrading of staff's knowledge and skills is required to support occupational therapy services in the changing health care environment. Areas of concern must first be targeted. In many cases educational strategies such as inservice education sessions, seminars, professional meetings, and college courses can effectively address these concerns.

References

1. Kotter JP, Schlesinger LA, Sathe V: *Organization: Text, Cases, and Readings on the Management of Organizational Design and Change*. Homewood, IL: Richard D Irwin Inc, 1979, p 1
2. American Occupational Therapy Association: Uniform terminology for reporting occupational therapy services and occupational therapy product output reporting system. In *Reference Manual of the Official Documents of the American Occupational Therapy Association*. Rockville, MD: American Occupational Therapy Assocation, 1983
3. American Occupational Therapy Association: Entry-level role delineation for OTRs and COTAs. In *Reference Manual of the Official Documents of the American Occupational Therapy Association*. Rockville, MD: American Occupational Therapy Association, 1983
4. Heneman HG, Schwab DP, Fossum JA, et al: *Personnel/Human Resource Management*. Homewood, IL: Richard D Irwin Inc, 1980, pp 85–109, 166, 237–263
5. American Occupational Therapy Association: Guide for supervision of occupational therapy personnel. In *Reference Manual of the Official Documents of the American Occupational Therapy Association*. Rockville, MD: American Occupational Therapy Association, 1983
6. American Occupational Therapy Association:

Classification Standards for Occupational Therapy Personnel. Rockville, MD: American Occupational Therapy Association, 1985

7. Metzger N: *The Health Care Supervisor's Handbook.* Rockville, MD: Aspen Systems Corp, 1978, pp 33–43, 45–54
8. Strauss G, Sayles RL: *Personnel: The Human Problems of Management*, 3rd edition. Englewood Cliffs, NJ: Prentice-Hall Inc, 1972, p 268
9. Vroom VH: *Work and Motivation*. New York: John Wiley & Sons Inc, 1964
10. Bullard M: A needs assessment strategy for educational planning. *Am J Occup Ther* 37:624–629, 1983

Section VI

Evaluating

Section VI treats the important managerial function of evaluating, that is, determining the extent to which programs are achieving the goals and the objectives established for them and using that information as necessary to modify activities. Two chapters constitute the section, "Program Evaluation" and "Quality Assurance." The first of these, Chapter 13, describes the sixteen elements of an outcome model of program evaluation. Figures are included to show the interrelationships of these elements and to display sample forms for collecting data and reporting outcomes. The chapter also discusses the many uses of a program evaluation system and the data it generates, from enhancing relationships between an organization's administration and governing board to improving benefits for patients/clients.

In Chapter 14, the historical roots of quality assurance are summarized, and the concept is explained in terms of its five basic elements: identification of a problem, verification of the problem, formulation of a plan to correct the problem, implementation of the plan, and measurement to determine if the problem was corrected. Thirteen methods of implementing the concept are briefly described. An example of a quality assurance study on prescribing and obtaining Medicaid reimbursement for wheelchairs is also presented, to help managers understand how quality assurance programs not only pinpoint problems but remedy them.

Chapter 13

Program Evaluation

Kenneth J. Shaw, CWA, CUE

It has become increasingly apparent in human services that a mechanism is needed for evaluating the outcomes of the services being provided to individuals. In part, the need results from the attitude that there are limits to almost everything, including funds for purchasing human services. This attitude has produced what some call the age of accountability. For most human service organizations the most likely form of accountability is program evaluation.

Program evaluation is an outcome-monitoring system that describes the impact of programs and services on individual patients/clients by defining the desired results of service delivery and comparing them with actual outcomes. Data on outcomes are always related to a change in patient/client status (1). They can be expressed as the percent of patients/clients who have reached a predetermined goal or goals, shown a reduction in particular problems, or experienced a change in circumstances as a consequence of service.

The primary assumption underlying the development and dissemi-

Kenneth J. Shaw conducts training in program evaluation for Goodwill Industries of America. He has published a how-to manual on the subject and developed a computerized model for implementing program evaluation.

[1]The section of this chapter titled Outcome Model of Program Evaluation is adapted from R. A. Haller and K. J. Shaw, *Program Evaluation Manual*. Bethesda, MD: Goodwill Industries of America Inc, 1984.

nation of a program evaluation system is that, with appropriate use in an organization, individuals will obtain more effective benefits, the cost of services can be reduced or at least controlled, and the organization will be able to generate community support on the basis of the quality of results obtained (2).

Program evaluation is described by the United Way of America as "the process of delineating, obtaining, analyzing and providing relevant information for better decisions by policy-makers and service providers (3, p 1). The Commission on Accreditation of Rehabilitation Facilities defines program evaluation as "a systematic procedure for determining the effectiveness and efficiency with which results are achieved by clients following rehabilitation services. These results are collected on a regular or continuous basis rather than a periodic sampling (2, p iii). When these definitions are understood and accepted, the arguments for application are overwhelming. Program evaluation encourages a systematic assessment of organizational and program performance to meet the challenges of public accountability and improved community services.

In more practical terms, program evaluation is an effective tool for decision makers. A properly designed system generates objective information about current activities or performance that should enhance the quality of future decisions. Program evaluation, then, represents a process for identifying (a) what services are provided, (b) who is served, (c) what the services are intended to achieve, (d) the effectiveness and efficiency of the services, and (e) changes needed to improve performance (4).

Managers and administrators find program evaluation an essential tool for—

1. Improving the quality and the responsiveness of organizational planning and decision making.
2. Increasing the rationality of decision making in the allocation of resources.
3. Strengthening an organization's ability to present an effective year-round case for continued public support.
4. Stimulating the development of clear policies and practices for improving productivity, efficiency, and effectiveness.
5. Justifying to contributors, in concrete terms, the outcomes of programs and services.

OUTCOME MODEL OF PROGRAM EVALUATION

This chapter focuses on the outcome model of program evaluation (as opposed to the process model). Four basic criteria must be followed to maintain consistency across an organization's programs and ensure the programs' integrity to the evaluation system:

1. Program evaluation measures what happens to all people whom a program serves. The system that is developed must therefore track both successful and unsuccessful patients/clients.
2. The outcome model of program evaluation measures outcomes following the discontinuation of treatment. Therefore, the system that is

developed must measure what happens after a patient/client has completed a program.

3. Reports on results are produced continually. Therefore, consistent and regular measures must be taken and reported.

4. Reports tell an organization whether its performance is acceptable according to standards that it has set. The organization must therefore have predetermined standards for outcomes, with which actual results can be compared.

An outcome-oriented program evaluation system should consist of the 16 elements listed below. In the following pages each element is explained briefly.

1. Program structure
2. Influencers
3. Purpose statement
4. Admission criteria
5. Program goals
6. Services provided
7. Patients/clients served
8. Patient/client descriptors
9. Objectives
10. Relative importance
11. Measures
12. Who is measured
13. Time of application of measures
14. Expectancies
15. Management reports
16. System review mechanism.

Program structure. Program structure differs from the administrative structure of an organization in that the administrative structure can usually be displayed as an organization chart. Program structure, in contrast, arranges the organization into distinct service elements for the purpose of evaluation. This structure helps the organization determine the degree to which it is accomplishing the goals it has set for patients/clients.

It is easiest and most useful to layout the structure and the organization of the program evaluation system in a flowchart such as appears in Figure 1. The major structural elements on this form include influencers, purpose statement, admission criteria, program goals, services provided, and patients/clients served.

Influencers. These are groups or individuals that affect the development and continuation of specific programs within the organization. Influencers that have a direct impact on the organization should be identified—for example, consumer groups, funding sources, regulatory authorities, and public officials.

Purpose statement. The purpose statement of an organization is a capsule declaration of the organization's mission, the services it provides, and the population(s) it serves. The statement needs to be sufficiently broad to cover all of the programs included in the program evaluation system, yet specific enough so that the organization cannot be confused with other service providers in the community. The statement should—

1. Specify who is served.
2. Describe the services provided.
3. State the expected outcomes.
4. Distinguish the organization from other agencies.
5. Enable the setting of goals and objectives.
6. Identify the geographic area of service.

FIGURE 13–1
Sample Program Structure Chart

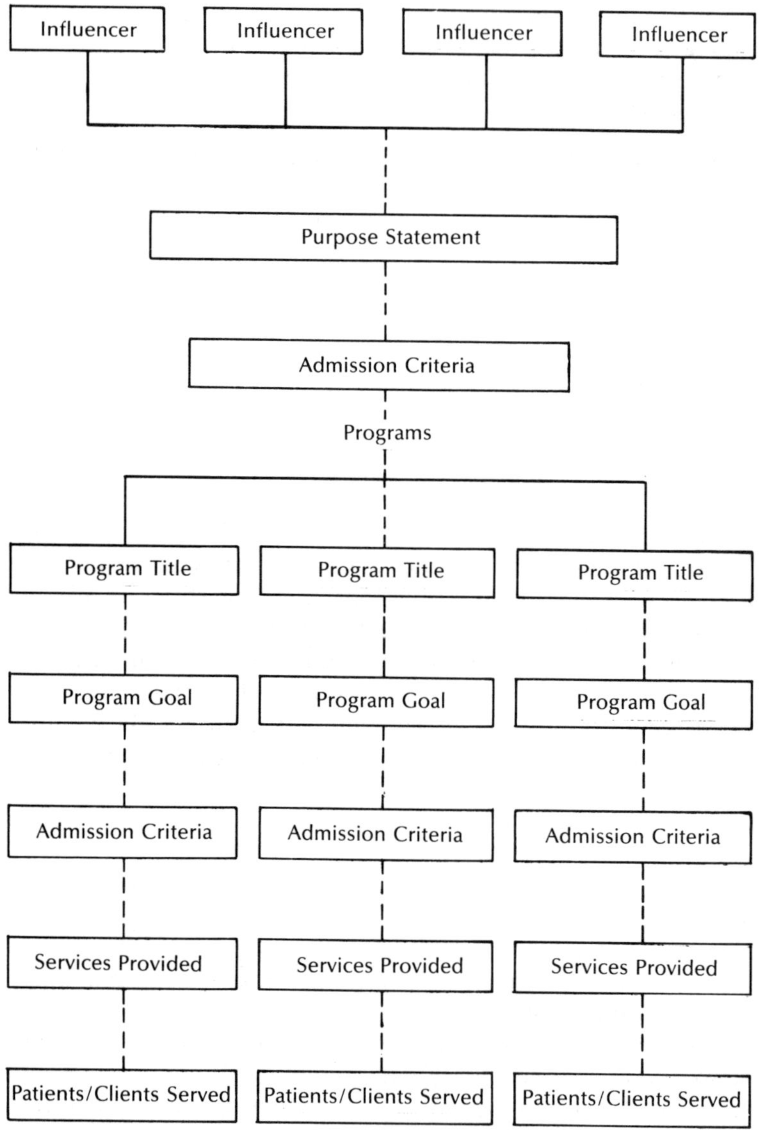

Note: Adapted from RA Haller, KJ Shaw, *Program Evaluation Manual*, Bethesda, MD, Goodwill Industries of America Inc, 1984, p 10.

Admission criteria. An organization must identify the capabilities and characteristics that a person must possess to be admitted to its programs. These criteria should assist in determining if the organization is serving the people for whom its programs are intended.

If more than one program is offered, two sets of admission criteria should be established: one set for admission to the general facility, requirements that must be met by everyone who is accepted into any of an organization's programs; and a second set, or series of sets, for acceptance into specific programs.

Program goals. Program goals, expressed in a statement, clearly articulate the components and characteristics of each program to individuals in and outside an organization. If an organization has no plans beyond what it is already doing, and has only one program, the purpose and goal statements are identical. Most organizations have more than one goal, however, and should prepare statements for each program that articulate more specifically who is served by it, what services are offered, and what it is designed to accomplish. If more than one goal statement is needed, then the achievement of all goals should lead to the accomplishment of the overall purpose. Goal statements should be specific enough that program objectives and measures can be derived from them. Also, it should be possible to logically assume from the wording of the statements that the services provided will accomplish the goals.

Services provided. The services provided are the activities available to each person admitted to a program. The identification of a service requires that an outline of the process used in delivering the service be completed, that specific staff be assigned to carry out the process, and that the service be related to the achievement of the goal. It is not necessary for all patients/clients to receive all services. There should, however, be a logical relationship between the patients/clients, the services, and the program goal, and the services should be appropriate to the accomplishment of the goal.

Patients/clients served. The types of patients/clients for whom an organization provides services should be listed in terms of disabilities and demographic characteristics. The list should be developed to link directly with the goals and services identified in the previous elements. Examples of patients/clients served are, by type of disability, the orthopedically disabled, the spinal cord injured, the neurologically disabled, and the developmentally disabled; and, by demographic variables, males, Hispanics, welfare recipients, and high school dropouts.

Patient/client descriptors. Patient/client descriptors define the populations being served in terms of the severity of problems or the barriers to success. The descriptors are monitored regularly in management reports to indicate changes in patient/client populations that may affect results. These data are important because knowledge of who is served is essential in assessing an organization's and a program's performance. Figure 2 gives examples of some types of descriptors that might be used.

Objectives. Objectives are the critical elements in a program evaluation system. They are expressed as specific statements of the results a program aims to achieve. The objectives for each program should be consistent with its goal. If all the objectives are achieved, then the program should have accomplished the goal.

Objectives are the statements from which measures are derived and therefore must be cast in terms of the outcomes for patients/clients in each program. They must reflect both effectiveness and efficiency. Effectiveness is how successful a patient/client has been in achieving the

FIGURE 13–2
Sample Patient/Client Descriptors

Sex
1. Male ____
2. Female ____

Age
3. Under 21 ____
4. Over 55 ____

National Origin
5. White ____
6. Black ____
7. Hispanic ____
8. American Indian ____
9. Asian ____

Severely Disabled
10. Severely disabled ____

Disability
11. Multiply disabled ____
12. Emotionally disabled ____
13. Mentally disabled ____
14. Visually disabled ____
15. Hearing disability ____
16. Orthopedic disability ____
17. Circulatory disability ____
18. Neurological disability ____

Form of Support
19. Own earning ____
20. Public assistance ____
21. Disability payment ____
22. Family ____

Education Level
23. Less than high school ____
24. High school diploma ____
25. GED ____
26. Post high school ____

Work History
27. No previous employment ____
28. Unemployed 50% or more of last 12 months ____

Referral Source
29. State VR ____
30. Blind agency ____
31. Schools ____
32. Job training programs ____
33. Worker's Comp ____
34. Title XX ____
35. Veterans Administration ____
36. Developmental disabilities ____

Mental Health Services
37. Prior institutionalization ____
38. Receiving mental health services ____
39. History of substance abuse ____
40. Public offender ____

Marital Status
41. Single ____
42. Married ____
43. Separated ____
44. Divorced ____

Transportation
45. Own auto ____
46. Public transportation ____

Living Arrangements
47. Independent ____
48. Dependent ____
49. Institution ____

Rehabilitation History
50. Previous rehabilitation services ____

Note: Adapted from KJ Shaw, *Program Evaluation Guidelines*, Bethesda, MD, Goodwill Industries of America Inc, 1982.

benefits of a program. Efficiency is how successful a program is in minimizing cost and time. Every program must have at least one effectiveness and one efficiency statement.

System developers must be able to discriminate among three types of objectives:

1. *Outcome objectives*, which are required in a system and specify the status of an individual after the provision of services. They should reflect a program's benefits for patients/clients.

2. *Process objectives*, which may be needed as internal monitors of an individual's progress through an extended program. Generally, process objectives are intermediate steps toward the achievement of outcome objectives.

3. *Management objectives*, which reflect the activities that management

FIGURE 13–3
Sample Objectives Chart

____

Program

Rank	Objectives	Measures	Time of Measure	Data Source	Expectancy
1.					
2.					
3.					
4.					
5.					

Note: From KJ Shaw, *Program Evaluation Guidelines*, Bethesda, MD, Goodwill Industries of America Inc, 1984.

intends to undertake for the good of the organization. They generally relate to establishing new services or programs, expanding existing programs, or making the best use of resources.

Five basic principles apply in writing objectives:

1. Objectives should be measurable.
2. Objectives should be achievable.
3. If all the objectives are accomplished, the goal should be achieved.
4. The close relationship between goals, objectives, and measures should be kept in mind.
5. Objectives should be ranked in order of importance, with the most important objective listed first.

Figure 3 is a sample objectives chart for use in relating the following data elements: the relative importance (rank) of an objective; the objective; the measure of the objective, including who is measured; the time of application of the measure; the data source; and the expectancy.

Relative importance. As noted earlier, the objectives within each program should be ranked in order of importance. This enables a management reviewer of a program's outcome to determine the level of importance of the various objectives that are achieved. An organization can thus tell how well it is doing in relation to the program priorities it has established.

Measures. Measures indicate how an organization will determine if an objective has been achieved. They should be reliable (that is, they should yield the same results regardless of who is doing the measuring or when it is being done) and they should be applied after the provision of services. Measures are generally stated in terms of numbers, averages, percentages, time, or money. There should be no gray areas in the establishment of measures; an individual should either meet the criteria or not.

Who is measured. This is a statement indicating the groups of patients/clients whose results are being calculated for a specific measure—for example, "Those who complete the service" or "Those not achieving Objective #2."

Time of application of measures. The time of application of measures is the point when the outcome information is collected. It should be related to a program and a specific objective. Some measures are taken as patients/clients leave the program whereas others are applied an extended period after completion. The latter must occur within a reasonable amount of time, however, to ensure that the outcome being measured is a result of the program.

Expectancies. Expectancies are the degree to which each objective is to be achieved or the criteria against which actual performance is measured. Obtaining performance data is the first step in determining pro-

FIGURE 13–4
Sample Form for Comparing Outcomes and Expectancies

____
Program

Month__________ **Cumulative Period**__________

Rank	**Objectives**	**This Month**			**Cumulative**		
		Data	**Amount**	**Expectancy**	**Data**	**Amount**	**Expectancy**
1		achieved / to be measured					
2							
3							
4							

Note: From KJ Shaw, *Program Evaluation Guidelines*, Bethesda, MD, Goodwill Industries of America Inc, 1982.

gram performance. To take action based on data describing outcomes, an organization should compare these data with some explicit criteria or expectancies. Expectancies should be expressed in numerical terms that are readily measurable. Most are stated in averages, percentages, time, or money.

Management reports. Management reports relate program performance. They include data on the achievement of goals and objectives and on the characteristics of patients/clients. Various management reports can be generated to communicate with specific populations or influencers by developing a narrative summarizing the actual outcomes relative to the expectancies. Figure 4 illustrates a form for comparing outcome data with expectancies. It can be used in conjunction with a narrative.

The sample form in Figure 5 is used to relate outcomes for each objective according to patient/client descriptors. This information describes the characteristics of patients/clients who are most likely to achieve specific objectives.

System review mechanism. This is an organized procedure for the regular review of the program evaluation system to monitor its effectiveness and reliability. The mechanism enables an organization to update or improve the program evaluation system as needed. The system is, perhaps, more vulnerable to change than any other aspect of an organization since any modifications in a program will affect the evaluation system. To ensure that the evaluation system is able to accomplish its purpose, it must reflect program alterations. A review committee should be established, which could be the same group used originally to establish the program evaluation system. This committee should review at least annually the system's effectiveness. Following are some basic questions that could be reviewed by the committee:

1. Does the system adequately and accurately describe the organization?
2. Do the outcome objectives accurately measure the results the organization strives to achieve? Are there management reports for all programs, and are they provided regularly?
3. Are problems being encountered collecting any of the data, and what are strategies to overcome the problems?
4. Have outcome data been used to improve program performance?
5. Have outcome evaluation data been used to enhance community relations?
6. Are reasonable steps taken to minimize reporting bias?

USES OF PROGRAM EVALUATION

Program evaluation has multiple uses. Not every organization will employ it in all the ways described here. However, at different points an organization may focus on one or another of the applications. Some of the more common uses of program evaluation are enhancing the relationship between an organization's administration and governing board, communicating with third-party groups and organizations, assisting in marketing, containing costs, adding new programs, and increasing benefits to patients/clients.

FIGURE 13–5
Sample Form for Reporting Outcomes of Objectives by Descriptors

____
Program

Month__________ **Cumulative Period**__________

Closed Clients Meeting Objectives

Descriptors	Objective #1				Objective #2			
	Month		Cumulative		Month		Cumulative	
	Data	%	Data	%	Data	%	Data	%
Male								
Female								
Under 21								
Over 55								
White								
Black								
Hispanic								
American Indian								
Asian								
Severely Disabled								
Multiply Disabled								
Emotionally Disabled								
Mentally Disabled								
Visually Disabled								
Hearing Disability								

Note: From KJ Shaw, *Program Evaluation Guidelines*, Bethesda, MD, Goodwill Industries of America Inc, 1982.

Enhancing Administration and Board Relationships

Program evaluation enhances administration and board relationships in several ways. First, it gives those who are responsible for policy making and administration some tools for orientation and education. Program evaluation will result in a well-defined structure of services and programs as well as a clear determination of the populations that are served by an organization. Second, program evaluation will generate information critical to the policy-making and planning responsibilities of the administration and the governing body. In many cases, program evaluation data will provide these groups with their first objective basis for making long-range decisions. Third, many organizations use board members to raise funds because of their stature in the community. Often these individuals are able to raise funds when no one in the organization itself can. Program evaluation gives them specific outcome data to use in explaining benefits to the funding source.

Communicating with Third-Party Groups and Organizations

Program evaluation can also be used very effectively in communicating with third-party groups and organizations. For example, it has been blended successfully with regulatory agencies' requirements for accreditation and quality assurance. It can address the five components of a quality assurance effort by (a) identifying problems occurring in individual patients/clients or specific groups of them; (b) providing an objective assessment of the causes of problems and their scope, and setting priorities for further problem definition; (c) determining whether or not a planned intervention solved a problem; (d) reassessing unsuccessful interventions so that another method can be developed; and (e) developing information that describes the effectiveness of programs.

Recently, consumer groups have become very active in advocating quality services for their constituents. Program evaluation develops straightforward answers to the questions often posed by these groups. For example, the data generated from a comprehensive system can identify which patients/clients in a program achieve benefits. Further, the system can provide answers to why some individuals cannot leave a program or need extended time in it to benefit.

Outcome data can also be used in developing contracts with third parties, for example, for reimbursement or referrals. Such information as who is served, the expected results, and the projected cost per result can easily be extracted from a system. The ready information that program evaluation provides is essential as accountability gains in importance.

Another use of outcome data is in working with planners in a community. Often, planning sessions focus on generalities rather than on concrete data that will support long-range planning for specific populations or types of programs.

Assisting in Marketing

There is an abundance of organizations providing services and a shortage of dollars to meet the needs of all people. Consequently program evaluation has been a useful tool for organizations in promoting their programs. "Marketing by results" involves presenting programs to potential funding sources not in terms of services, but in terms of outcomes that can be achieved (5). Data can also be targeted at special groups, indicating how well the program responds to their needs. Because program evaluation maintains demographic information on individuals by program, presenting pertinent outcome data is relatively easy.

Program evaluation can also be used to develop new markets. In a presentation to potential funders, managers can describe how an evaluation system will inform them whether a program has been efficient and effective for the dollars spent. Programs testing new markets can be set up for a fixed duration, and evaluation results can be used to decide whether to continue the program.

Containing Costs

In all human services, cost containment has become a paramount issue. Most service providers as well as funding sources are becoming increasingly sensitive to the issue of ensuring the most gain for the least expenditure. Because program evaluation defines an acceptable objective, it will provide feedback on the actual versus the expected cost of individual programs. This feedback, coupled with the identification of a program's outcome, can help management determine whether the program is cost-effective.

Another advantage of program evaluation data is that they can track a program's use as opposed to its defined capacity. Use is one of the major elements in determining cost efficiency. With adequate data to determine the actual use of a program, managers can decide whether to increase marketing efforts or reduce costs.

Program evaluation also has the flexibility to isolate particular data (e.g., positive outcomes by age or sex of patients/clients) and relate them to cost. Consequently, if a program is achieving positive results but its cost effectiveness is less than desirable, specific activities or elements of the program can be reviewed to determine which have the greatest effect on positive outcome at what cost. Managers can use the resulting data to decide whether to maintain or eliminate the activities.

Another application of program evaluation cost data comes in helping an organization determine what services or programs might best be provided through a contractual arrangement with another agency as opposed to the organization's providing the service itself. Often a particular service is expensive for one organization to operate because of its low rate of actual or projected use, whereas another organization may have sufficient volume to provide the service more cost-effectively. An organization could thus offer the array of services necessary to achieve benefits, but not provide all of the services itself.

Adding New Programs

Frequent changes in the marketplace, the priorities of funding authorities, and concerns of consumer organizations require continual review and monitoring of existing services and programs with an eye to contraction or expansion. A primary use of program evaluation data is to analyze the prospects of a new venture before embarking on it. Outcome data can determine effectively who is not benefiting from existing programs. If a sufficient pattern of problems or a sufficient number of people can be identified as needing a service, and if appropriate funding sources can be found, a reasonably safe decision can be made regarding the development of a new program or the expansion of an existing one.

One of the most cost-effective mechanisms available to organizations is to replicate services and programs that have demonstrated their effectiveness and efficiency. An organization looking to implement a new program might review program evaluation data on similar programs in like organizations.

Increasing Benefits to Patients/Clients

Finally, program evaluation can increase benefits to patients/clients. One way in which it does this is by identifying the types of people most likely to gain from a program. The organization can then develop procedures to ensure that the program admits only those who both need and can benefit from the services. Many programs accept everyone who is referred, regardless of the expected outcome. Unfortunately, with patients/clients who are not expected to benefit, this policy communicates ineffectiveness to referral sources and often results in a frustrating and negative experience for the patient/client.

A program evaluation system also supplies information to hold the staff accountable for obtaining results. Studies show and organizations confirm that a considerable increase in benefits occurs when information on outcomes is communicated to the people who provide a service. In effect, the feedback suggests clearly that staff are responsible and in most situations they respond by trying to achieve performance standards (5).

As mentioned in the previous section, program evaluation also lends itself to the development of specialized data. Essentially, a system can be constructed to track a specific type of person or specific groups of people through a particular program. The results can assist an organization in responding to the unique problems of types of people or programs.

IMPLEMENTING PROGRAM EVALUATION

For an organization to realize the obvious and long-range benefits of program evaluation, a system must be implemented and used. Four major factors influence implementation and use: commitment, accountability, productivity planning, and readiness.

Commitment. Commitment to the concept seems to be the major influencing factor in whether a system is developed and used. The need for program evaluation must be recognized at the very top of an organization, and the system must be mandated throughout. To add credibility, responsibility for the system should be vested in a high-level staff person.

Accountability. Accountability is both a positive and a negative force in the implementation of program evaluation. In holding people responsible for their actions, it can improve results. But who specifically should be held accountable for outcomes? Often, many staff members are involved in providing a service and they may have varying degrees of accountability. The staff who are most accountable could attempt to manipulate the results for their own benefit and thereby undermine the validity of the system. The systems that work best do not look for accountability in individual service providers so much as they hold department managers or program heads accountable for the results of their unit.

Productivity planning. Implementation and use of program evaluation yield very positive results in productivity planning. Recognizing that a program evaluation system will generate information about weaknesses in a program, most organizations that have a system develop intervention strategies to attend to problems as they arise. Generally, when unsatisfactory outcomes of a program are identified, productivity planning uses the staff involved in the program to recommend alternatives. Often a program evaluation system is the first useful tool that managers have had to identify and objectively define problems.

Readiness. Effective program evaluation cannot take place until an organization is ready for it. Readiness includes staff awareness of the design of the system and its expected results and a clear understanding of their responsibilities in ensuring consistency in the system. Consequently, appropriate training must occur to inform staff about purposes, procedures, and their own and others' responsibilities.

SUMMARY

Program evaluation is an outcome-monitoring system that describes the impact of programs and services on individual patients/clients by defining the desired results of service delivery and comparing them with actual outcomes. Data on outcomes are always related to a change in patient/client status. A properly designed system generates objective information about current activities or performance that should enhance the quality of future decisions.

In an outcome model of program evaluation four basic criteria must be followed: (a) measurement of all patients/clients, (b) measurement after the discontinuation of treatment, (c) continual reporting, and (d) preset standards for outcomes. Sixteen elements comprise the model:

1. Program structure—arrangement of the organization into distinct service elements. The components of the structure are influencers, purpose statement, admission criteria, program goals, services provided, and patients/clients served.
2. Influencers—groups or individuals who affect the development and the continuation of specific programs.
3. Purpose statement—a capsule declaration of the organization's mission, services, and patient/client populations.
4. Admission criteria—the capabilities and characteristics that a person must possess to be admitted to an organization's programs.
5. Program goals—the components and characteristics of each program.
6. Services provided—the activities available to patients/clients.

7. Patients/clients served—types by disabilities and demographic characteristics.
8. Patient/client descriptors—characteristics according to severity of problems or barriers to success.
9. Objectives—the results a program aims to achieve.
10. Relative importance—a ranking of the objectives within each program.
11. Measures—the standards with which outcomes are compared.
12. Who is measured—the groups of patients/clients whose results are being calculated for a specific measure.
13. Time of application of measures—the point when outcome information is collected.
14. Expectancies—the degree to which objectives are to be achieved.
15. Management reports—narratives summarizing the actual outcomes relative to the expectancies.
16. System review mechanism—a procedure for monitoring the program evaluation system.

Program evaluation has multiple uses. The most common ones are enhancing the relationship between an organization's administration and board, communicating with third-party groups and organizations, assisting in marketing, containing costs, adding new programs, and increasing benefits to patients/clients.

Four major factors influence the implementation and use of program evaluation in an organization: commitment, accountability, productivity planning, and readiness.

References

1. *Assessing and Enhancing the Quality of Services: A Guide for the Human Services Field*. Boston: Human Services Research Institute, 1984
2. *Program Evaluation in Rehabilitation Facilities*. Tucson, AZ: Commission on Accreditation of Rehabilitation Facilities, 1977
3. Lindeman DJ, Hesselbein FR, Hall PR, et al: *Evaluation Concepts and Agency Self-Evaluation Methods: A Handbook*. Alexandria, VA: United Way of America, 1981
4. Haller RA, Shaw KJ: *Program Evaluation Manual*. Bethesda, MD: Goodwill Industries of America Inc, 1984
5. *Program Evaluation: A Guide to Utilization*. Tucson, AZ: Commission on Accreditation of Rehabilitation Facilities, 1982

Chapter 14

Quality Assurance

Barbara E. Joe, MA

As demands for accountability have grown, quality assurance has come into its own as a necessary and recognized component of health care. Yet because it is a relatively recent addition to the health care lexicon, many occupational therapy personnel—clinicians and students alike—lack a clear understanding of its role and importance in the health care system. *Peer review, patient care evaluation, audit, outcome assessment, health accounting*—all of these increasingly familiar terms are encompassed under the more general rubric of *quality assurance.*

Quality assurance lies at the heart of the basic purpose of health care. That purpose, generally stated, is to improve human well-being, function, and longevity. The existence of, or the desire to avoid, a health problem (as defined by society and by patients/clients) is what leads patients/clients to seek care. Quality assurance is a system of enhancing the benefits that are the *raison d'etre* of intervention. People would not submit to treatment nor pay its costs, even indirectly, unless they expected benefits. How health care achieves and increases these benefits is what quality assurance is all about.

Quality assurance is a problem-solving system. It is like the system used with individual patients/clients, but it applies to aggregates of patients/clients with similar diagnoses and characteristics. Quality assurance asks and answers questions such as the following: Is the care being provided to a given group of patients/clients having the expected or desired effect? If so, to what extent? If not, what changes are likely to produce the intended outcomes? Are these changes feasible? Is this an

---

Barbara E. Joe is a quality assurance and program evaluation specialist at AOTA, where she has worked for three years. In her job she teaches, writes about, and consults on program evaluation.

area in which expenditures of effort and resources are apt to produce considerable improvement, or might these be better directed to some other, more fruitful area? If a plan for improvement has been implemented, has it actually been successful?

All the basic elements of quality assurance are implied in the above questions:

1. Identification of a problem through an apparent failure to achieve a standard of quality based on the desired or expected outcomes of the care provided.
2. Verification of the problem through measurements showing that desired outcomes are not being achieved.
3. Formulation of a plan to achieve such outcomes that is both feasible and cost-effective.
4. Implementation of the plan for improvement.
5. Measurement to determine if the problem has been solved (i. e., if the standard of quality has been met).

This process, with its emphasis on measurement, provides checks at two critical junctures. First, there is initial measurement to make sure the problem identified actually exists. This may seem obvious, yet such initial measurement often shows that the standard is already being achieved. Therefore, there is no problem after all. Second, when a problem has been verified, a measurement is made *after* the intended improvement to make sure the problem has actually been solved. Unless this final step is included, it may be blithely assumed that a new procedure has taken care of the problem when actual measurement would reveal this not to be so. In such cases the improvement action must be reformulated, or, in rare instances, the standard itself must be reevaluated to make sure it is achievable.

HISTORICAL PERSPECTIVES AND PRESENT REGULATIONS

Early Pioneers

Before the elements of quality assurance are explored in greater depth, it is instructive to look at how a concern with health care quality evolved, from a set of implicit and unquestioned beliefs in the value of health care, to the explicit, formal, and objective system called quality assurance.

Throughout history and in much of the world today, folk remedies have predominated, and only the wealthy have enjoyed the privilege of medical treatment. Even among the latter, probably few questioned whether the treatment they were receiving actually worked.

Society has come a long way from the days when healers had magical status and absolute authority, yet the patient's/client's trust in the practitioner contributes to health improvement. Although health care today remains art as well as science, science has been in the ascendancy ever since the sixteenth century, when Harvey, Willis, and other prominent physicians shocked their contemporaries by dissecting the human body to discover its workings firsthand.

In the 1860s, Florence Nightingale (1) observed and reported on the deficiencies of health care services provided to those wounded in the war. The first person to collect and compare mortality statistics from different hospitals, she saw the death rate in military hospitals during the Crimean War plunge from 42 percent to 2.2 percent (p 117). Her efforts were continued by Abraham Flexner, a physician whose 1910 report on the poor quality of medical education (2) was instrumental in closing 60 of 155 U. S. medical schools then in existence. Another key pioneer was E. A. Codman, who in 1912 initiated "end-result" assessment to improve hospital care (3).

On November 15, 1912, The Third Clinical Congress of Surgeons of North America put forth a resolution that was both prophetic and revolutionary: "Some system of standardization of hospital equipment and hospital work should be developed, to the end that those institutions having the highest ideals may have proper recognition before the profession, and that those of inferior equipment and standards should be stimulated to raise the quality of their work" (as quoted in 4, p 476). Several years later, the American College of Surgeons initiated the process of hospital accreditation. Of 692 hospitals covered in their first survey, only 90 (12.9 percent) were approved (5, p 7).

Quality Assurance Requirements of the Joint Commission on Accreditation of Hospitals

The Joint Commission on Accreditation of Hospitals (JCAH) was established in 1951 (see Chapter 19). Most states now mandate JCAH accreditation for licensure, and most third-party and government payers require it for reimbursement.

The quality assurance program of JCAH has been evolving over the years. In 1955, JCAH first began to stress the importance of medical audits. By 1974, hospitals were required to audit medical records and make quarterly reports. In 1981, judging that the audit system was producing good medical records, but not necessarily better care, JCAH began urging the introduction of additional monitors (measures of important outcomes of patient/client care) and a focus on problem resolution.

The JCAH has included the following elements in its guidelines for quality assurance plans: problem identification, priority setting, problem assessment, problem resolution, and problem-monitoring follow-up (6). Also included are concerns about how the quality assurance plan is developed and carried out, such as designating responsibility, assuring representation of all disciplines involved in patient care, and establishing quality assurance reporting procedures (6).

Quality assurance, according to the most recent JCAH policy statements, is concerned with monitoring and evaluating the quality and appropriateness of patient care. Quality assurance covers all clinical activities, using continuous monitors or indicators selected according to criteria identified in the literature or by experts and professional associations. Data sources can include patient records, as in the audit days, but should go beyond them. JCAH gives the following examples of data sources for monitoring quality assurance: medical records, incidence reports, laboratory reports, generic screening, patient bills, staff surveys, patient surveys, direct observation, and credentialing reports. The most essential monitors should be selected first, such as those dealing with life and death. Monitors may be continually added, and those no longer needed may be discarded. Quality assurance monitors in health care must have a direct impact on patient care; thus, administrative concerns are excluded unless such an impact can be demonstrated.

In addition to measuring important aspects of patient care, monitors must be comprehensive in scope, ongoing, and continuous, according to JCAH. Routine, systematic monitoring initially identifies problems and subsequently verifies that remedies continue to be effective. In sum, quality assurance monitors must be important, routine, and comprehensive, and must directly affect patient care. Dealing with discrete problems no longer satisfies JCAH's quality assurance standards. However, when the monitoring process picks up a problem, if appropriate, it may be dealt with separately by a special quality assurance study (7, 8).

Designing a quality assurance monitor requires designation of the activity, its objectives, measurable criteria, data sources, frequency of monitoring, and responsibility for monitoring and reporting. Specific reporting intervals are not mandated by JCAH, but must be appropriate to the situation.

In occupational therapy, monitors could assess whether or not treatment goals are being met. Cost and efficiency concerns such as promptness, frequency, and length of treatments could be included, as long as they were also related to treatment outcomes. Standards could be established for such variables as functional ability at discharge, or discharge dispositions for various diagnoses, or groups of patients. Failure to achieve the standards would signal the need for improvement. These standards have implications not only for patient/client well-being, but for cost, with higher function and discharge to home likely to be related to cost savings.

Peer Review

In 1965 the federal government began requiring JCAH accreditation for hospitals participating in Medicare. It initiated another formal check on health care quality in 1972 with the establishment of professional standards review organizations (PSROs). These were groups of locally organized physicians and other health care representatives authorized to perform a continuous form of peer, nonbureaucratic, grass roots review of the quality of care being provided to Medicare patients/clients. Organized medicine initially opposed PSROs as an infringement on professional prerogatives. However, many physicians eventually swung behind the program, which was designed to improve care, correct deficiencies, and contain costs.

Professional standards review organizations were an innovative idea intended both to protect patients/clients and to assure that federally financed care was appropriate in quality and cost. Proponents estimated savings beyond the program's cost of $144 million per year (9). However, opponents disputed these claims and characterized PSROs as a costly and complicated layer of bureaucracy.

Eventually, cost pressures led to the Peer Review Improvement Act of 1982, a reformulation of peer review that called for the replacing of PSROs by peer review organizations (PROs). According to federal regulations, each state was required before the end of 1984 to designate a single PRO to act on its behalf in monitoring the quality of care for Medicare beneficiaries under a two-year contract with the federal Health Care Financing Administration (HCFA). The law gave preference in designing PROs to physician-sponsored organizations. Other professions, including occupational therapy personnel, can volunteer to serve on state PRO advisory boards.

Peer review organizations' quality objectives must be expressed in numerical or percentage terms. They include reduction of unnecessary surgery, patient/client deaths, inappropriate admissions, and readmissions due to prior substandard care.

It is too soon to evaluate the specific contributions of PROs. However, a comment about PSRO from quality assurance theoretician Avedis Donabedian (10) may also pertain to PROs: "In time, the records of the PSROs may create historical archives into which the antiquary of quality assessment may wish, mole-like, to burrow" (p 375).

Other Quality Assurance Mechanisms

Some commentators include credentialing, licensure, and practice standards or protocols under quality assurance because the aim of these measures is to assure or improve the quality of care. In addition, program evaluation, the system used by the Commission on Accreditation of Rehabilitation Facilities (CARF) (treated in the previous chapter) is sometimes considered a tool or a method of quality assurance (11).

In practice, quality assurance and program evaluation are sometimes merged. Some occupational therapy departments use program evaluation as their monitoring system for identifying quality assurance problems, and a number of rehabilitation programs have both program evaluation and quality assurance programs in place.

States may require either JCAH or CARF accreditation for rehabilitation programs, and sometimes both. States may also have their own requirements related to quality of care, usually adapted from the standards and procedures of these two accrediting bodies.

DEFINITIONS AND DISTINCTIONS

Measuring Quality

According to quality assurance expert John W. Williamson (12), health care "demands a continual objective appraisal of outcomes so as to seek and achieve the highest benefit consistent with the patient's needs within constraints set by society and current health care technology. This continual reassessment of the outcomes of one's performance (that is, quality assurance) is an indispensable and integral part of providing care." (p 275) Failing to take time for quality assurance, Williamson (12) maintains, "is equivalent to a pilot's being too busy flying the plane to have time to check his compass to see where he is in relation to where he wants to be" (p 275).

The term *quality* ultimately rests not on objective facts, but as Williamson (12) indicates, on values, the values of health care practitioners, patients/clients, and society. Sometimes there is agreement on these values, such as the value of a life saved or a death postponed. Sometimes there is disagreement, such as whether abortion is a desirable medical procedure. In other cases, values about the continuance of life conflict with values about its quality. Does the maintenance of physical life through extraordinary measures take precedence over maintaining a "meaningful" life, and how is the latter defined?

In quality assurance, determinations such as these must be made by a broad spectrum of professionals, along with patient/client representatives. There should be a fairly high consensus on what constitutes quality and therefore on what constitutes a problem, because lack of agreement, by definition, puts the existence of a problem in doubt and undermines solution.

However, once standards of quality are established—such as what percentage of stroke patients can be expected to improve one level in activities of daily living after a given number of treatments—measurement of how well these standards are being achieved can be fairly objective, a matter of numbers and statistical sampling. Although quality assurance measures are objective, "subjective" feelings of well-being and satisfaction—whether expressed by patients/clients or staff—can be surveyed (for example, through questionnaires). Quality assurance makes certain that quality, once defined, is measured, improved, and then maintained.

The term *quality assurance*, with its implication of promises for the future, is perhaps more accurately rendered as *quality confirmation*. This is because the judgment that patient/client outcomes actually meet standards of quality can only be made after measurement of the results of a particular health care intervention.

Cost Effectiveness as a Component of Quality

Usually a distinction is made between health benefits and costs, the latter referring to the individual's or society's sacrifice in providing such benefits. Quality assurance attempts to blend these sometimes antagonistic themes into a single formulation, transforming Bentham's "greatest good for the greatest number" into "the best care at the least cost." According to the Institute of Medicine, quality assurance is a system "to make health care more effective in improving the health status and satisfaction of a population within the resources which society and the individual have chosen to spend for that care" (13).

The cost component is not something new in quality assurance; it has always been part of the quality equation. However, it is now receiving renewed emphasis and is an explicit concern. As Donabedian (10) has expressed it, "Quality consists in a precise matching of services to needs, without excess or deficit" (p 116). He contends that "the net benefit to health must exceed the monetary cost incurred in obtaining that benefit. Unfortunately, our estimates of the benefits, harm, and cost of care are often very imprecise" (p 5). Donabedian (10) goes on to argue that "the schemes of management used in actual practice may embody more efficient strategies than those incorporated in norms that presuppose almost unlimited resources" (p 139), and that even when "attention to cost may lower the standards of care below the optimal, . . . one could argue that the new standards merely represent an attempt to optimize the attainment of a broader set of social objectives" (p 204).

Williamson (12), the father of a problem-oriented approach to quality assurance, defines quality assurance in terms of both effectiveness and efficiency, thereby recognizing "that quality assurance encompasses both the traditional concept of quality (that is, a high degree of effectiveness in providing care) and cost containment (that is, an efficient use of resources)" (p xvii).

Williamson (14) also distinguishes between *efficacy*, which is the benefits of health care intervention under ideal or experimental conditions, *effectiveness*, which refers to health care benefits under the ordinary circumstance of clinical practice, and *efficiency*, which means the extent to which health care benefits are achieved with a minimum of unnecessary expenditure and effort.

Relation to Research

Although quality assurance relies on research in setting standards and borrows some of its measurement techniques, quality assurance is not research. As a practical matter, most clinicians are not able to set up controlled trials, to control variables, to collect data on sufficient numbers for valid research, or to draw conclusions applicable beyond their own organization. However, as part of their regular clinical duties, they are able to conduct quality assurance that has no control groups as such, though patients/clients measured *before* and *after* an improvement action do function as a type of control for themselves.

This does not make quality assurance just a poor cousin of research. The basic difference between quality assurance and research is one of purpose, not of technique. Research shows *what* happens, whereas quality assurance is concerned with *making* a particular thing happen. In very crude terms, research shows what is possible, and quality assurance applies research findings in actual clinical situations.

For example, research shows that early occupational therapy intervention results in earlier hospital discharge and greater functional improvement for stroke patients (15, 16). A hospital desiring to achieve earlier discharge and better functional gains for stroke patients initiates early occupational therapy services, then determines whether it has actually achieved the results research has shown to be possible. Even in the absence of research data, quality assurance can show measurable improvement in meeting preestablished standards in a given setting and can also point the way to areas for further research.

Criteria, Norms, Standards, and Outcomes

It is easy to become entangled in a semantic tie-up over the distinction between *criteria*, *norms*, and *standards*. The *1974 PSRO Program Manual* (17) defines *medical care criteria* as predetermined elements of care developed by professionals, based on professional expertise and the literature, which in turn define quality care. *Norms* are numerical or statistical measures of usual or observed performance, that is, statements of what is actually occurring apart from any evaluation of quality. *Standards* are professionally developed expressions of the permissible range of variation from either criteria or norms (17). Therefore, standards, like criteria, carry a quality or value component, whereas norms are merely statements of averages.

C. M. Jacobs (18), commenting on JCAH's Performance Evaluation Procedure (PEP), defines a criterion as an element of care of major consequence and a standard as a percentage that attaches to each criterion. In a recent book Donabedian (10) skirts the issue of distinguishing between standards and criteria, but seems to favor concentration on criteria, reserving the term *standard* for a broader measure, based on percentage or numerical measurement, of a cluster of criteria. Along these lines, quality assurance theoretician Nancy Graham (19) defines criteria as the important elements of health care being measured or monitored, with standards being numerical or percentage expressions of the acceptable level or range of criteria expression. Thus, among quality assurance experts criteria seem to be items that define the broader standards, which are expressed in percentage terms.

Donabedian (10) goes on to point out that "criteria sets can be distinguished by whether they consist primarily of elements of structure, process, or outcome" (p 90). Observing that the lines between these three types of criteria are fuzzy and sometimes arbitrary, Williamson (20) has attempted to clarify matters, at least between process and outcome standards or criteria, by defining outcomes broadly as "any characteristics of patients, health problems, providers, or their interaction in the care process that results from care provided or required, as measured at one point in time" (p 26).

SOME RECOGNIZED METHODS OF QUALITY ASSURANCE

Following are some established methods of quality assurance.

Comprehensive Quality Assurance Systems (CQAS). In CQAS, two practitioners (21) carefully review a small number of medical records to identify problems in patient care. They present their results to a quality assurance committee, which selects the most important ones and sets standards of care for them. All, or most, medical records are reviewed to determine whether the standards for these problems are being met. CQAS rely heavily on process criteria and medical record documentation and can be time-consuming because of the levels of review involved (21).

Concurrent Quality Assurance (CQA). CQA is a method of quality assurance that is carried out while patients are still under care. For selected diagnoses, a panel of experts determines process criteria for diagnosis, documentation, and treatment. Errors found are corrected immediately, without waiting for outcomes. Assessment is specifically disease oriented and not geared to more generic problems (22).

Criteria Mapping. Criteria Mapping is based on medical records, evaluated according to clinical decisions made at various junctures. The basis of evaluation is a "map" that offers potential alternative decisions and criteria at each critical branching of the road. This system is well geared to evaluation of individual patients (23).

Medical Management Analysis. This is a risk management system based on generic screening criteria. It involves review of medical records while care is in process to reveal patterns of substandard care. However, it yields relatively little information about infrequent events or the possible causes of a problem (24).

Performance Evaluation Procedure. PEP is an outcome-based, retrospective method of reviewing patient records selected for diagnostic or procedural commonalities. The system can be adapted to verify the existence and extent of a problem and its probable causes. One of the first quality assurance systems developed by JCAH, it still has applicability (25).

Periodic Medical Review (PMR). This is a quality assurance system designed to find patterns of deficiency in patient care based on a fairly lengthy questionnaire to be filled out by a reviewer for individual patients (26).

Problem Status Index-Outcome (PSI). PSI is a system of assessing the outcomes of care from the patient's viewpoint, using a questionnaire. Patients'/clients' reported outcomes are correlated with process information in medical records. The response rate to the somewhat complicated questionnaires has been low. That is unfortunate, because PSI is one of the few methods of health care evaluation that is specifically patient/client oriented (27).

Profile Analysis. This is a retrospective review of patient, practitioner, or institutional profiles, either individually or in groups. It is similar to tracers (see below), except that instead of tracking a problem, it follows a patient/client through a hospital stay. A wealth of data is generated, which then must be further analyzed to find solvable problems. Profile analysis can be costly (28).

Quality Assurance Monitor (QAM). QAM is a continuous-monitoring technique that incorporates a system of priorities for investigation. It was a forerunner of JCAH's current system of continuous monitoring for detection of problems (29).

Staging. Staging is an outcome-based method of assessing both inpatient and outpatient care for conditions at various levels of severity and at different stages of treatment (30).

Sentinel Health Events. These are negative health events, such as unnecessary disease, avoidable disability, and untimely death. Measuring the incidence of these events gives a baseline for improvement (31).

Tracers. Tracers are selected diagnoses (such as cerebrovascular accident and rheumatoid arthritis) that are studied when they occur as a sole diagnosis. They are followed through the health care system and presumably represent how the system works in general (32).

California Medical Association/California Hospital Association Educational Patient Care Audit. This system has largely been incorporated into present quality assurance methods. It requires professionals to be involved in choosing evaluation criteria and in setting "thresholds for action," that is, minimum percentages that must meet preestablished criteria before care can be considered acceptable. Failure to achieve the minimum signals the need for corrective action (33).

Many of these quality assurance approaches are still used, either singly or in combination. A given health care situation might be most appropriately measured and dealt with by one method, whereas another aspect of care might best be measured by a different method. Many of the approaches are not sufficient in themselves for full-scale quality assurance activities, but are effective as problem-solving tools within a broader plan.

PROBLEM-BASED QUALITY ASSURANCE

As quality assurance becomes more widespread, adherence to basic elements takes on more importance than particular quality assurance strategies. Regardless of the particular system used, there are five key steps in quality assurance problem solving, paralleling those in clinical problem solving for individual patients. These steps, not necessarily in order of occurrence, are (a) problem identification and standard setting, (b) problem measurement, (c) improvement planning, (d) implementation of an improvement plan, and (e) measurement to determine whether standards have been met.

The new JCAH continuous-monitoring system automatically fulfills the first two steps through the choice and implementation of continuous monitors. Likewise, the last step, measuring improvement, is picked up by continuous monitoring. However, improvement planning and implementation often need to be broken out separately.

A generic quality assurance approach compatible with other methods is problem-based quality assurance, originally called health accounting, a formalization of the five steps already mentioned. Developed by Williamson, it has been successfully field-tested in more than 80 studies. Although quality assurance experts may quibble about the relative merits of process versus outcome criteria, Williamson has opted to concentrate on outcomes, considering them the most direct avenue to problem identification.

Williamson (12, 34) has developed agendas and procedures to guide problem-based quality assurance. The American Occupational Therapy Association (AOTA) also has publications available adapting the approach to occupational therapy (14, 35). These AOTA publications, developed to assist members with quality assurance, provide detailed, step-by-step guidance beyond what is offered here.

EXAMPLE OF A QUALITY ASSURANCE STUDY

A brief description of an actual quality assurance study may serve to highlight aspects of problem-based quality assurance. The Occupational Therapy Department of Santa Clara Valley Medical Center, a northern California rehabilitation and acute care facility, conducted a problem-based quality assurance study related to the ordering of wheelchairs. The Quality Assurance Committee felt that Medicaid (known as Medi-Cal in California) had been denying or deferring prescribed wheelchairs at an excessive rate. When a third-party payer such as Medicaid denies reimbursement for the purchase of a wheelchair, a patient/client is forced to obtain his or her own funding. For the majority of patients/clients involved, this is impossible, so they must go without wheelchairs.

The committee considered the problem of selecting and obtaining reimbursement for wheelchairs for Medicaid patients/clients to have high ABNA, an acronym coined by Williamson to stand for *achievable benefits not achieved*. In other words, the committee thought that the identified problem was not only important and solvable, two requisites for going ahead with a quality assurance study, but also one with much room for improvement.

Before it could determine whether, in fact, a problem existed, the team designated to conduct the study had to set a standard for obtaining reimbursement. It was agreed that patients/clients and wheelchairs had to be matched within the Medicaid cost ceiling. After consulting the literature and experts, the team decided that 95 percent of Medicaid patients/clients for whom a wheelchair was prescribed should receive coverage. (Because of the contingencies of ordinary clinical circumstances, quality assurance standards are almost never set at 100 percent.) Quality assurance concentrates on problems and their solution, so the standard was expressed in negative rather than positive terms, with a denial or deferral rate of 5 percent or less defining success. The term for this negative standard is *maximum acceptable standard* (MAS), and it represents the maximum rate of error, or noncontrol of the problem, that can be tolerated. It is important to note that this standard of 5 percent denials or deferrals in no way implied that an occupational therapist's actual recommendations and measurements would be in error. Rather, it reflected limitations in the reimbursement system.

The team estimated that the actual rate of denials and deferrals *before* starting any improvement was 25 percent and that the 5-percent standard could be met *after* action was taken to improve the situation. There was some initial doubt on the latter estimate because of uncertainty about the response of the reimbursing agency. The estimate, however, indicated high ABNA or high potential for improvement because of the discrepancy between expected findings before and after improvement.

The team then measured actual performance and found the rate of denials and deferrals to be exactly what it had anticipated. This coincidence of actual measurement and clinical judgment served to increase the team's confidence in future judgments and decisions, as well as its investment in this particular study and the quality assurance program as a whole.

The team next designed and implemented a plan for improvement involving not only the occupational therapy department, but Medicaid physician reviewers. Seminars were provided for the Medicaid field office staff on criteria for ordering a particular type of wheelchair, as well as the need for custom wheelchairs for certain disabilities or clinical problems. A resource liaison in the occupational therapy department was established for the physician reviewers to contact with questions or concerns regarding equipment orders. The department also developed a wheelchair-ordering packet to serve as a guideline for therapists in making recommendations. The packet analyzed features of wheelchairs, from lightweight to electric, and related them to disability, cost, clinical picture, psychological status, and other factors.[1] Finally, training was offered to occupational therapy staff to improve their skills in writing wheelchair justifications or prescriptions.

---

[1]This packet is available from the Occupational Therapy Department, Santa Clara Valley Medical Center, 751 South Bascom Avenue, San Jose, California 95128.

FIGURE 14–1
Results of Quality Assurance Study on
Wheelchair Ordering

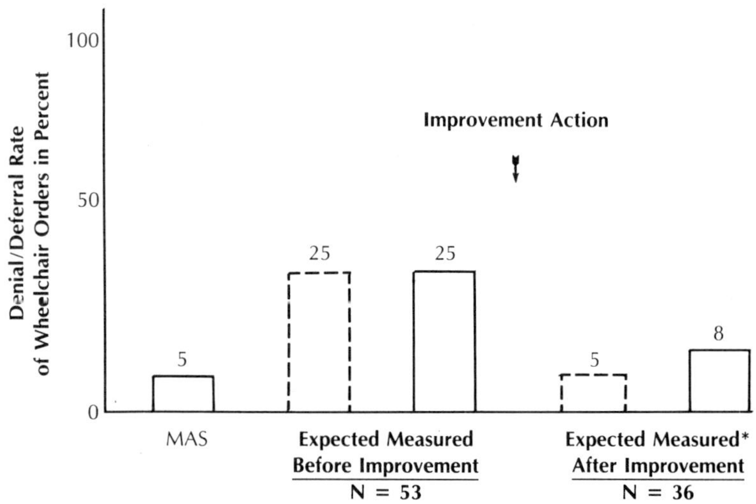

*This final figure represents denials only.
MAS, maximum acceptable standard.

After the plan was implemented, three out of thirty-six wheelchair orders were denied (8 percent), and no deferrals were pending (see Figure 1). This rate, although not quite reaching the MAS of 5 percent, indicated a significant improvement from the original 25 percent rate, with a consequent and direct impact on patient/client care and well-being. Efforts have continued to bring the rate down to or below 5 percent. Not all problems require a full-fledged quality assurance study such as this. Sometimes mere identification of a problem results in improvement. Other examples of quality assurance studies relevant to occupational therapy are available from various sources (36–38).

OVERCOMING OBSTACLES TO QUALITY ASSURANCE

There has been resistance to quality assurance on several grounds. One has been the fear of malpractice suits or, conversely, the fear of lawsuits from colleagues judged to be providing substandard care (39). Other significant barriers have been health professionals' expectations of autonomy (40), habitual and established systems of behavior and interaction, psychological inflexibility, investment in current procedures, the financial impact of change, and entrenched official policies (41).

Rachelle Kaye, who calls quality assurance "a strategy for planned change," observes that there are three stages in the change process:

unfreezing of current attitudes and behaviors, change, and "refreezing" (42, p 157). The latter represents a new equilibrium. However, in quality assurance, as in life, this equilibrium is only temporary. Solution of one problem leads to discovery of another, and the process of change goes on.

An example from occupational therapy bears this out. A quality assurance study identified, measured, and then solved the problem of occupational therapists failing to respond to referrals within twenty-four hours. Once the standard response time had been routinely achieved, a new problem was discovered and tackled through quality assurance: initial evaluations being given patients/clients within the specified time limit were not always complete; that is, standards for quality evaluations were not being met.

Quality assurance, therefore, like health care itself, is evolving. Occupational therapy personnel are continually adding to the course of development and to the body of knowledge and practice in this vital area.

SUMMARY

Quality assurance is an expression of the new demand for accountability and cost containment in health care. It offers a method for solving either treatment or cost problems for aggregates of patients/clients with similar diagnoses and characteristics. There are five basic elements in quality assurance:

1. Identification of a problem through an apparent failure to achieve a standard of quality based on the desired or expected outcomes of the care provided.
2. Verification of the problem through measurements showing that desired outcomes are not being achieved.
3. Formulation of a plan to achieve such outcomes that is both feasible and cost-effective.
4. Implementation of the plan for improvement.
5. Measurement to determine if the problem has been solved.

The quality assurance program of the JCAH has been evolving over the years. According to the most recent JCAH policy statements, quality assurance is concerned with monitoring and evaluating the quality and the appropriateness of patient care. Data sources used in monitoring can include patient records, incidence reports, laboratory reports, generic screening, patient bills, staff surveys, patient surveys, direct observation, and credentialing reports. Designing a quality assurance monitor requires designation of the activity, its objectives, measurable criteria, data sources, frequency of monitoring, and responsibility for monitoring and reporting. Monitors must have a direct impact on patient care. They must also be comprehensive in scope, ongoing, and continuous. Dealing with discrete problems no longer satisfies JCAH's quality assurance standards. However, when the monitoring process picks up a problem, it may be dealt with separately by a special quality assurance study.

Quality assurance attempts to blend the sometimes antagonistic themes of health benefits and low costs into a single formulation, "the best care at the least cost." Unlike research, which shows what happens, quality assurance is concerned with making a particular thing happen. There are many established methods of quality assurance. A given health care situation might be most appropriately measured by one method, whereas another aspect of care might best be measured by a different method. Many of the approaches are not sufficient in themselves for full-scale quality assurance activities, but are effective as problem-solving tools within a broader plan.

There has been resistance to quality assurance on several grounds: fear of lawsuits, health professionals' expectations of autonomy, habitual and established systems of behavior and interaction, psychological inflexibility, investment in current procedures, the financial impact of change, and entrenched official policies.

References

1. Huxley E: *Florence Nightingale*. New York: Putnum, 1975, p 117
2. Flexner A: *Medical Education in the United States and Canada*. New York: Carnegie Foundation, Merrymount Press, 1910
3. Codman EA: The product of a hospital. *Surg, Gynecol Obstet* 18:491–496, 1914
4. Davis L: *Fellowship of Surgeons: A History of the American College of Surgeons*. Springfield, IL: Charles C Thomas Publisher, 1960
5. Graham N: Historical perspective and regulations. In *Quality Assurance in Hospitals*, N Graham, Editor. Rockville, MD: Aspen Systems Corp, 1982, pp 3–13
6. Joint Commission on Accreditation of Hospitals: *The QA Guide*. Chicago: Joint Commission on Accreditation of Hospitals, 1980, pp 177–181
7. Roberts JS, Walczak RM: Toward effective quality assurance: The evaluation and current status of the JCAH QA standard. *QRB* 10(1):11–15, 1984
8. Joint Commission on Accreditation of Hospitals: *Accreditation Manual for Hospitals*. Chicago: Joint Commission on Accreditation of Hospitals, 1984
9. Kurtz H: Three medical study units in area lose funds. *Washington Post*, November 5, 1981
10. Donabedian A: *Explorations in Quality Assessment and Monitoring*, vol 2: *The Criteria and Standards of Quality*. Ann Arbor, MI: Health Administration Press, 1982
11. Michnich ME, Shortell SM, Richardson WC: Program evaluation resource for decision making. In *Organization and Change in Health Care Quality Assurance*, RD Luke, JC Krueger, RE Modrow, Editors. Rockville, MD: Aspen Systems Corp, 1983, pp 263–279
12. Williamson JW, Barr DM, Fee E, et al: *Teaching Quality Assurance and Cost Containment in Health Care*. San Francisco: Jossey-Bass Inc Publishers, 1982
13. National Academy of Sciences, Institute of Medicine: *Assessing Quality in Health Care: An Evaluation*. Washington, DC: National Academy of Sciences, 1976
14. Ostrow PC, Williamson JW, Joe BE: *Quality Assurance Primer*. Rockville, MD: American Occupational Therapy Association, 1983
15. Garraway WM, Akhtar AJ, Prescott RJ, et al: Management of acute stroke in the elderly: Preliminary results of a controlled trial. *Br Med J*, April 12, 1980, pp 1040–1043
16. Smith ME, Garraway WM, Smith DL, et al: Therapy impact on functional outcome in a controlled trial of stroke rehabilitation. *Arch Phys Med Rehabil* 63:21–24, 1982
17. American Medical Association: *PSRO Program Manual*. Chicago: American Medical Association, March 15, 1974, chap 7
18. Jacobs CM, Christoffel TH, Dixon N: *Measuring the Quality of Patient Care: The Rationale for Outcome Audit*. Cambridge, MA: Ballinger Publishing Co, 1976, pp 51–52 ff
19. Graham N: Criteria development. In *Quality Assurance in Hospitals*, N Graham, Editor. Rockville, MD: Aspen Systems Corp, 1982, pp 43–53
20. Williamson JW: *Assessing and Improving Health Care Outcomes: The Health Accounting Approach to Quality Assurance*. Cambridge, MA: Ballinger Publishing Co, 1978
21. Kellogg RL: The Comprehensive Quality Assurance System. In *Ambulatory Medical Care Quality Assurance*, GA Giebink, NH White, ES Short, Editors. LaJolla, CA: LaJolla Health Science Foundation, 1977, pp 141–167
22. Sanazaro PJ, Worth RM: Concurrent Quality Assurance in hospital care. *N Engl J Med* 298:1171–1177, 1978
23. Kaplan SH, Greenfield S: Criteria Mapping: Using logic in evaluation of processes of care. *QRB* 4(1):3–9, 1978
24. Craddick JW: The Medical Management System:

A professional liability warning medicine. *QRB* 5(4):2–8, 1979

25. Joint Commission on Accreditation of Hospitals: *The PEP Primer*. Chicago: Joint Commission on Accreditation of Hospitals, 1974
26. Pierson D: Periodic Medical Review (PMR). In *Marketing for Mental Health Service*, Winston WJ, Editor. New York: The Haworth Press Inc, 1984, pp 139–166
27. Mushlin AI, et al: Quality assurance in primary care: A strategy based on outcome assessment. *J Community Health* 3:292–305, 1978
28. Remmlinger E: Profile analysis. In *Quality Assurance in Hospitals*, N Graham, Editor. Rockville, MD: Aspen Systems Corp, 1982, pp 219–237
29. Lowe JA: Pasport. *QRB* 3(8):20–23, 1977
30. Gonnella JS, et al: Use of outcome measures in ambulatory care evaluation. In *Ambulatory Medical Care Quality Assurance*, GA Giebink, NH White, ES Short, Editors. LaJolla, CA: LaJolla Health Science Foundation, 1977, pp 91–125
31. Rutstein D, Berenberg W, Chalmers TC: Measuring the quality of medical care. *N Engl J Med* 294:582–588, 1976
32. Kessner DM, Kalk CE, Singer P: Assessing health quality: The case for Tracers. *N Engl J Med* 288:189–194, 1973
33. California Medical Association/California Hospital Association: *Educational Patient Care Audit Manual*. San Francisco: CMA/CHA, 1975
34. Williamson JW, Hudson JI, Nevins MM: *Principles of Quality Assurance and Cost Containment in Health Care*. San Francisco: Jossey-Bass Inc Publishers, 1982
35. Williamson JW, Ostrow PC, Braswell HR: *Health Accounting for Quality Assurance*. Rockville, MD: American Occupational Therapy Association, 1981
36. Kuntavanish AK, Ostrow PC: The outcomes of back conservation education. *QRB* 6:22–26, 1980
37. Ostrow PC, Kuntavanish AK: Improving the utilization of occupational therapy: A quality assurance study. *Am J Occup Ther* 37:388–391, 1983
38. Williamson JW, Ostrow PC: *Improving the Impact of Occupational Therapy*. Rockville, MD: American Occupational Therapy Association, 1980
39. Fifer W: Integrating quality assurance mechanisms. In *Organization and Change in Health Care Quality Assurance*, RD Luke, JC Krueger, RE Modrow, Editors. Rockville, MD: Aspen Systems Corp, 1983, pp 217–230
40. Rosenberg EW: What kind of criteria? *Med Care* 13:966–975, 1975
41. Luke RD, Boss RW: Barriers limiting the implementation of quality assurance programs. *Health Sci Res* 16:305–314, 1981
42. Kaye R: Quality assurance: A strategy for planned change. In *Organization and Change in Health Care Quality Assurance*, Luke RD, Krueger JC, Modrow RE, Editors. Rockville, MD: Aspen Systems Corp, 1983, pp 157–169

Section VII

Communicating

Chapter 15, the first of three chapters on the manager's role of communicating, addresses basic concepts and principles of effective one-to-one communication, be it manager to employee, manager to manager, or manager to superior. Communication is interpreted as an interactive process, rather than the mere imparting of facts, and the importance of feedback and clarification is stressed. To reinforce and illustrate its points, the chapter uses many examples and anecdotes, some humorous, some poignant. Attention is given to professional image and all the ways in which it is projected—for example, dress, office decor, and manager-employee relationships.

Chapter 16, "Targeting Communications," expands communication to creating an image for one's occupational therapy organization in particular and the profession in general. The chapter stresses the importance of defining the audience for a given communication and tailoring the communication to the needs and the interests of that audience. Two tables are included to aid managers in analyzing their publics and selecting appropriate methods of communication. Also, a sample promotion plan is developed around a hypothetical scenario.

Chapter 17 addresses the coupling of communication and facilitation skills in a particular model of practice, consultation. The model, which also calls for a strong clinical background and entrepreneurial talent, is particularly attractive in today's changing health care environment, as new and different opportunities open up for occupational therapy personnel.

Chapter 15

Principles of Communication

Elizabeth B. Devereaux,
MSW, ACSW, OTR/L, FAOTA

Meanings are not in words, meanings are in people, the saying goes. Therein lies the primary barrier to clear communication, for each person interprets the meanings of words in terms of his or her own unique life experiences. The sender of a message may intend to communicate something quite different from what is actually perceived by the receiver. True communication results in comprehension and understanding. Neither the sender nor the receiver of a message can assess the accuracy or the level of understanding until a dialogue ensues that includes feedback, clarification, and verification relative to intentions, perceptions, and comprehension.

THE STRUCTURE OF MEANING

When a word or a phrase is seen or heard, when a concept is expressed, people immediately try to make it fit with something they already know, so that they can understand it and put it in some perspective. If a person has never seen nor heard of a zebra, *zebra* is not in that person's structure

---

In her current position on the faculty of the department of psychiatry at Marshall University in Huntington, West Virginia, Elizabeth B. Devereaux teaches principles of communication daily to medical students, patients (individually and in groups), and staff. She has also studied communications as a graduate student and in continuing education experiences over the last 20 years. She is often called upon as a consultant in management communication.

of meaning. But if the person has seen a horse, and a zebra is described as an animal similar to a horse, but with black and white stripes on its body, the mental image evoked by the word *zebra* begins to approximate reality, and the person can respond to *zebra* with some comprehension. *Zebra* then is in that person's structure of meaning and would "fit" in his or her comprehension as "something like a horse with stripes."

However, if the horse with black and white stripes is in the person's image the height of a pony or a large draft horse rather than the four to four-and-one-half feet of the average zebra, the person has a distortion in perception of the intended message. This distortion is not critical to most people, but if the message is a program concept for which the receiver is to develop a written proposal, distortion can result in wasted time and frustration for both the sender and the receiver.

Generally speaking, the more varied life experiences and knowledge the receiver has, the more readily he or she can find a fit for the message, and the greater precision there will be in the integration. When the sender *and* the receiver have many life experiences in common, they more nearly speak the same language, and understanding is less cluttered with gaps or distortions of perception. Combs et al (1, p 249) explain,

> Communication is a function of common meanings, the overlapping of the perceptual fields of communicator and communicatee. It is a matter of acquiring common "maps" so that the meaning existing for one person may exist for the others as well . . . When meanings overlap we have the feeling of understanding or of being understood. When meanings fail to overlap, communications break down and misunderstandings occur.

An example follows of the kind of distortion and misunderstanding that can occur when meanings do not overlap and the receiver attempts to make information fit with what he or she already knows: A woman tearfully revealed to an occupational therapist friend that the doctor had diagnosed her illness as cystic fibrosis. On probing further, the friend learned that the doctor had actually said "fibrocystic disease."

Effects of Emotion

Because humans are all thinking *and* feeling beings, one or the other of these capacities sometimes gains ascendancy. When thinking (cognition) comes to the foreground, feeling (emotion) fades to the background, and vice versa. Communication between hierarchical levels, such as between manager and staff, often prompts emotion to move to the foreground. The closer the dialogue or situation moves to the individual's self-interest, the more the individual cares about the outcome and the more emotionally involved he or she becomes.

Professionals are familiar with the phenomenon of being quite able to problem-solve with friends and patients/clients, yet unable to do so for themselves. This reflects the distance-closeness quotient, or the amount of emotional investment. Communication to, with, or from a boss produces an increase in emotion in most people.

Emotion increases in response to threat, actual or perceived. As emotion increases, so does stress. Paradoxically, in stressful situations, when a person most needs to think clearly, the body's automatic physiological reaction called the stress response makes this least likely to happen. Basically, when it is threatened, the body prepares a "fight or flight" response. Verbal, logical, and analytical faculties give way to the brain's more primitive functions of organizing the musculoskeletal system for survival (2). This explains delayed brilliance, in which a person thinks of the perfect response fifteen minutes or so after a confrontation has ended.

Effects of Stress

Stress blocks communication. The greater the stress the receiver of a message is experiencing, the greater the deterrent to his or her hearing, integrating, and comprehending what the sender is saying. The message need not be a negative one to trigger the stress response because the body does not discriminate between good news and bad news in its initial response. When the body returns to a calmer state, generally within a few minutes, the brain is ready to process the message as usual.

Although this information has numerous implications for the everyday interactions of staff, it also has direct applicability to communications with patients/clients. The woman with "cystic fibrosis" is an example. When patients/clients are in pain, not feeling well, apprehensive about the unknown, in a strange treatment setting, or all the above, their ability to understand and retain instructions related to their treatment regimen may be impaired in varying degrees. This affects their compliance. To reinforce verbal instructions, patients/clients are often also given written instructions. This two-step system is generally helpful. However, in one primary care clinic where it was being used, it did not appreciably improve the compliance rate. The staff seemed startled when a consultant asked if their problem patients could read. Assuming that there is a comfortable relationship between a therapist and a patient/client, which also has a direct effect on patient compliance, a helpful technique for the therapist is to interrupt the discussion and ask what the patient/client has heard, or to ask that instructions be repeated or demonstrated. This works best when it is done periodically throughout the session rather than at the end.

Effects of Threat

Sometimes a person's perception of the message he or she is being given is distorted because he or she feels threatened by some aspect of the interchange. It does not matter if the threat is real or imagined. The individual's defense mechanisms are aroused by the sense of threat. He or she begins to defend his or her position and hears only what he or she wants to hear. If the sender of the message responds in like fashion, the dialogue will escalate, until both are defending their narrow positions and neither really hears the other. People who are threatened are very emotionally involved in their position and are saying, in essence, "Don't bother me with the facts!" They resist any information that does not agree with their perceptions. This is a time to remember that one cannot deal rationally with irrational people.

Use of Another's System and Language

In attempting to create understanding through communication, it is necessary to address an individual's system, in his or her own language. To enhance communication, an example or an anecdote can be used, or a situation can be discussed symbolically. For instance, if a staff member's rigid personality is interfering with his or her job performance, and that staff member has skill in constructing splints, the supervisor might begin a discussion of the situation by asking the staff member to explain why splints are not worn twenty-four hours a day, but removed periodically. The discussion can then be continued using the splinting process symbolically in relation to the personality issue. In addition, many a tense situation has been defused, many a point has been made, through the use of a story, particularly a humorous one.

TIMING AND LEVELS

With the information explosion affecting every aspect of life, it is important to distinguish between communication and information. Drucker maintains that "communication and information are different and indeed largely opposite—yet interdependent. Where communication is perception, information is logic. As such, information is purely formal and has no meaning. It is impersonal rather than interpersonal" (3, p 487). Communication deals with factors such as feelings, values, expectations, and perceptions, which demand that the individual believe or do something or become a particular kind of person. Information at its purest is factual, specific, without the human qualities inherent in communication (3).

The Need to Know and Timing

A manager may think he or she is communicating with a coworker when in fact the manager is merely imparting information. The manager may give the message too fast, may say too much, or may discuss a subject that is not relevant to the immediacy of the need to know. In such cases the receiver will block the information out completely or give it brief attention then ignore it, but not retain it. For instance, if a therapist is reviewing equipment catalogs to select the most appropriate feeding aids for a particular patient/client, a simultaneous discussion of psychotropic medications is unlikely to penetrate his or her concentration barrier.

Another example relates to the numerous tire ads that appear in almost every newspaper. One barely registers their presence until one has to buy tires. Then there is an immediate need to know the information provided in the ads.

Sensitivity to the timing of communication is also important to its effectiveness. For example, on the morning before she had to teach an afternoon class, a faculty member in the occupational therapy department neither received nor responded to communication. However, after the class she was very relaxed, attentive, and receptive to problem solving or other types of communication.

A very effective learning experience for many seventh- and eighth-grade students occurred some years ago during a two-year experiment in Parkersburg, West Virginia. The students participated in a program called Integrated Studies, in which all courses related to common themes. For instance, for a while, the theme was early state history. In art class, students were expected to make scale drawings of one of the state's historic mansions. To do so, they needed the math they were learning. In history class they read books on the development of science in the state, so that in science class they could replicate the experiments. The speed and pacing of communication and information were determined by their need to know. Unfortunately this is not often true in the average work setting, but occupational therapists have the knowledge and skills to structure such an experience in their work setting as well as in patient/client task-centered groups.

With today's information explosion and resulting information overload, it is remarkable that humans do not experience "data arrest" as well as cardiac arrest. A manager can control much of the pressure from information overload by attention to the immediacy of the need to know, the speed and spacing of communication and information, and sensitivity to others' ability to process messages. One person may thrive on juggling and processing six projects at once; another may need to focus on a project at a time to work most effectively.

Qualities of a Good Communicator

According to Bandler and Grinder in their book about neurolinguistic programming, *Frogs into Princes*, one needs three abilities to be a good communicator:

1. "You must know what outcome you want."
2. "You must have flexibility in your behavior. You need to be able to generate lots and lots of different behaviors to find out what responses you get."
3. "You need to have enough sensory experience to notice when you get the responses that you want."

"If you have those three abilities, then you can just alter your behavior until you get the responses that you want" (4, pp. 54–55).

An additional quality that affects communication is intensity, which is expressed in the *amount* of emotion included. Enthusiasm, love, hate, anger, irritation, caring, disagreement are but a few examples of the emotions expressed through intensity and the gradations of intensity that are possible in communicating. Intensity may also be expressed in tone of voice and amount of time spent talking with someone.

Nonverbal Language

People often assume that others experience various emotions the same way they do, and they try to understand others through themselves. This can be an erroneous assumption. Emotional reaction is related to basic personality type. One person may react to his or her anger with a flood of feeling and have to fight tears, whereas another person may shut off all feeling and become icy calm. Such differences in reaction may be most apparent in an individual's nonverbal communication. Are there discrepancies between what a person is saying and the look in his or her eyes? Is the person making eye contact or avoiding it? Is the person smiling, expressing pleasure with a new job assignment, yet clenching his or her fists? Many books have been written about body language and nonverbal communication that may be helpful to read.

TWO-WAY COMMUNICATION

Communicating understanding is the responsibility of the sender of a message. If the receiver does not understand, the sender must express the message another way—for example, demonstrate it or use an example. But communication is an interaction, so the sender must receive feedback from the receiver(s), in the form of dialogue or body language, to gauge the reception of the message. The receiver has the responsibility to clarify the message with replies such as "I'm not sure I understand what you're saying," "Could you say that another way?" or "Could you give me an example?" Paraphrasing the message also helps to clarify it: "Are you saying that . . .?" If the receiver does not take the responsibility of checking his or her understanding of the message, the sender should not assume that understanding has occurred, or interpret feedback, without verifying it. The sender could respond, "You look puzzled. Would you like me to say it another way?" This kind of comment gives the receiver the opportunity to agree with or to correct the sender with a reply such as "I'm *not* puzzled by your message, but I *am* puzzled about how your plan would work."

Closing the Communication Loop

One of the problems in communications, particularly in organizations, is that often a communicator (frequently a manager) is so absorbed in sending a message that he or she gives little or no attention to what employees need to know, want to know, or are interested in. An effective communicator/manager solicits this information from subordinates as well as bosses. Messages from the top down, from a manager to subordinates, are simply that—messages. No communication occurs, as understanding is created through interaction. Open communication channels emphasize messages being sent from the bottom upward, and the manager's responding, thus avoiding one-way communication and closing the communication loop. An effective manager encourages open communication and listens and responds to employees' suggestions and complaints.

Drucker (3) says that when a manager makes a decision, organized feedback through the communication channels is needed in the form of reports and figures, but these alone are not enough. The manager must also check the data by talking with the staff and observing for himself or herself. A manager should not rely for accurate feedback on the employee to whom an assignment was given. It is not that the manager should not trust the employee; the manager should distrust the employee's perceptions; and thus the accuracy and reality of the communication. This is akin to the concept of "management by walking about" or "management by wandering around" described by Peters and Waterman in their book about the best-run companies in America (5, p 122).

Opening Communication Channels

Opening communication channels by making information about a system readily available can also facilitate decision making by those lower in the hierarchy. The people who work in a system need to know its characteristics. Information such as salary ranges, meeting minutes, budgets, and the laws of responsibility for various decisions is knowledge essential to staff if the manager wants their help and their commitment to making the system work. Often this type of information seems to be withheld for no good reason (6). "*Access to operating data* and formerly restricted information is a must, furthermore, for any decentralized or team-oriented system" (6, p 279).

COMMUNICATING VALUES

"Values are beliefs, preferences, or assumptions about what is desirable or good for man. An example is the belief that society has an obligation to help each individual realize his fullest potential. They are not assertions about how the world is and what we know about it, but how it *should* be" (7, p 38). Just as individuals have values, so do systems or organizations and professions. One of occupational therapy's values has always been the belief expressed in the preceding quotation. Occupational therapists reflect their belief in that value every day in their work with patients/clients and also when they request payment for the treatment they provide. They would be communicating disbelief in that value if they labeled a patient/client hopeless. Hopeless in relation to what? At an Easter Seal Center in Parkersburg, West Virginia, one of the greatest obstacles the occupational therapy staff had to overcome was when parents would bring their child for treatment and say, "Doctor so-and-so told us our child was hopeless." The manager's standard reply was, "Hopeless for what? If we can help your child learn to sit up, isn't that hope? If we can help your child learn to dress and feed herself, isn't that hope? May be she will never be President of the United States, but there is definitely hope that she can do some things she is not doing now, and that is worth our working on."

Organizations have values, although they are not always articulated. These values constantly serve as reference points for decision making, whether the decisions are big or little, and are most effective when everyone involved in an organization knows what they are. If an organizational value is that of providing quality care to patients/clients at the lowest possible cost, then a purchasing agent knows to order not the lowest-cost supplies, but the lowest-cost supplies that contribute to quality care. Similarly a physician in this system knows to request no laboratory test without justification, but to ask for any tests that are clearly needed. Each decision made consistent with a value of the organization reinforces that value throughout the organization and to that organization's public.

STYLE OF COMMUNICATING

A manager's style of communicating is influenced by many factors, such as his or her personality, his or her approach to management, the organizational structure, the physical environment, and the size, complexity, culture, and values of the organization. Most of these subjects are addressed in greater detail in other chapters in this book. Some brief comments about the ways in which such factors may enhance or block communication are appropriate here. A much fuller treatment of the subject can be found in an outstanding book, *In Search of Excellence: Lessons from America's Best-Run Companies* by Peters and Waterman (5). It is basically a book about the process and results of facilitating organizational communications.

Formal and Informal Communications

Both formal and informal communications are needed in any organization. A manager must decide which communications should be formal and which informal on the basis of the outcome desired. For example, if a system operates with management by objectives, formal communications would be used to disseminate the objectives. They need to be written and widely distributed so that all employees know what they are and can measure progress toward their achievement. In the same system, however, a manager with an informal communication style might create a small task group to address a problem, to discuss its recommendations with him or her, to get verbal modifications of its plan, and then to try the plan. In a formal system this same group would have to write a report to the manager and await a written reply before acting. In either type of system, however, the task group might be composed of those who have the power to implement the changes directly.

The point is that there are many different configurations for problem solving and decision making. An organization or a communication system works best when each situation is analyzed as possibly different from the others and the management style is flexible enough to deal with it differently. If a situation is important enough to be studied, action should follow the study.

Physical and Other Barriers to Effective Communication

Occupational therapists are very knowledgeable about analyzing and altering physical structures and architectural barriers so that the physically handicapped can function in a given space. Using those same skills to identify and alter physical and procedural barriers to communication in one's work setting can support efforts to create an open, informal communication system. Are the desks or offices of staff who need to confer regularly adjacent? Must staff always make an appointment through the secretary to see the manager?

Culture of an Organization

The culture of an organization reflects ideas and customs that have developed over time, and it often sanctions behaviors that are accepted and expected. It is probably not policy but organizational culture that "the women never wear slacks here" or "the men always wear ties." Culture may dictate that one always go through the chain of command with an issue rather than going directly to the person who has the information one seeks. The most elementary mode of informal communication, the gossip network, is probably culturally derived in organizations. Certainly the peer culture sustains it, and its level of accuracy is generally very high.

EFFECTIVE COMMUNICATION

Blocks to Communication

Most people like to talk with others to whom they do not have to explain things, with whom they have something in common. When occupational therapy personnel talk among themselves, they can use jargon as shortcuts to communication and be confident that they are understood. However, when they use occupational therapy jargon with someone else, it becomes a block to communication.

Several barriers or blocks to communication are discussed earlier in this chapter. Another category is "put-offs" or excluding behavior. People are sometimes unaware of it. When an employee goes into a manager's office to talk, does the manager go on writing or doing whatever he or she was doing and keep glancing at the clock? Does the manager take any telephone calls that come through? If so, the manager is saying to the employee that *anyone* else is more deserving of the manager's time and attention. Such behavior also creates an awkward situation for the employee, who does not know whether to exit discreetly or stay when the manager takes a call.

There are just a few examples of excluding behavior, which can be modified for a more satisfactory outcome. For example, if a visit is unexpected, the manager might stop what he or she is doing, welcome the visitor, say right away that he or she has *x* minutes until the next appointment or meeting, then ask the secretary to signal at the end of that time, or set a timer.

Red Flags

Another area that warrants careful monitoring is "red flag" issues or phrases. "You must" or "you will" are often red flag phrases. With some thought, the point can be stated another way that is less anger producing. When people are angry, they do not hear. Managers can often defuse red flag issues by discussing them very openly and calmly before they are brought up by staff in anger. Generally, red flag issues provoke anger because they produce fear or in some way threaten individuals or groups. They are frequently a mixture of fact and rumor.

Missing the Level of Communication

Missing the level of communication is also a barrier to understanding. A mental image of this block is that of one person sending a message straight to a second person, and the second person sending a reply that goes into left field. For example, if a person says something like "My dog just died," and the reply is, "How's the weather outside?" the reply missed the level of communication in the message. Communication is enhanced when the reply is on the same emotional level as the message.

FACILITATING COMMUNICATION

In communicating, sending clear messages is not enough. Careful listening and responding are necessary to create understanding and convey comprehension.

The Art of Listening

Much has been written about the art of listening. Just a few comments are made here. When an employee knows that he or she has the complete attention of a manager, that the manager is focusing on his or her message, then the employee feels that what he or she has to say is important and that he or she as a person is important. This feeling leads to a relaxing of barriers and more open communication. Such listening by a manager also involves hearing the feelings *behind* the words, because sometimes words and feelings do not match; they are incongruent. For true communication to occur, it is occasionally necessary to ignore the stated content and instead to study facial expressions and gestures and the tone of words.

Dealing with the Feelings Behind the Words

Most people have had the experience of attending a meeting at which decisions are made, leaving the meeting, and finding participants clustered in small groups discussing and disagreeing with the decisions. In group decision making, dealing with the *emotions* attached to issues is necessary to reach decisions that most participants will back. The communication within a group needs to be safe enough and open enough for people to express in a meeting what they say so eloquently in the halls.

Hidden Agendas/Messages

"He's not talking about what he's talking about" captures the sense of a listener's frustration at the circuitous remarks of someone who has a hidden agenda or a hidden message. This happens most often in meetings and sometimes can be spotted when a person keeps hammering at the same issue but never quite comes to the point. Careful listening and attention to the phrases the person keeps coming back to often enable the listener to realize what the real message is.

If nobody is making mistakes in a system, then nothing is happening. For an organization to grow, people need to take risks, try new approaches, attempt fresh ways of solving problems. Open communication helps to keep risks and mistakes manageable. "Management by walking about" (5, p 122) is a very useful technique in this regard.

COMMUNICATING A PROFESSIONAL IMAGE

In all areas of communication, a manager should be a professional communicator and strive to communicate that he or she is a professional. Part of being a professional is being responsible for one's lifelong education. Besides books and articles, many educational courses, seminars, and workshops can assist a professional in refining his or her skills as a manager and a communicator. "Communication in organization . . . is not a *means* of organization. It is the mode of organization" (3, p 493).

Words are one type of symbol used to communicate; bumper stickers, dress, behavior, and letters are some others. Managers must be concerned with developing, maintaining, and projecting a professional image. All behavior is motivated; it is not accidental.

Choice of dress communicates many messages, some subtle and some not so subtle. People tend to use clothes to say, "This is who I am," "This is how I feel about myself." In health care,

> uniforms are tempting. Rather than agonize "Is this appropriate?" it's easier to slip into something prescribed, be it blue pinstripe or blue denim . . . however, professional no longer means impersonal. As we rise in the corporate ranks, we are realizing that "what's right for the office" is what's right for our style—our own style (8, p 65).

There is no single set of rules for appropriate dress at the office. The only good guideline is the kind of image one wants to project. If that is a professional image, one's appearance should be consistent with it.

The professional image that one projects extends to tone of voice and telephone manners. It also extends to one's office, verbal and written reports, letters, and supervisor-employee relationships. A manager's office can express his or her tastes and still be an office. Even if everyone with the same status has identical furniture, a few pictures, plants, and desk accessories can reflect an individual's image and make the office a more comfortable place in which to work. Everyone has more papers than he or she can hide most of the time, but a cluttered office may project the image of a cluttered mind, of indecisiveness and inattention to details, even though this may not necessarily be true.

The content of reports and letters is discussed in Chapter 16. It is important to remember that the appearance of these items ". . . contributes greatly to the attention the report is given" (9, p 818). Also, missing dates, improper headings, lack of identification of the author, and similar oversights or errors cause enough difficulty when reports and letters are fresh. They may be extremely problematic five years later when the correct information is critical. If a message is sufficiently important to put in writing, doing it properly is worth the extra time.

The manager-employee relationship is different from a peer relationship. The manager must keep at least a fine line between himself or herself and staff. This can be communicated by dress and behavior as well as through decision making and other responsibilities. The relationship can be comfortable, but being a manager is not the same as being an equal member of the group.

SUMMARY

True communication results in comprehension and understanding. Neither the sender nor the receiver of a message can assess the accuracy or the level of understanding until a dialogue ensues that includes feedback, clarification, and verification relative to intentions, perceptions, and comprehension.

When people hear or see a word, they try to make it fit with something they already know. The more and the more varied life experiences and knowledge a person has, the more readily he or she can find a fit for a word or a message. When the sender and the receiver of a message have many life experiences in common, they more nearly speak the same language, and understanding is less cluttered with gaps or distortions of perception.

Emotions affect communications, especially between hierarchical levels, such as between manager and staff. Emotion increases in response to threat, actual or perceived. As emotion increases, so does stress. Stress too blocks communication.

In attempting to create understanding through communication, it is necessary to address an individual's system, in his or her own language. Examples, anecdotes, symbolism, and humor can help accomplish this and enhance communication.

It is important to distinguish between communication and information. Communication deals with factors such as feelings, values, expectations, and perceptions, which demand that the individual believe or do something or become a particular kind of person. Information at its purest is factual, specific, without the human qualities inherent in communication.

The immediacy of the need to know and timing are important variables in communication. A manager can control much of the pressure from information overload by attention to immediacy of the need to know, the speed and pacing of communication and information, and sensitivity to others' ability to process messages.

To be a good communicator, a manager must know what outcome he or she wants, be able to generate many different behaviors, and have enough sensory experience to notice when he or she gets the desired response. The response may be nonverbal as well as verbal. Nonverbal communication provides important cues to what a person is truly feeling.

Communication is an interaction, so the sender must receive feedback from the receiver to gauge the reception of the message. An effective manager pays attention to what employees need or want to know. Open communication channels emphasize messages being sent from the bottom upward, and the manager's responding, thus avoiding one-way communication from the top down. Making information about an organization readily available also keeps communication channels open and facilitates decision making by those lower in the hierarchy.

Just as individuals have values, so do systems or organizations and professions. An organization's values constantly serve as reference points for decision making.

A manager's style of communicating is influenced by many factors, such as his or her personality, his or her approach to management, the organizational structure, the physical environment, the size, complexity, culture, and values of the organization. Both formal and informal communications are needed in any organization. A manager must decide which communications should be formal and which informal on the basis of the outcome desired.

The use of jargon is often a barrier to communication. So is excluding behavior, such as a manager's taking telephone calls when an employee has come in to talk. Red flag phrases or issues can provoke anger. Sometimes the receiver misses the level of communication in the sender's message.

Careful listening requires giving complete attention to the speaker and also being alert to the feelings behind the words. In group decision making, dealing with the emotions attached to issues is necessary to reach decisions that most group members will back. Hidden agendas can often be detected through close attention to words and gestures.

Managers must be concerned with developing, maintaining, and projecting a professional image. This is accomplished through dress, voice, telephone manners, the appearance of one's office, verbal and written reports, letters, and supervisor-employee relationships.

References

1. Combs A, Avila D, Purkey W: *Helping Relationships: Basic Concepts for the Helping Professions*. Boston: Allyn & Bacon Inc, 1971, p 249
2. Albrecht K: *Stress and the Manager: Making It Work for You*. Englewood Cliffs, NJ: Prentice-Hall Inc, 1979, pp 74–75
3. Drucker P: *Management: Tasks, Responsibilities, Practices*. New York: Harper & Row Publishers Inc, 1973, pp 480, 487–488, 493
4. Bandler R, Grinder J: *Frogs into Princes: Neuro Linguistic Programming*. Moab, UT: Real People Press, 1979, pp 54–55
5. Peters T, Waterman R: *In Search of Excellence: Lessons from America's Best-Run Companies*. New York: Warner Books Inc, 1982, p 122
6. Kanter R: *Men and Women of the Corporation*. New York: Basic Books Inc, 1977, pp 278–279
7. Pincus A, Minahan A: *Social Work Practice: Model and Method*. Itasca, IL: FE Peacock Publishers Inc, 1973, p 38
8. Segal A, Sutton T: Ready to wear. *Savvy*, September 1984, p 65
9. Baum C: Management of finances, communications, personnel, with resources and documentation. In *Willard and Spackman's Occupational Therapy*, 6th edition, H Hopkins, H Smith, Editors. Philadelphia: JB Lippincott Co, 1983, p 818

Additional Resources

Berne E: *Games People Play: The Psychology of Human Relationships*. New York: Grove Press Inc, 1964

Blanchard K, Johnson S: *The One Minute Manager*. New York: Berkley Publishing Corp, 1981

Bramson R: *Coping With Difficult People*. Garden City, NY: Anchor Press/Doubleday & Co Inc, 1981

Howard J: *Please Touch*. New York: McGraw-Hill Book Co, 1970

Jourard S: *The Transparent Self*, 2nd edition. New York: Van Nostrand Reinhold Co, 1971

Rogers C: *Freedom to Learn*. Columbus, OH: Charles E Merrill Publishing Co, 1969

Rogers C: *On Becoming a Person*. Boston: Houghton Mifflin Co, 1970

Stevens J: *Awareness: Exploring, Experimenting, Experiencing*. Moab, UT: Real People Press, 1971

Chapter 16

Targeting Communications

Wendy Krupnick, MBA, OTR

Communicating successfully with a mechanic, an accountant, or a bank loan officer can be difficult and is often further complicated by the use of jargon. Mechanics speak in terms of plugs, points, and batteries; accountants in terms of interest rates and negative amortization; and loan officers in terms of credit history and payback periods. The consumer ends up with a large car bill for service he or she cannot understand, or a bank loan whose interest rate never seems to stop changing.

The key to successful communication is being able to deliver a message in a form that is meaningful to its audience. The message should be packaged in language that attracts attention and has meaning for the recipient. Demands on the profession and within the present health environment require the ability to communicate effectively with a diverse number of audiences. Occupational therapy personnel do not operate in a vacuum. As professionals within a large health care system, they must be able to deliver their message to physicians, administrators, insurance providers, patients/clients, and families.

To ensure that a message is understood, the sender must segment the audience into smaller publics or targets (to the extent that this is possible). Each target should consist of homogeneous segments of the larger

---

Before joining AOTA's staff as the director of public affairs, Wendy Krupnick had several years of business development experience in the private sector and, before that, experience as a clinician. Her master's degree is in marketing.

audience. This segmentation allows the structuring of the message to meet the information needs of each target. For maximum impact the target's background, interests, and needs should be taken into consideration.

For example, an occupational therapy manager is interested in increasing referrals to the occupational therapy department in a teaching hospital. He or she targets physicians as potential referral sources. To convey the merits of occupational therapy adequately, he or she needs to segment physicians further into pediatricians, neurologists, orthopedic surgeons, and residents. Each group has specific information needs and concerns that can be addressed in different ways. A pediatrician needs to know which children may benefit from occupational therapy intervention, what difference intervention can make with these children, the kinds of evaluations an occupational therapist performs, the scope of an occupational therapist's knowledge about development, and the recommended frequency of treatment. A resident may need to know about the occupational therapy staff's credentials, scope of practice, and skills for treating a variety of patient/client populations.

Although the ultimate message is that occupational therapy is cost-effective, the delivery of that message must be customized so that each target pays attention and makes referrals. After delivering the message, it is important to get feedback from the targeted group to determine if the message was received as it was intended. Individuals listen to and remember only that which is relevant to them, either personally or professionally. The occupational therapy manager's job is to make occupational therapy relevant to many targets.

MAKING COMMUNICATIONS WORK

Defining the Message

One of the important responsibilities that an occupational therapy manager has is ensuring that the department or program functions at a productive capacity, provides quality services, and is respected by other health professionals. (This is true for members of the staff as well as for managers.) The relationship that one establishes with members of the health team will influence the reputation of the occupational therapy organization. The objective, of course, is to influence health professionals positively by presenting accurate, timely, and relevant information on a regular basis.

For example, a manager is interested in increasing the number of referrals for occupational therapy. He or she notes that several types of patients/clients could benefit from occupational therapy but are not referred, and that some referrals come right before a patient/client is scheduled for discharge. The manager has to convince several groups within the hospital system that patients/clients and referral sources would benefit from occupational therapy. The success of the plan depends on what is said, to whom, and when.

The manager's first step is to gather information from other health team members to strengthen his or her position. The department's statistics on use should be helpful at this stage, that is, the number of patients/clients evaluated, the number treated, the number on waiting lists, the number discharged to home health, and so forth. The information the manager wants from other health professionals includes their perception of what occupational therapists do, their opinion of how well it is done, the kinds of patients/clients who were and were not referred for occupational therapy, the length of stay of those individuals, and readmission rates. Once the manager has these data, he or she can identify the problem and its cause, and work toward developing a sound strategy. In this case the manager needs to determine why the department is not getting referrals and to consider whether lack of information about the types of patients/clients who are treated in occupational therapy contributes to the problem.

The challenge to the manager is to convey specific information to several groups so that the result is overwhelming support of his or her position. Of course, he or she has to address the target's needs, the value individuals place on the goals set in occupational therapy, and their willingness to work with occupational therapy staff in establishing a mutually beneficial relationship. Information needs to be presented in a way that is most useful to the particular public being addressed. In other words, it is important to demonstrate to referral sources that occupational therapy intervention can benefit patients/clients; to the nursing team that occupational therapy assists a patient/client in becoming independent; to hospital administrators that occupational therapy helps in the early discharge of patients/clients and can continue in the home setting; and finally, to all, that occupational therapy works.

Defining Occupational Therapy's Publics

The art of successful communication relies heavily on presenting the right message to the right public. As professionals, occupational therapy personnel should identify the diverse groups to which they must appeal and recognize that they need to communicate to these groups in different ways.

For example, *patients/clients* can be segmented into two groups: current and potential. Current patients/clients need to know what occupational therapy can help them accomplish. Members of the community or potential patients/clients need consumer information on specific areas of occupational therapy practice, such as stroke, arthritis, developmental disabilities, and mental health. Providing them with this information will stimulate awareness of the role of occupational therapy and enhance the potential referral network.

Referral sources are another public that can benefit from information. They need to know how occupational therapy can help affect the early recovery of specific patients/clients. Other health team members, in particular, should be helped to understand why a timely occupational therapy consultation is useful.

Administrators are concerned with revenue and need statistics on the length of stay, cost of service, quantity of treatment, and capability of occupational therapy to generate income.

Insurance providers work with information regarding the cost effectiveness of occupational therapy and its record in reducing the number of readmissions.

Principals and *school superintendents* need to know how occupational therapy enhances learning for handicapped or learning-disabled children, and enables them to benefit from the educational system.

Legislators and other public officials who influence legislation and regulations affecting occupational therapy are an important target. These officials should be made aware that occupational therapy helps return disabled people to work, thus reducing their dependence on public funds and increasing their contribution to society.

In general, in defining a particular target or public, one should think about three issues:

- What action he or she wants from that public;
- What information or action that public wants from occupational therapy;
- What means of communication is best for reaching that public.

Table 1 presents analyses of three publics in terms of these issues.

SELECTING COMMUNICATION METHODS

Communication between occupational therapy personnel and other members of the health care system is critical to the growth and acceptance of the profession. Through exchange of information and ideas with other groups, occupational therapy personnel gain the exposure that is necessary for achieving understanding, awareness, and respect.

Selecting the appropriate method of communication largely depends on the message and the public. Communication can be formal, as in letters and reports, or informal, as in displays and conversation. Every method has its positive and negative characteristics. One should choose the method that best suits his or her needs.

Many avenues of communication are open to therapists. Sometimes an informal phone call will suit their needs. A phone call provides immediate feedback, although the message can easily be forgotten. Contact by letter is more formal and furnishes written documentation of the communication. However, it does not allow for immediate feedback nor does it ensure that the message was actually delivered to the individual for whom it was intended.

Table 2 is a checklist that categorizes the most frequently used communication methods and indicates their various uses. Some methods are better for reaching targeted audiences, whereas others are useful for distributing general information.

Internal Communication

Internal communication generally refers to communication among people within an organization. It can take place over lunch, at an exercise class, on the way to a meeting, or in the parking lot. Interactions at such moments help to build support systems and are often more important than external communications. The image of a department or a program depends on the effectiveness of its internal communications. For ex-

TABLE 16–1
Analyzing Occupational Therapy's Publics

Public	What Occupational Therapy Providers Want from the Public	What the Public Wants from Occupational Therapy Providers	Communication Method
Referral source	• Steady referral base • Appropriate types of referrals • Good working relationship • Good understanding of occupational therapy	• Timely scheduling of patients/clients • Effective treatment techniques • Current treatment methods • Caring, professional environment • Communication concerning individual's progress	• Written progress and discharge notes • Open houses • Fact sheets/ brochures • Observation of individuals during therapy • In-service presentations • Phone calls • Rounds • Case conferences
Patient/client	• Understanding of occupational therapy treatment • Potential referrals	• Prompt professional care • Methods of coping with pain, fear, and disability • Identification of support groups and resources • Caring and courteous attitude • Accessible and cost-effective treatment • Efficient use of time	• Educational forums • Orientation programs • Open houses • Media coverage • Fact sheets/ brochures • Therapeutic relationship, one-to-one communication
Community	• Public support and understanding • Use of occupational therapy consultant services to develop/improve community resources	• Meeting of community's therapy and education needs	• Participation in community events • Health fairs • Talks at civic and senior citizens meetings • Open houses • Media coverage • Educational forums • Volunteering • Communication through family of patient/client

Note: From Public Relations: A valuable and inexpensive tool! *Course of Action*, May 1984. © 1984 by Sherry Reed. Reprinted, with adaptations, by permission of the publisher. (Address: 2420 Brookside Way, Carson City, NV 89701)

TABLE 16–2
Sample Checklist for Assessing Communication Methods

	General Occupational Therapy Information	Information About Specific Occupational Therapy Service	Teaching Opportunity	Public Information/ Awareness	Personal Contact
Types of Internal Communication					
• Organization's employee newsletter	X			X	
• Organization open house	X			X	X
• Inservice training, seminars, workshops		X	X	X	X
• Progress notes, memos, reports		X		X	
• Case conferences		X	X		X
• Participation in activities sponsored by organization	X			X	X
Types of External Communication					
• Organization's community newsletter	X			X	
• Annual reports		X		X	
• Suburban newspapers	X			X	
• Direct mail		X		X	
• Seminars/workshops		X	X	X	X
• Health fairs and exhibits	X			X	X
• Scholarly articles		X	X	X	
• Participation in community/charitable/religious organizations (newsletters, fund-raisers, volunteer program)	X			X	X
• Guest speeches at community programs	X	X	X	X	X
• Presentations at professional conferences		X	X	X	
• Speakers bureau		X	X	X	X
• Personal visits	X		X	X	X

ample, with effective internal communications, other staff members, including the receptionist, would know something as simple, yet vital, as the location of the occupational therapy department.

The staff of an educational or health care organization have many commonalities. Thus, numerous opportunities are available to build rapport, share information, and educate others about the world of occupational therapy.

Internal Communication Methods

An organization's employee newsletter. An employee newsletter provides many opportunities for sharing information about occupational therapy with colleagues. Such a newsletter is distributed to all staff, from support to technical to professional. Consequently information must be general in nature, have major public appeal, and be interesting to read. The idea is to attract attention to occupational therapy programs. For example, an article might describe occupational therapy in terms of patient/client successes, new equipment or services, new staff, clinic activities, or available in-service materials. Pictures of staff engaged in activities with patients/clients might be included. Help in writing or placing an article can usually be obtained from an organization's public relations or personnel department, whichever is responsible for employee relations.

An organization open house. The open house is another way to display the whys and hows of occupational therapy. The audience will comprise persons passing by who stop because the occupational therapy display attracts their attention. Once they have stopped, more detailed information can be offered. An open house provides personal contact and allows information exchange. Some excellent methods of describing occupational therapy include posters depicting occupational therapy practice, statistics on the kinds of patients/clients treated in occupational therapy, and displays of treatment modalities and equipment with the reasons why particular activities were selected. To get the most attention, information should be simple, in lay terms, and illustrated graphically as often as possible.

In-service training, seminars, and workshops. Continuing education programs allow specific information on occupational therapy to be delivered to a targeted group. Occupational therapy personnel can volunteer to present a topic and invite individuals who would benefit from and be interested in the information. Topics can range from occupational therapy evaluations for a psychiatric patient/client to the care and treatment of burn patients. Each topic should be tailored to the projected audience's needs and designed to educate participants on the benefits of occupational therapy to their patients/clients. In this way you can depend on having the audience's individual attention and can more thoroughly cover a topic. Advanced preparation and time are required, but once the materials are collected, the program can be repeated, with modifications for different audiences.

Progress notes, memos, and reports. These types of communication tools also provide information about occupational therapy to those who read them. Progress notes should be concise and descriptive so that the reader understands the purpose, the method, and the results of the occupational therapy intervention. Ideally written after each treatment, they should, over time, serve to document change in a patient's/client's condition. Memos should be short and have a clear objective—for example, responding to a request, confirming a meeting, outlining the results of a meeting, informing people about new staff and practice hours, or announcing new services.

Reports are good tools for making the administration aware of occupational therapy services. For instance, a manager might write a report about the growth of the occupational therapy department over the last six months or about the outcomes of an occupational therapy in-service program for teachers. Reports should always begin with an introductory paragraph and then proceed to specific information. Content might cover the number of referrals received each month, the types of referrals in relation to the length of patient/client treatment, and the revenue generated by the program versus the cost of services (staff salaries, equipment, etc.). The report should conclude with a summary of the essential points for people to remember. These might include a statement identifying occupational therapy as one of the important factors in reducing readmission rates or further disability.

Case conferences. In case conferences occupational therapy personnel report on patient/client progress more comprehensively than they do in progress notes. These conferences provide opportunities to describe occupational therapy principles to other health personnel and to members of the patient's/client's family, and to educate them about occupational therapy's benefits.

Participation in activities sponsored by the organization. One way of getting recognition for a department or a program is to participate in volunteer efforts sponsored by the organization, such as fund drives, talent shows, and community service projects. Working with others provides an opportunity for informal dialogue. People assume different roles and relate to one another as peers collaborating on a task. Conversation can turn to occupational therapy's relationship to the project or its role in the organization. Either way, this informal method will make a lasting impression because of the personal contact.

External Communication

Contact with individuals outside an organization is defined as external communication. Some of the characteristics associated with internal communication apply to external communication. One of the main differences is a focus on the profession of occupational therapy rather than on an occupational therapy department or program. Many opportunities are available for influencing people's perceptions and generally raising the public's awareness of the existence and the need for occupational therapy. Through external communication the profession can be promoted in the community.

External Communication Methods

An organization's community newsletter. This publication is distributed to people who reside within an organization's service area. Included are current and potential patients/clients, members of the business community, educators, community leaders, and general residents of the community. Just as in an organization's employee newsletter, the information in this publication must be general in order to appeal to its diverse audiences. These audiences relate best to stories about people or to information that may be personally useful, such as parenting hints, screening information for school-age children, and tips on dealing with holiday stress.

An organization may produce other publications targeted at the community, such as information brochures about services and announcements about community education opportunities. Therapists can volunteer to present consumer information in these publications about an area of occupational therapy practice such as learning disabilities, stroke, or stress management. This will enhance both the organization's and occupational therapy's community image.

Annual reports. Such reports provide opportunities to highlight a department's or program's strengths. An annual report can record the past, interpret the present, and project the future. It can identify trends and reinforce a department's image. An organization's annual report is distributed to many publics, most often to representatives of the community. The manager should make sure that occupational therapy is mentioned in it, either by picture and caption or written paragraph. The report provides an opportunity to highlight new equipment, services, clubs (such as a stroke club for patients/clients and their families).

Suburban newspapers. These have the highest readership of all newspapers. That is, more people read more of the information in these publications than in major city and daily newspapers. Suburban newspapers are also community oriented and eager to print information about local people and businesses. Particulars about activities to which the public is invited (such as open houses and health fairs in malls) should be provided to these papers. Additionally, they should be notified about staff changes and promotions and occupational therapists' presentations at conferences or seminars. Suburban newspapers also feature stories on businesses, organizations, and service programs. They are ideal for reporting exceptional patient/client success stories. Through this medium occupational therapy practices and purposes can be described in a way that easily captures the public's interest.

Direct mail. This term is applied to the targeted distribution of information via the mail. For example, if a department wants to expand its occupational therapy services to include evaluation and treatment of learning-disabled children, information about the new service would be distributed to the people who might make referrals. This could be in the form of a letter, a fact sheet, or a brochure. Targets might include guidance counselors, pediatricians, social workers, special education teachers, parents of learning disabled children, and so forth. Direct mail ensures that a message is received by the people who are most likely to act on the information.

Seminars and workshops. Continuing education programs offered to community residents provide increased visibility for occupational therapy. Every time that the profession appears in the public eye means additional exposure. Workshops should be customized to the needs of the community and the staff's areas of expertise. If the community has a large elderly population, a seminar on maintaining the elderly in the community would be appropriate. If the major work in the community is service related (as opposed to industry), a workshop on stress might be conducted. Parenting workshops might be presented through the local health department, the YMCA/YWCA, and adult education programs. Such presentations not only bring occupational therapy to the public's attention; they serve to strengthen its public image.

Health fairs and exhibits. These are excellent means of providing general information about occupational therapy to consumers. Occupational therapists can team up with other health professionals in their own or another organization, or plan their own exhibit. Contracting with a mall to display information on occupational therapy is a good way of recruiting people for the profession or demonstrating the diverse areas of occupational therapy practice. Adaptive devices, splinting supplies, sensory stimulation materials, crafts, and testing equipment make for interesting displays. Exhibits should be of interest to the people who visit a mall on a weekend afternoon—mainly parents and young families, teenagers, and older adults. The goal, once again, is general occupational therapy exposure to raise people's consciousness.

Scholarly articles. An important way to generate professional exposure for occupational therapy is to publish scholarly articles in the journals of other professions. The content of an article would be dictated by the readership of a journal. For example, to educate psychologists on the role of occupational therapy in the evaluation and treatment of developmentally delayed children, a paper could be written for one of the journals of the American Psychological Association. Similarly, to reach psychiatrists, a paper on occupational therapy in mental health might be submitted to a journal produced by the American Psychiatric Association. The *Journal of Rehabilitation* is a good placement for articles on occupational therapy program development and research. The idea is to reach a specialized group and present specialized information.

Participation in community, charitable, and religious organizations. Community, charitable, and religious organizations are made up of individuals whose special interest is to support the group's cause. These individuals represent some of the community's interests and are potential occupational therapy patients/clients or referral sources. Occupational therapy personnel who volunteer their participation in these organizations have a unique opportunity to establish valuable contacts and promote the profession. The contacts they make could result in improved access to the media, inclusion in other groups' long-range plans, and exposure to community members who might influence the expansion of coverage for occupational therapy. Occupational therapy personnel could benefit from being seen as members of the community, as people who are understanding and enthusiastic, and who will align themselves with a beneficial cause. References to occupational therapy should not be self-serving; rather, the profession should be portrayed as fulfilling a health care need.

Guest speeches at community programs. This is another method of increasing occupational therapy's visibility. Speeches can be made at programs offered by hospital groups, senior citizens centers, youth organizations, political gatherings, the county or state health department, and groups concerned with education. Timely topics for presentations are health prevention, safety in the home, occupational therapy in home health, and day care for the elderly. Promoting independence in the elderly, another possible topic, is an important concern in every community as the aging population grows and health care funds shrink. Occupational therapy speakers could also guide families in choosing a nursing home, provide suggestions for adapting the home environment to promote safety and independence, or offer help in understanding the psychological changes accompanying aging. The importance of early treatment for learning disabilities could generate such topics as identifying when a child needs professional help, how children learn, and how parents can tell if children are developing normally.

Presentations at professional conferences. Presentations at the conferences of other professional organizations, such as the American Public Health Association, the Association for Counseling and Development, the American Psychiatric Association, and the Group Health Association of America (the trade organization for health maintenance organizations), are another means of promoting occupational therapy. It is useful to provide fact sheets and written materials as handouts. Information on where to obtain occupational therapy evaluation and treatment should be included in all materials.

Speakers bureau. The state or district occupational therapy association can organize or participate in a speakers bureau. Developing and promoting a roster of speakers can reach and influence a variety of audiences and can help to establish an image of occupational therapy as a profession with competence in a wide variety of practice areas. As an organization of occupational therapy professionals, the state or district association already has the necessary ingredients for a successful speakers bureau. The task is to identify speakers and topics through the association's newsletter and professional network. In choosing the speakers to be included in the bureau, individuals should be identified who have the skills and interest to relate material to consumer audiences, and who are dynamic public speakers. Professional competence does not necessarily make a person a good public speaker; someone who cannot tailor information to a non-health-profession audience may leave listeners confused.

A plan for promoting a speakers bureau should include contact with civic, religious, and fraternal organizations that welcome suggestions for speakers. Consideration should also be given to support groups, such as those for stroke and heart attack victims, families of the mentally ill, and parents of disabled children. The local Chamber of Commerce can often provide lists of organizations in the community. Schools, colleges, and parent-teacher organizations, as well as radio programs that attract particular audiences, should be among the groups and the agencies that are informed about the speakers bureau.

Personal visits. With some publics, one-to-one communication is essential. For example, to be certain that legislators and other public officials have sufficient information to make favorable decisions on issues of concern to occupational therapy and its consumers, occupational therapy personnel should pay personal calls on them. Slide-tape shows, fact sheets, brochures, and a promotion piece such as an occupational therapy calendar can help to make a point during and even after such visits. Public officials' understanding of occupational therapy can also be influenced by timely features in the broadcast and print media.

EXECUTING A COMMUNICATIONS PROGRAM

The following scenario is an example of a situation that would benefit from a communications program: Referrals to the occupational therapy organization and the number of treatments per patient/client have declined as a result of early discharges and changing patterns of payment for services.

Define Specific Objectives

In the scenario a particular concern has been identified within the occupational therapy organization, and now a specific goal must be set. Through investigation and analysis the occupational therapy manager determines that developing and providing home health services will expand the organization's revenue base. These services will also compensate for the decrease in referrals and patient/client treatment hours brought on by early discharges and changing patterns of payment for services. The objectives of the program will be to maintain the continuity of follow-up care, which will aid in improving patients'/clients' rate of recovery and decrease hospital readmissions. A goal of 10 home health referrals per month, or 120 per year, is set.

Prepare a Communications Plan

A plan must now be developed for reaching the goal. A primary concern is to disseminate information to referral sources. As discussed earlier, the steps are defining the message, defining the publics, and selecting appropriate communication methods.

The message needs to address *who* can be served in a home health setting, *what kind* of occupational therapy treatment will be provided; *when* the treatment should be provided (e.g., immediately on discharge for approximately *x* weeks); *where* the treatment will be provided, if applicable; and *why* occupational therapy treatment will be effective.

The publics would include physicians, social workers, nurses, hospital discharge planners, community agencies, support groups, religious groups, senior citizens centers, community media, the county medical society, and other health organizations.

Select Communication Methods

The manner in which information is provided will influence the success of the plan. The message should be tailored to the particular audiences, to what each one would want and need to know. Whenever a new service is instituted, it should be kicked off with an open house. This provides a good opportunity to introduce or refamiliarize guests with occupational therapy. If the correct people are invited, such as physicians, administrators, and discharge planners, the open house will provide personal contact with referral sources. Printed information about the service should be made available. This can be done with inexpensive fact sheets that address the who, what, when, where, and why in a clear and attractive format.

A new service also has news merit, so it should be announced in the organization's publications and in the local newspapers. The style or health editors of suburban newspapers are generally interested in printing information about health, fitness, leisure, coping strategies, and so forth, and often describe personal and professional community resources that can assist individuals in dealing with contemporary living.

Speaking engagements for staff of the new service should be sought through the health department, the local library, the Chamber of Commerce, and community health groups and clubs. Printed information should be posted on community bulletin boards, in libraries, in supermarkets, and in the waiting areas of health care facilities. A list of physicians might be obtained from the county or state medical society, and a direct mail information piece might be sent to them. Various facilities that might be interested in developing an occupational therapy service could also be contacted.

The final plan should take timetables and budgets into consideration. A realistic schedule for completing activities, gathering materials, and assigning responsibilities should be included.

Follow-up

Once a contact has been made with potential referral sources, it is important to recontact them and follow up with additional information. This could be in the form of a quick phone call or a letter repeating the home health service's hours, costs, and therapy components. A brief description of the types of patients/clients who have been treated recently could be included to encourage similar referrals.

After a referral has been received and an initial evaluation has been completed, it is useful to keep the referral source informed of significant progress. To accomplish this, a form can be developed with the service's name, address, phone number, and hours as a heading.

Evaluation

To determine the success of the communications plan, promotional activities must be evaluated. How were referrals obtained—from an inservice presentation, an article in the organization's newsletter, word of mouth, or direct contact by an occupational therapist? All referral sources should be asked how they heard of the new service. This information will assist not only in evaluating the effectiveness of the communications outreach but also in planning the initial communications outreach.

The plan should be reviewed after there has been ample time to implement it. Usually six months later is a reasonable time for assessment. Was the overall goal of ten referrals per month achieved? Were the timetables realistic? What unanticipated problems developed? Did the program lead to unexpected benefits?

The overall evaluation will help to fine-tune goals and activities. Activities that were ineffective should be eliminated, and those that gave positive results should be repeated.

SUMMARY

Providing effective occupational therapy services is only part of the puzzle. One must also be able to let others know about those services and about the purposes and results of interventions. To do so, one must be able to communicate with others meaningfully. The message should be packaged to attract attention, be comprehensible, and be useful.

To ensure that a message is understood, the sender must segment the audience into smaller publics, or targets (to the extent that this is possible). This segmentation allows the structuring of the message to meet the information needs of each target. Information must be presented in a way that is most useful to the particular public being addressed.

As professionals, occupational therapy personnel should identify the diverse groups to which they must appeal and recognize the need to communicate to these groups in different ways. Among occupational therapy's publics are patients/clients, referral sources, administrators, insurance providers, principals and school superintendents, and legislators and other public officials. In general, in defining a particular target or public, one should think about (a) what action he or she wants from that public, (b) what information and action that public wants from occupational therapy, and (c) what means of communication is best for reaching that public.

Selecting the appropriate method of communication largely depends on the message and the public. One should choose the methods that best suit his or her needs. Internal communication is interaction among people within an organization. Methods include an organization's employee newsletter, open houses, in-service programs, progress notes, memos, reports, case conferences, and participation in activities sponsored by the organization. Contact with individuals outside an organization is defined as external communication. Among the methods in this category are an organization's community newsletter, annual reports, suburban newspapers, direct mail, seminars and workshops, health fairs and exhibits, publication of scholarly articles, participation in local organizations, guest speeches at community programs, presentations at professional conferences, a speakers bureau, and personal visits.

In executing a communications program, a manager should first define a specific objective, then prepare a plan to reach it. Once contact has been made with the targeted audiences, there should be follow-up to keep them informed. Also, the success of the communication plan should be evaluated.

Resources

Ackey DS, Editor: *Encyclopedia of Associations, vol 1, National Organizations of the United States, 17th edition.* Detroit: Gale Research Co, 1983

Barach JA: Applying marketing principles to social causes. *Business Horizons,* July–August 1984

Bateman JC: Public relations for the business and

professional organization. In *Lesly's Public Relations Handbook, 2nd edition,* P Lesly, Editor. Englewood Cliffs, NJ: Prentice-Hall Inc, 1978, pp 230–244

Brawley EA: *Mass Media and Human Services: Getting the Message Across.* Beverly Hills, CA: Sage Publications Inc, 1983

Engel JF, Warshaw MR, Kerinear TC: *Managing the Marketing Communications Process: Promotional Strategy.* Homewood, IL: Richard D Irwin Inc, 1979

Fox KFA, Kotler P: The marketing of social causes: The first 10 years. *J Marketing* 44:24–33, 1980

Public relations: A valuable and inexpensive tool! *Course of Action,* May 1984 (Address: S. M. Reed, Publisher, 2420 Brookside Way, Carson City, NV 89701)

Public Relations Resource Guide, 3rd edition. Rockville, MD: American Occupational Therapy Association, Division of Public Affairs, 1984

Ross RD: *The Management of Public Relations: Analysis and Planning External Relations.* New York: John Wiley & Sons Inc, 1977

Scott SJ, Acquaviva JD: *Lobbying for Health Care: A Guide Book for Professionals and Associations.* Rockville, MD: American Occupational Therapy Association, Government and Legal Affairs Division, 1985

Straus IL: Pointers to help you get your message across. *Assoc Manage,* June:91–94, 1972

Ten steps to a winning marketing plan. *Course of Action,* July 1983

Use the marketing process to cope with DRG prospective payment. *Course of Action,* September 1984

Where to Speak and Publish: Developmental Disabilities, Gerontology, Mental Health, Physical Disabilities, Sensory Integration. Rockville, MD: American Occupational Therapy Association, 1984

Winston W, Editor: *Marketing for Mental Health Services.* New York: Haworth Press Inc, 1984

Chapter 17

Consultation: Communicating and Facilitating

Cynthia F. Epstein, MA, OTR, FAOTA

Consultation and private practice models of service delivery began to grow significantly in the mid-1960s as health care providers and planners started advocating preventive health services, moving from an illness- to a wellness-oriented, holistic model of care (1). Expansion of community services outside traditional institutions was therefore encouraged. Concurrently, occupational therapy personnel began receiving more recognition in community health settings and assuming more autonomy as health care providers. The shift in focus and the growth in autonomy, combined with the ever-present shortage of occupational therapy personnel and an expanded marketplace, have led to increased use of consultation services.

Consultation is a process by which expertise is communicated to others who need assistance in solving existing or potential problems. Key elements in consultation, in addition to competence in occupational therapy, are an understanding of systems, organizational theory, and be-

Cynthia F. Epstein is the president and the director of Occupational Therapy Consultants, Inc., in Somerville, New Jersey. She has over 20 years of experience as a consultant, practicing in such diverse areas as vocational rehabilitation research and program development, adult day care, wheelchair management, and specialized programming for the institutionalized elderly.

havior; an ability to communicate and to listen effectively; and a capacity to diagnose a problem and recommend appropriate strategies for resolving it (2).

Occupational therapy consultation may be sought by individuals, groups, educational programs, human service agencies, or industrial corporations, and may involve a brief intervention or a continuing relationship. The consultee—that is, the person seeking help—usually works with patients/clients or employees and uses consultation to improve planning and interaction with them. The consultant must be able to help the consultee mobilize internal and external resources that allow for change and problem resolution (3).

The major role of the occupational therapy consultant is to effectively communicate new elements, information, concepts, perspectives, values, and skills, thereby facilitating the consultee's ability to deal with change (4). To do this, the consultee's problems must be viewed from a broad perspective, using skills in analysis to view the system through "OT glasses" (5). This allows consideration of the total system, including its environmental, psychosocial, and economic aspects, as it relates to the specific problems presented by a consultee.

Occupational therapists are known as the people who make doing possible, helping patients/clients help themselves. Consultation is also viewed as a helping process. Occupational therapy personnel often consult colleagues and peers for advice on a problem. Students (6), entry-level personnel (7), and staff therapists have the potential to perform a consultative function (1, 8). Occupational therapy personnel at all levels should take advantage of opportunities to participate in consultation. By doing so, they will begin building the skills necessary for more extensive, higher-level consultation, in which the helping process extends into a larger system.

AN EXPANDING MARKETPLACE

Legislation, economic issues, personnel shortages, and the spread of technology have had a profound influence on the growth of consultation and private practice. The consultant, at the leading edge of practice, initiates occupational therapy services in new markets. As an evaluator, a clarifier, and a trainer, the consultant may help solve specific problems for human service personnel and the systems in which they function. As a facilitator and program developer, the consultant may pave the way for occupational therapy to become a permanent part of the organizational structure.

An example can readily be seen in the phenomenal growth of occupational therapy programs in school systems. Public Law 94-142, enacted in 1975, mandated the inclusion of occupational therapy as a related service for handicapped children who need it to benefit from the special education experience. The demand for services swelled, and consultants began working with school personnel to develop programs. Although many school systems still use a consultation model, 18 percent of all registered occupational therapists (OTRs) surveyed in 1982 reported being employed by schools. This was a 7.3 percent increase over the 1973 figure (9).

Similarly, health care legislation in the 1960s and 1970s increased funding for maternal and child health programs, and expanded benefits for the elderly through Medicare, Medicaid, and the Older Americans Act. As a result, the demand for rehabilitation (10) and health promotion services in community settings rose. From 1973 to 1982, occupational therapy services delivered in the community grew by 17 percent (9).

Occupational therapy's chronic problem, insufficient personnel to meet market demands, became more acute in the late 1960s and remains a dominant issue today. The profession has searched for methods to expand its numbers and make more efficient use of existing personnel, as illustrated in *Occupational Therapy Manpower: A Plan for Progress* (11). Programs preparing technical-level assistants have been developed, reactivation programs have been implemented, and therapists have been trained to assume consultant roles (12–14). Therapists working as consultants and private practitioners continue to forge new directions for practice, creating jobs that may then be filled by entry-level and reactivating occupational therapists or occupational therapy assistants. In many instances the consultant remains available to provide expertise and support to the agency and to occupational therapy personnel.

As the profession looks toward the end of the twentieth century, demands for occupational therapy services and opportunities in new markets continue to increase. Deregulation and cost containment legislation have spurred privatization in the health care industry, creating the "health care entrepreneur" (15). Occupational therapy entrepreneurs can be found in health clinics, fitness centers, day-care programs, and holistic health centers, working collaboratively within these settings or establishing and owning them. The changes in health care delivery models, combined with an older population that is growing rapidly, have helped occupational therapy become one of the nation's twenty fastest-growing occupations, with a projected growth rate of 60 percent between 1982 and 1995 (16).

The need for consultants and private practitioners working at the forefront of practice will increase dramatically in future years. In recognition of this expanding need, occupational therapy conferences, workshops, texts, and official publications now routinely include topics pertinent to consultation and private practice. Building a core of expert therapists capable of performing consultation functions begins with an expanded knowledge base. The information presented in this chapter is intended to widen the perspective of occupational therapy students and personnel regarding the practice of consultation.

CONCEPTS OF CONSULTATION

The word *consultant* brings to mind such synonyms as *expert*, *adviser*, and *professional*. A consultant may also be thought of as a change agent, a counselor, a reflector, a health advocate/agent, a diagnostician, and a facilitator. Concepts of consultation are drawn from many fields of study.

Within each field the emphasis and the perspective may vary, but the essentials are generic.

General Views

Caplin (17, p 19), a psychiatrist whose special concern is community mental health, defines mental health consultation as

> a process of interaction between two professional persons—the consultant who is a specialist, and the consultee, who invokes the consultant's help in regard to a current work problem . . . which . . . is within the other's area of specialized competence. The work problem involves the management or treatment of one or more clients of the consultee, or the planning or implementation of a program to cater to such clients.

An essential part of the consultation process, according to Caplin, is that the professional responsibility for the patient/client remains with the consultee. Treatment is not part of consultation. Equally important is teaching and/or education. As the consultee becomes more knowledgeable, he or she will apply what has been learned to similar problems.

Bennis, Benne, and Chin are behavioral scientists who have written extensively in the field of planned change. Discussing its evolution, they point out:

> The roots of planned change can be seen developmentally as representing three sets of entangled issues: the role of the expert in practice and action; the uses of knowledge of man and his relationships, including knowledge of change and changing; and newly emerging definitions of the collaborative relationship between the change agent and those being changed. (18, p 13)

They view the consultant as an agent of planned change:

> The change agent uses his own person and the relationship that he jointly builds, adapts and terminates with the client system he is seeking to help, as major tools in liberating, informing and empowering the client to deal more aptly with itself . . . and its . . . worlds. (18, p 371)

These theorists emphasize the important consultant roles of educator and facilitator. They believe that the consultant must elicit and transmit needed information and knowledge through training that involves participative decision making. The assumption is that as the consultee gains knowledge, behavioral changes will follow. Recognizing that there are noncognitive factors that can support or prevent change, the consultant must also help consultees explore the validity of their attitudes, processes, and values in relation to their problems.

Lippitt and Lippitt (3), behavioral scientists and educators, view consultation as a collaborative problem-solving process in which the consultant, or the helper, has as much chance to learn as those who are helped. The helper may be employed in the same system as the consultee and be termed an *internal consultant*, or may come from outside the system and offer the more removed perspective of an *external consultant*.

In contrast with Caplin's view, Lippitt and Lippitt perceive the consultee and the client as the same. The help sought by the consultee does not necessarily pertain to management or treatment of a third party. Rather, the consultant is asked to help a person, a group, or a system deal with one or more problems. Lippitt and Lippitt see a role not only for the professional consultant, but for helping-consulting teams created by pairing trained volunteers and paraprofessionals with professionals.

Lewin (19), the great social psychologist, stresses that behavior is a function of both environment and personal characteristics. Thus, the consultant must be aware of both physical and social environmental factors that may impede or foster change. An organization's mission and goals, its policies and procedures, the availability of funding, use of role modeling, and socialization are examples of environmental factors of a nonphysical nature.

The force-field analysis conceptualized by Lewin helps one look at behavior in a group, an institution, or a community, not as a static pattern but as a dynamic balance of forces working in opposite directions. Behavior is stabilized when the restraining and the driving forces are equalized. Lewin terms the balance a "quasi-stationary equilibrium." An imbalance occurs when change is taking place. That is, either the driving or the restraining force takes over. This unfreezes the situation, allowing movement and change. Eventually the forces become equalized again, with the change incorporated into the environment.

For example, limitations in health care reimbursement through the Prospective Payment System of Medicare have demanded higher productivity from existing staff. Occupational therapy personnel have been forced to examine and change treatment methodologies and schedules to accommodate this driving force. Their feelings of anger and frustration, combined with stress and anxiety, have become the restraining forces to the mandated change. During the period of instability, administrators and staff must work together to find ways of balancing their needs so that the change can be incorporated successfully.

Power and its use in the consultant-consultee relationship must also be considered. Leopold (20) speaks of this in relation to the consultant's need for sanction. The consultant obtains sanction through a sponsor, the person/authority who has asked for or authorized the consultation. To be effective, the consultant must know the degree of power and influence held by the sponsor. The greater the sponsor's power, the more easily the consultant can move into the system.

Although power is usually discussed as part of the consultee's role (i. e., the consultant recommends, the consultee decides), it is also part of the consultant's role. Gaupp (21) notes that power elements seem to be present in all consultation, on both formal and informal levels. Informally the consultant is assumed to have power. Formally the consultant may have power through legislation, through issues of reimbursement, or, as in the case of state consultants, through the organization that brings them into the consulting relationship. An example is the legislative mandates at both ends of the developmental spectrum that have expanded the need for occupational therapy services. Early discussion between the consultant and the consultee of the factors of authority, influence, and control will help clear the air and set the stage. It will also help in building a relationship of trust and confidence, which is necessary for effective communication.

The several authors and theoreticians whose views are discussed here concur that consultation is a task-oriented, interactive process in which consultant and consultee focus on a specific problem. The relationship is coordinate, even though the final decision rests with the consultee.

Recognizing the complex nature of consultation, the theoreticians advocate using various approaches and techniques in a structured process to reach the goal of problem resolution.

Occupational Therapy Views

Consultation has enabled occupational therapy to broaden its sphere of influence and make better use of its personnel. As advocates of activity and as experts in the use of occupation to improve health, occupational therapy personnel have gradually expanded their services into the community (22, 23). In this setting, the importance of promoting health and preventing disability, combined with occupational therapy's holistic view of individuals' performance of occupation in a world fraught with change, has increased the demand for consultation as a model of service delivery.

Moving into the constantly changing arena of community health, occupational therapy personnel have become increasingly aware of their need to understand and apply specific concepts. West (24), Wiemer (25), and Finn (26) point out that to be effective in community health, occupational therapy personnel must develop more knowledge of and concern for health and preventive care. Discussing prevention, West notes that it is the first component on the continuum of comprehensive health care. Weimer views the occupational therapist in community health as an advocate who alerts the public to the relationship between health and occupations that challenge the use of hand and mind. By creating public awareness and sensitivity to the effect that occupation has on health, the advocate can help the community plan and implement preventive programs. Finn identifies crucial elements needed for successful practice in the community, including a knowledge of agencies and their systems, the ability to articulate and develop occupational therapy intervention strategies that are appropriate in community settings, the development of risk-taking skills, and the establishment of effective communications. All three authors view consultation as an effective method of practice in community settings.

Recognizing the importance of preventive health care and community programming, Grossman (27, p 351) discusses the concepts of primary, secondary, and tertiary prevention and their application to practice. She points out that occupational therapy personnel "have a commitment to primary and secondary health care, to reduce the incidence and duration of disorder." Their role in tertiary prevention, the rehabilitation phase, is well recognized. The techniques in primary and secondary prevention require further emphasis. On a primary level these include consultation to, education of, and collaboration with the community to help forestall dysfunction. Here services focus on activities to help the consumer and the planner take a more active role in maintaining health. In secondary prevention the focus is on early identification and detection in populations at risk. Through timely diagnosis and treatment more complex and chronic dysfunction can be prevented or retarded. Working in primary and secondary prevention means being comfortable operating in a model of indirect service such as consultation. This approach requires collaboration, self-confidence, and an awareness of the social, economic, and political conditions that interfere with health and may be beyond the professional's control.

Mazer (28, p 419) supports the need for a preventive focus in consultation. Her "action model" views the consultant as an enabling leader, collaborating with the consultee to influence changes in community attitudes and functioning. "The new role of the occupational therapist consultant may well be that of therapist to the community, rather than to individual patients," she observes. In this role the consultant can influence changes in community attitudes and functioning, thereby affecting a much larger number of people.

Jaffe (29, p 49) stresses that community consultation must be "responsive to and responsible for, the needs of consumers in [the] community." This approach has its basis in a cultural-enhancement model of consultation, "derived primarily from the principles of environment, with emphasis on the social and cultural issues indigenous to the community through a multidisciplinary approach to the problem" (pp 48–49).

Rogers (30, p 117) discusses consultation from an occupational behavior viewpoint:

> Personal changes in occupational behavior . . . will not necessarily carry over to the environments of daily life. Occupational therapy intervention must also be directed toward the client's environments. Consultation is the mode through which environmental intervention is accomplished.
>
> Consultation is an indirect service . . . expert knowledge, skills, and attitudes are transmitted to someone other than the client for the purpose of benefiting the client.

Consultation in the school system is viewed by Llorens (31, p vi) as "a work-centered, problem-solving, helping relationship . . . to remediate education-related problems through the use of occupational therapy." She sees the consultant as "a change agent, helping to identify problems, proposing solutions, and suggesting alternatives." In the educational setting, the relationship between the consultant and the consultee calls for mutual respect and recognition of each other's knowledge, background, and skills.

Gilfoyle (32, p 582), looking at the directions in which practice is headed, indicates that "new service delivery patterns involving consultation and monitoring, and collaborative programming will be imperative." She points out the importance of occupational therapy's move into the educational arena. The school consultant brings "certain expertise [to the educational system] that can facilitate a student's adaptation process so that the student can function more effectively . . ." (33, p 19).

According to these authors, occupational therapy consultants in community settings need to understand and effectively use concepts of prevention. Boundaries and systems in these settings may appear more diffuse, requiring skillful negotiation of the environment, accurate and appropriate evaluation of the setting, and effective communication. The occupational therapy consultant brings a special perspective and competence to the community setting. Working in a collaborative and helping role, he or she must understand and be comfortable with the indirect nature of the service.

CURRENT CONSULTATION PRACTICE

Understanding today's consultation practice requires identifying current practice settings where occupational therapy functions include consultation, and reviewing the varied environments in which consultation is sought. Further examination of the role of the consultant will clarify some of the differences and identify the commonalities between consultation, supervision, and treatment.

Consultation Settings and Environments

Occupational therapy consultants can be found in private practice, in public and private school systems, in industry, in occupational therapy departments of hospitals and rehabilitation centers that have community outreach programming, and in schools of occupational therapy whose faculty provide community consultation. A small number serve as administrative consultants (34) for state and federal governments, national health organizations, insurance companies, accrediting agencies, and other national groups concerned with health issues.

The spectrum of consultation environments is as varied as the imagination allows. Some of the more unusual ones include prisons, Indian reservations, programs dealing with abuse of children and the elderly, and women's crisis centers. The most familiar settings are school systems, community mental health centers, and nursing homes, where the emphasis is on secondary and tertiary models of prevention rather than on primary models. Consultants also work in community and health planning programs, advise architects and designers, and develop rehabilitation and occupational therapy programs for acute care, outpatient, and rehabilitation settings. In industry they analyze the occupational performance of employees to help plan more appropriate and efficient work environments.

Consultant Roles

Although each setting may demand variations, in current practice the consultant is seen in these roles:

- An adviser, a helper, a facilitator with occupational therapy expertise, who is invited into a system
- An outsider, with no formal authority in a system
- A change agent, using knowledge of the system, its goals, and its objectives to effect positive change
- An evaluator-diagnostician, focusing on identified problems
- A clarifier, helping a consultee analyze and understand a problem objectively
- A trainer, providing opportunities to learn skills that will aid in the development of short- and long-term goals
- A planner, collaborating with the consultee to develop or modify long-range plans
- An extender, providing occupational therapy assessment and developing maintenance programs to be carried out by the consultee when direct treatment services are not feasible or appropriate.

What seems to create the most role confusion and difficulty for occupational therapists is functioning as both a consultant and a therapist, and sometimes also as a supervisor. That is, a consultant may be asked to perform a consultative function (indirect service), a therapeutic function (direct treatment service), and possibly a supervisory function for an occupational therapy assistant or an entry-level or reactivating occupational therapist. The contrasts and parallels among these roles are detailed in Table 1.

Frequently consultants are asked to both consult and supervise in a human service agency that employs an occupational therapy assistant as the primary provider of occupational therapy treatment. Here the consultant performs the direct service functions of assessment and treatment planning, and gives the occupational therapy assistant the professional support necessary to carry out the occupational therapy program. In so doing, the consultant maintains an obligation to the administrator or other management personnel to provide consultation services. The differences in these roles must be clarified for all concerned for the consultation process to be effective.

The role of extender also causes much concern. Working in community settings, such as schools, day-care centers, and nursing homes, the consultant collaborates with a team of consultees, identifying and assessing a problem, and then develops a program plan that can be carried out by the consultees with specific follow-up provided by the consultant. In this role the consultant is effectively extending the use of occupational therapy services into community settings that might otherwise be without them.

Gilfoyle (33, pp 22–23) discusses this role as monitoring, which she defines as

> the training and supervision of other persons involved with the implementation of occupational therapy [in the school system]. Persons assisting may include classroom teachers, aides, parents, the student and volunteers. Although another person may be performing the actual service program, the [occupational therapist] is both professionally and legally responsible for the program and its outcomes.
>
> The roles of assessment and program planning *must* be carried out by the [occupational therapist] . . . Therefore, [these] are not considered part of the monitoring delivery pattern . . . Monitoring includes training and ongoing supervision of others, provided by the [consultant] for the intervention aspects of direct services.

Similarly, consultants providing service in long-term care facilities perform assessments and develop program plans that will be carried out by facility staff. Many restorative nursing programs (35) are established through occupational therapy intervention and are monitored by the consultant at specified intervals.

The varied environments in which consultation is practiced call on consultants to use flexibility and creativity as part of their role. To meet today's pressing demands for occupational therapy service, and in anticipation of continued growth, greater numbers of therapists will need to assume consultant roles. As they do, they may find it helpful to recall Mazer's action model of consultation, which suggests "that community consultation in occupational therapy must mean using professional expertise to enable people to grow and heal other people more effectively" (28, p 420).

THE CONSULTATION PROCESS

Effective consultation requires careful planning and an understanding of the process. This may be viewed in stages: (a) initiation and clarification, (b) evaluation and communication, (c) interactive problem resolution, and (d) termination.

Initiation and Clarification

Having identified a need or a problem relating to occupational performance, a consultee requests occupational therapy consultation services. To enter the consultee's system in the role of a change agent, the consultant must obtain sanction from an administrative source within. In

(*text continued on page 310*)

TABLE 17–1
Consultation, Supervision, Treatment: Contrasts and Parallels

Consultation	Supervision	Treatment
1. The purpose of consultation is to enable the consultee to work through a problem that is of concern to the consultee.	1. The purpose of supervision is to direct staff to do a job effectively.	1. The purpose of treatment is to resolve a problem.
2. Consultation is offered.	2. Supervision is given.	2. Treatment is both offered and given.
3. Consultation is a mutual learning and problem-solving process.	3. Supervision is a directing and instructional process.	3. Treatment is a directing/instructional, assisting process.
4. The essential characteristic of consultation is catalytic and facilitative in decision making.	4. The essential characteristic of supervision is responsibility for decision making.	4. The essential characteristic of treatment is improving individual functioning.
5. The consultee has the freedom to initiate, refuse, interrupt, modify, or terminate the process.	5. The process starts when the work relationship is established. The supervisee does not have the freedom to refuse, interrupt or terminate the process as long as the work relationship exists. However, he or she may make suggestions.	5. The patient/client has the freedom to accept, refuse, or interrupt the treatment process.

6. The consultant may withhold consultation.	6. The supervisor may not withhold supervision.	6. The therapist may withhold treatment.
7. To be effective, the consultant must possess technical knowledge and skills that are valued by the consultee.	7. To be effective, the supervisor must possess technical knowledge and skills that are seen as necessary to the job by the supervisee.	7. To be effective, the therapist must possess technical knowledge and skills that are effective in the alteration of a problem.
8. The consultant must establish rapport with the consultee. To do this, one must have insight into one's own feelings about giving consultation and about the consultee, and be sensitive to how the consultee feels.	8. The supervisor must establish rapport with the supervisee. To do this, one must have insight into one's own feelings about giving supervision and about the supervisee, and be sensitive to how the person feels.	8. The therapist must establish rapport with the patient/client. One must have insight into feelings about giving treatment and be sensitive to the patient's/client's feelings.
9. To utilize consultation, it is necessary that the consultee possess some degree of skill and technical competence. Competence may be equal, even superior, to that of the consultant.	9. It is not necessary for the supervisee to possess technical or professional competence in order to utilize supervision.	9. It is not necessary for the patient/client to have technical professional competence to benefit from the treatment process.
10. It requires some self-confidence to give and receive consultation.	10. It requires some self-confidence to give and receive supervision.	10. It requires some self-confidence to treat and some motivation to receive treatment.
11. Consultation is adapted to the needs of the consultee; the consultant deals with the consultee's agenda.	11. Supervision is geared to the demands of the job. The extent to which the needs of the supervisee may be met are limited by the demands of the job and capabilities of those involved.	11. Treatment is adapted to the needs of the patient/client. The extent to which these needs may be met is limited by abilities of the therapist and the motivation of the patient/client.

Note: Adapted from EM Gilfoyle, Editor, *TOTEMS: A Competency-Based Educational Program*, Rockville, MD: American Occupational Therapy Association, 1980, vol 3, pp 70–71 initial meetings with the administrator and/or the consultee, the consultant's knowledge and experience are delineated, and the consultee presents an overview of the system and enumerates the desired outcomes of the consultation. During these interactions there is an opportunity to clarify roles, expectations, and goals. Clear communication and understanding are essential when establishing a collaborative relationship. The stage culminates in the drawing up of a contract, which is signed by both parties. This formal document defines the purpose of the consultation and the qualifications of the consultant, identifies the obligations and expectations of both parties, and delineates procedures, time constraints, and the method and amount of compensation.

Evaluation and Communication

Once the contract has been formalized and open communication established with the administrator or other source of power within the system, the consultant begins to assess the problem, drawing on professional knowledge, experience, and resources in conjunction with an in-depth study of the consultee's system. As part of data gathering, the consultant uses the consultee's competence and knowledge. Equally important, the consultant becomes familiar with the special terminology and/or procedures used in the setting, to ensure effective communication. External sources of power such as regulatory agencies, funding sources, and community consumer groups also need to be considered, for they may have direct impact on the system and the problem at hand.

Having clarified roles and opened communication during the initial stage, the consultant should continue this process in the evaluation stage. Through communication and sharing of knowledge, the consultee and other members of the system develop greater understanding and appreciation of the occupational performance perspective used by the consultant. During the data-gathering stages, the consultant meets and works with a variety of individuals who are concerned with the problem at hand. These occasions provide further opportunities to observe the system in action and consider possible solutions. The consultant must be constantly aware of the needs of those working in the system and the difficulties presented when change is being considered.

During this stage the consultant needs to identify sources for feedback and reflection. As a stranger, or an outsider, the consultant may not always perceive and interpret actions and information accurately. Using a variety of techniques that may include interviews, surveys, group discussions, and documentation, the consultant should verify information.

Interactive Problem Resolution

Having thoroughly studied the situation, the consultant begins the process of problem resolution. The data gathered must be analyzed carefully, perhaps using several perspectives, to ensure the validity of the diagnosis. Decisions remain the province of the consultee. Therefore, if the consultant wishes to help effect change in the system, work must be done with and through the consultee. Interactive problem resolution presumes that the consultant is committed to helping the consultee effect change through collaborative strategy development. This collaborative development has a basis in the consultant's role as trainer, facilitator, educator, communicator, and resource person. Participative decision making allows the consultant to facilitate identification of multiple strategies for consideration. The consultant must also demonstrate a commitment to confidentiality and an adherence to professional ethics. A relationship of mutual trust and respect is built, establishing an open environment. The consultee can then creatively and comfortably consider change strategies, using the perspective and knowledge offered by the consultant.

Termination

With information in hand and recommendations identified, the consultant writes a final report for the administrator or other identified sponsor. Before this, an exit or summary conference may be held. This conference is usually attended by system personnel who will be responsible for implementing change. It provides an opportunity for clarification, feedback, and discussion of any remaining areas of concern.

The final report should include the following information: dates of service, individuals/departments involved, plan of action and methodology used, findings, assessment, collaborative strategy development, and recommendations. In occupational therapy consultation, a recommendation for follow-up is often included. This provides an avenue for further communication as needed.

A Continuing Process

The process as presented here implies that consultation is a short-term, problem-specific intervention. This is not always the case. In some environments consultation is provided at specified intervals or on a continuing basis, as needed. Examples of this type of continual consultation can be found in school systems, community mental health settings, nursing homes, and adult day-care centers. Here the availability of occupational therapy services is often mandated by law. In these settings direct service providers may be an occupational therapy assistant, a nurse, a teacher, an aide, an activities coordinator, a volunteer, or another care giver working with individuals who have deficits in occupational performance. The consultation process is the same as previously outlined, with some modification. The consultant still receives authorization to enter a system through an administrator, but the more direct consultee is the care giver, who will provide the hands-on service, using the training and guidance obtained through consultation.

When services are requested in these settings, often a consultant must also provide direct treatment. To avoid confusion and misunderstandings in this dual role, the consultant-therapist must carefully plan and clarify. Should an occupational therapy assistant be on the staff, the consultant may also have to assume supervisory functions. In all cases it is helpful to keep in mind the contrasts and parallels between consultation, supervision, and treatment, previously pointed out in Table 1.

CONSULTATION SKILLS AND KNOWLEDGE

The occupational therapy philosophy and orientation of helping others do for themselves carries over naturally into consultation. Knowledge and professional competence in occupational therapy, an understanding of professional ethics, and behavior that reflects it help provide a sound foundation for developing consultation skills. So do education and training in such areas as human development and group process. Then there is a need for professional experience as a supervisor and a manager, and for an expanded knowledge base.

Areas of knowledge critical in consultation have been identified by Lippitt and Lippitt (3). These include a thorough foundation in systems theory and behavioral sciences; developmental theory as it applies to individuals, groups, organizations, and communities; education and training methodologies, including problem solving and role playing; knowledge and understanding of human personality, attitude formation, and change; and knowledge of self.

Key skills that the consultant must possess are communicating, educating, diagnosing, and linking. To employ these skills successfully, the consultant must also be able to establish effective interpersonal relationships. Attitudes and attributes such as flexibility, creativity, maturity, and self-confidence help the consultant move successfully in varied environments.

Communicating

Communicating is a primary consultation skill. It encompasses more than verbal and written abilities. Body language, role modeling, use of analogies, reflection, and confrontation may all be incorporated into it. Similarly, the ability to listen to what is—and is not—said, and to how it is presented, provides valuable insight. The consultation environment communicates too. A working space with walls covered by lists of rules, regulations, and procedures conveys a very different message from one that has interesting artwork and growing plants.

Written and oral communication must take into consideration differences in language usage in the consultation setting. In school settings, industry, and day-care centers, for example, catchphrases or special terms may be used as part of the communication process. Outsiders, unfamiliar with this language, may feel cut off from meaningful dialogue. Occupational therapy personnel also use special terms and phrases that may not be easily understood in community environments. When consultants use professional terminology, they must define their terms in the consultee's language.

Educating

Training and educating are basic components of consultation. The consultant may use a variety of methods to help broaden the consultee's skills and further develop his or her abilities to effect change independently. Designing and leading workshops is one such method. Here the consultant is able to present new material, and the consultee is able to participate actively through experiential learning. Special audiovisual materials or computerized instructional programs may also be used, allowing the consultee to proceed at a comfortable pace, with built-in opportunities for feedback and discussion. The materials must be clearly presented and relevant for the consultee.

Diagnosing

Occupational therapists are most familiar with assessment technology as it pertains to the diagnosis and treatment of individuals who are dysfunctional. In consultation a more global perspective is required. Moving into a dysfunctional system, the consultant must gather data from a variety of sources in collaboration with the consultee. As the data are reviewed and assessed, feedback is obtained, which helps in verification and clarification before a final diagnosis or conclusion is reached. In diagnosing, Lippitt and Lippitt (3) point out, the consultant must have the ability to diagnose problems; to locate sources of help, power, and influence; to understand the consultee's values and culture; and to determine readiness for change.

Linking

Linking is a skill that comes very naturally to occupational therapy personnel. As proponents of adaptation, they are constantly identifying resources and alternative methods to help achieve a particular goal. The consultant links the consultee to appropriate resources both within and outside the consultation environment. A consultant, for example, may learn about new and competitive sources for equipment and supplies when consulting with one organization. These resources may then be linked to another consultee, when appropriate.

Effective Interpersonal Relationships

Establishing effective interpersonal relationships requires an understanding of the consultee's value system and attitudes, and the external and internal pressures of the system. These all have a bearing on the capacity to change. For example, pressured by time and environment, an aide finds it quicker, easier, and less frustrating to feed a child who is able to eat independently with adaptive equipment. Yet the aide also wants to further the child's independence. The consultant's task is to help the aide and other staff understand the importance of self-care so that it becomes a first priority. The task also involves working with the aide's supervisors, so that they will find methods of modifying time and environmental constraints and thus foster change in the aide's behavior. To develop such a collaborative relationship, the consultant must have a sincere interest in the consultees and must gain their confidence and respect.

Attitudes and Attributes

Consultation requires a high degree of self-direction, comfort with taking risks, and ease in working without a formalized support system. Satisfaction for a job well done comes through the success achieved by a consultee. This indirect type of gratification necessitates a strong sense of security and self-confidence on the part of the consultant.

Maturity, flexibility, a sense of humor and of timing are also important. At times, a crisis shunts the original consultation problem aside. The consultant may come prepared to deal with one problem and find the system's priority is quite different. At such a moment no one is amenable to considering "lesser" issues, and the consultant must help resolve the more pressing problem.

The consultant needs to make a realistic appraisal of his or her limitations and abilities. One cannot be expert at everything. When additional skills are required, the consultant should have the confidence to acknowledge this and to suggest other resources, one of which may be the consultee.

ON BECOMING A CONSULTANT

When forging into new and less secure settings, a consultant should follow the Scouting motto, "Be prepared." Current and future environments must be considered. Economic factors require careful study, and a market plan must be created (see Chapter 6 also). Resources must be developed and used appropriately. The "business of being in business" can then become a reality.

Consultation Environments

In addition to the already familiar consultation environments of schools, long-term-care facilities, community mental health settings, and industry, current health planning has finally moved toward firm support of a health promotion model of care. This emphasis on primary prevention can be seen in the growing use of health maintenance organizations (HMO) and their newer relatives, social/health maintenance organizations (SHMO). The HMO was created to provide all necessary medical care, including routine health screenings and other preventive measures, for a fixed yearly fee. Occupational therapy personnel providing services in HMO work in such areas as developmental screening, stress and pain management, energy conservation and work simplification, and environmental adaptation. The SHMO has been targeted at the older population, which is growing rapidly. In these settings social and health services are coordinated so that greater emphasis can be placed on primary prevention activities. Occupational therapy consultants are conducting health education classes at nutrition sites and in day-care centers, working with remodeling services and housing planners to revise and adapt home settings, and adapting communication equipment for use by the homebound elderly.

Today's technologically oriented information society requires occupational therapy consultants to be more knowledgeable regarding the use of robotics and computers. Their knowledge of the use of occupation as a health determinant and the effect that activity—or lack of activity—has on health will be important assets in the society of the future. The occupational therapy consultant's unique perspective will also help those experiencing deficits in occupational performance related to living and working in space, underground, or undersea.

Marketing Consultation Services

Occupational therapy consultation services can be used effectively in a variety of settings. The potential market is extensive. The problem is how to tap it. In some areas—for example, schools and skilled nursing facilities—federal regulations require that occupational therapy services be available as needed. The invitation to enter these systems exists; the consultant only needs to know how to contact the ready buyer. In most other instances the consultant must create the invitation. In all cases the consultant should thoroughly evaluate the situation before beginning a consultation practice. To do this, one must consider the potential needs in the geographic area, the cost and reimbursement factors, and the competition from other occupational therapists and other health care professionals.

On the other side of the coin, the consultant must have an accurate assessment of his or her skills, competence, and consulting style. By definition, the service depends on the individual provider's abilities, and no one person can be confortable in all environments. Similarly, economic, social, physical, and psychological factors that affect the consultant must be considered.

A consultation model of practice allows therapists to maintain a variety of roles, meeting their personal needs. This freedom may make it easier to blend the roles of parent, spouse, and therapist, or those of graduate student, skier, and therapist. Economically a consultation practice does not assure the individual of a steady income. The hourly rate may appear high, but the income can be erratic.

Having defined an area of competence and potential practice environments, and having considered economic and personal resources and needs, the consultant has a market plan and is ready to lay out a promotional plan. This requires knowing the target market and the potential for acceptance of the service. It means identifying all possible activities that can generate referrals or recommended clients. For example:

- Promoting one's services through such tools as professional brochures, letters, business cards, and yellow page listings
- Networking with fellow therapists, professionals in allied fields, and former patients/clients and agency personnel who are advocates of one's competence.
- Doing research, drawing on health planning reports, economic indicators of growing health services, local health classified ads, and state department of health listings of potential user agencies and organizations.

The potential consultant must be willing to contribute time and energy to community activities that focus on health concerns. Providing free lectures, assisting in planning and running special programs, and participating in committees and on boards not only heighten a consultant's visibility, they expand his or her knowledge base and resource network.

To become self-employed, a consultant must have access to funds during the start-up period. Initial expenses such as printing, mailing, office supplies, telephone, and transportation must be considered. If another source of income is not readily available, the amount needed must include the consultant's cost of living.

Developing a formula for reimbursement of services requires taking into consideration present earning potential, the range of competitive fees, and costs. One possible method of calculating charges (36) is to add present salary or earning potential (including fringe benefits) and professional overhead (rent, utilities, depreciation, transportation, printing supplies, etc.) and divide the sum by the number of chargeable hours, hours that one could work and hours that one should be paid for (sick days, vacation, and holidays).

$$\frac{\text{Present salary/earning potential} + \text{Professional overhead}}{\text{Chargeable hours}}$$

The figure obtained is the hourly rate. Factors that may warrant a downward adjustment of this rate include the learning opportunity that a particular consulting experience might offer, the possibility that a particular experience might promote more business, or the guarantee of a substantive number of work hours per week or month.

Another method of determining rates is to research the current market value for the service in the geographic area that has been targeted. Other consultants, private practitioners, or organizations providing service to the target population have established fees. Information regarding their range of fees can be helpful in realistically setting one's own. A warning in this regard: The antitrust laws prohibit competitors from fixing prices for services. Occupational therapists in consultation or private practice are in competition under the antitrust laws.

Developing and Using Resources

Developing the competence necessary to provide consultation services means devoting time, money, and creative energy to building up a "hip-pocket necessity"—resources. Not only are resources important in a given consultation setting; they also provide a natural support system for the consultant, who often practices in isolation. Included in this category are people, places, literature, educational experiences, and political and economic concerns.

One often hears, "It is not *what* you know, but *whom* you know." This statement needs modification for the consultant. "It is what *and* whom you know, that help make you successful." Experience alone, within a sheltered setting, will not expand one's knowledge base for consultation. Meeting other professionals within and outside occupational therapy helps broaden perspective and heighten awareness of important trends, and alerts one to changes affecting health care practice. Networking through professional organizations, locally and nationally, provides a method for building a natural support system. It also helps develop a roster of experts who may provide needed information, advice, or direction for a specific problem. Similarly, membership in community and other professional organizations, and participation in meetings and committees will extend the resource network. Field visits also stimulate information sharing and networking, and help provide perspective regarding geographic and socioeconomic differences that influence the responses of a given system.

Continuing education for the consultant includes extensive review of professional and related literature, as well as attendance at occupational therapy and multidisciplinary conferences and workshops. In addition to maintaining and improving competence, these activities help keep one abreast of changes, trends, and emerging issues affecting the health care market. Participation also helps increase familiarity with differences in language usage and terminology, thus helping communication skills.

Economics and politics play major roles in shaping the delivery of today's health care. Pending legislation, newly enacted laws, changes in reimbursement methodologies, and revised guidelines for service delivery all have significant implications. Continuing review of current publications and special newsletters such as AOTA's *Federal Report* helps keep the information base up-to-date.

Judicious use of resources helps maintain a broad and well-rounded knowledge base. This expanded perspective and support system encourages creativity and flexibility. A commitment to continued development of resources allows a consultant and a consultee to draw from a comprehensive and current pool of information.

The Business of Being in Business

Today's entrepreneur-therapist may be a self-employed individual, a partner in a group practice, or an owner or a part-owner of a corporation. Each of these options has particular legal, economic, and tax considerations. They also have different practice benefits with regard to sharing responsibilities, caseloads, resources, and support systems.

Self-employment. In a solo practice the therapist is responsible for all the work performed and has full control of the business. As a proprietor, he or she must keep detailed records of any and all income and expenses. Estimated taxes must be paid to make sure that income tax and Social Security obligations are covered. A portion of earnings can be set aside in a retirement plan.

Many tax deductions may be possible in maintaining a business. Any that are taken must be itemized and documented. Malpractice insurance is needed to protect the consultant from liability in a practice, and is an important deduction. Using a room in one's home solely for business may qualify that space for an office-in-home deduction. Other deductions may include travel expenses when away overnight, a per-mile rate for automobile mileage when a car is used to conduct business, professional dues and journals, fees and expenses connected with continuing education, the cost of uniforms, and child care expenses.

A self-employed therapist may hire other people. These individuals become employees, and the employer is responsible for making timely payroll deductions, providing benefits, and establishing written policies and procedures for the business.

Practicing alone allows for great freedom and control. It also means working hard to develop outside support systems and backup arrangements for those emergencies when a consultant is unable to meet an obligation.

Partnership in a group practice. In a group practice, in which a consultant participates as a partner, some expenses, such as overhead, are shared by all, whereas other expenses, such as transportation, are charged to the partner who incurred them. Income is allocated according to a formula agreed on by the partners. In general, the rules for individual proprietors apply to partnerships.

Professionally a partnership can have many rewards. It fosters mutual support, facilitates a sharing of ideas and expertise, builds in a backup system, and, by virtue of its size, offers expanded visibility and marketability.

Incorporation. Therapists who incorporate expect to generate a large volume of work and usually employ others. A major advantage of a corporation is that it is considered a legal entity. If the business goes under or a client sues, the corporation takes responsibility, not the officers. This does not preclude the need for therapist-owners to hold professional liability insurance. If money must be borrowed to set up the corporation or expand it, the corporation is the legally responsible party. Other advantages of a corporation include expanded pension and other fringe benefits, such as health insurance, continuing education, and limited personal liability. The company also can reimburse officers and employees for expenses incurred as part of the business, rather than their having to deduct the expenses from their income.

A decision to own and operate a business is a significant step for any therapist. The considerations and complexities of entrepreneurship require major commitments of time, energy, and money. Self-education, risk-taking abilities, and organizational and management skills are important prerequisites. A broad array of books, periodicals, and organizations are available as resources to those contemplating this step. Specific books, pamphlets, and articles detailing occupational therapy private practice (33, 37–42) should be reviewed during the preliminary planning period.

Being in business for oneself can be an exciting and rewarding experience. Although there are many risks, frustrations, and extensive commitments, this model of practice is attracting increasing numbers of therapists. The satisfaction of building a business, the opportunities offered in new markets, and the freedom of self-direction are among the many rewards.

CONCLUSION

Consultation and private practice are rapidly expanding areas of occupational therapy practice. As the pool of experienced therapists increases and as practice settings diversify and proliferate, entrepreneurs will play a major role in shaping future practice.

Therapists at every level of practice should take advantage of daily opportunities to build consultation skills. With greater experience, more complex consultation tasks can be attempted. As occupational therapists increase their visibility in this area, they must expand their knowledge of the health care system and the issues and trends that affect its growth. Maintaining and improving professional competence and quality assurance in service delivery are critical factors for the successful practice of occupational therapy consultants and private practitioners. Experience and competence are hallmarks of the community consultant who will continue to forge new roles and directions for the profession.

SUMMARY

Consultation is a process by which expertise is communicated to others who need assistance in solving existing or potential problems. Legislation, economic issues, personnel shortages, and the spread of technology have had a profound influence on the growth of consultation and private practice. As the professional looks toward the end of the twentieth century, demands for occupational therapy services and opportunities in new markets continue to increase.

Concepts of consultation are drawn from many fields of study. Within each field the emphasis and perspective may vary, but the essentials are generic: consultation is a task-oriented, interactive process in which consultant and consultee focus on a specific problem. The relationship is coordinate, even though the final decision rests with the consultee.

Within occupational therapy, various authors agree that occupational therapy consultants need to understand and effectively use concepts of prevention. Working in a collaborative and helping role, they must comprehend and be comfortable with the indirect nature of the service.

Occupational therapy consultants can be found in private practice, in public and private school systems, in industry, in occupational therapy departments of hospitals and rehabilitation centers, and in schools of occupational therapy. A small number serve in state and federal governments, national health organizations, insurance companies, and accrediting agencies.

In current practice the consultant is seen in many roles: adviser, helper, facilitator; outsider; change agent; evaluator-diagnostician; trainer; planner; and extender. The role of extender causes much concern. Working in settings that do not employ occupational therapy personnel, the consultant assesses a problem and develops a plan that is then carried out by the consultee. This requires ongoing monitoring and follow-up by the consultant. What seems to create the most role confusion and difficulty, however, is functioning as both a consultant and a therapist, and sometimes also as a supervisor. There are important contrasts and parallels among these three roles.

The consultation process may be viewed in four stages: initiation and clarification, in which the expectations of the consultation are established; evaluation and communication, in which information is gathered and assessed; interactive problem resolution, in which strategies are developed cooperatively; and termination, in which a formal plan is presented and the consultation completed. A fifth stage may involve follow-up consultation, at specified intervals or as needed.

Several areas of knowledge are critical in consultation: a thorough foundation in systems theory and behavioral sciences; developmental theory; education and training methodologies; human personality, attitude formation, and change; and knowledge of self. Key skills that the consultant must possess are communicating, educating, diagnosing, and linking. The consultant must also be able to relate easily and effectively to others. Attitudes and attributes such as flexibility, creativity, maturity, and self-confidence help the consultant move successfully in varied environments.

Becoming a consultant requires considering the potential markets for one's services in various settings now and in the future; assessing the needs of consumers, the cost and reimbursement factors, and the competition in those markets; and assessing one's own skills, competence, and style. The consultant must then develop a promotional plan, identifying all possible activities that can generate referrals or recommended clients. Practical matters also require attention, such as locating start-up funds and determining rates. A critically important activity is developing resources through such endeavors as networking, membership in other organizations, continuing education, and the monitoring of current economic and political developments.

A consultant may set up a practice alone, with a group, or as a corporation. These alternatives have different legal, economic, and tax considerations and different practice benefits. For example, in a solo practice the consultant has full control of the business but no built-in support system.

A decision to own and operate a business is a significant step for any therapist. The considerations and the complexities require major commitments of time, energy, and money. But being in business for oneself can be an exciting and rewarding experience.

Consultants have been and will continue to be at the leading edge of practice. Assuming a consultant role requires a high degree of professional competence, risk-taking ability, and self-confidence. A bright future filled with continued opportunities and challenges awaits those who choose this model of practice.

References

1. West WL: The occupational therapist's changing responsibility to the community. *Am J Occup Ther* 21:312–316, 1967
2. Yerxa E: The occupational therapist as consultant and researcher. In *Willard and Spackman's Occupational Therapy*, 5th edition, HL Hopkins, HD Smith, Editors. Philadelphia: JB Lippincott Co, 1978, pp 689–693
3. Lippitt G, Lippitt R: *The Consulting Process in Action*. San Diego, CA: University Associates, 1978
4. Gallessich J: *The Profession and Practice of Consultation*. San Francisco: Jossey-Bass Inc Publishers, 1982
5. Epstein CF: Directions in long-term care. *Gerontology Specialty Section Newsletter* 2(4):1, 4, 1979
6. Laukaran VH: Nationally speaking: Toward a model of occupational therapy for community health. *Am J Occup Ther* 31:71–74, 1977
7. American Occupational Therapy Association: Entry-level role delineation for OTRs and COTAs. In *Reference Manual of the Official Documents of the American Occupational Therapy Association*. Rockville, MD: American Occupational Therapy Association, 1985
8. Moersch M: The occupational therapist as a consultant, as a consultant, as a consultant, In *The Occupational Therapist as Consultant to Community Agencies: Conference Proceedings*, A Jantzen, R Anderson, K Sieg, Editors. Gainesville, FL: University of Florida, College of Health Related Professions, 1975, pp 15–29
9. Dataline: Where occupational therapists are employed. *Occup Ther Newspaper* 38(10):9, 1984
10. Jackson BN: The occupational therapist as consultant to the aged. *Am J Occup Ther* 24:572–575, 1970
11. *Occupational Therapy Manpower: A Plan for Progress*, Report of the Ad Hoc Commission on Occupational Therapy Manpower. Rockville, MD: American Occupational Therapy Association, 1985
12. Coffee D: *Teaching the Consultative Process*. Ithaca, NY: New York State School of Industrial and Labor Relations, Cornell University, 1966
13. American Occupational Therapy Association,

Council on Standards: *The Consulting Process for Occupational Therapists: Introductory Information.* New York: American Occupational Therapy Association, 1969
14. Jantzen A, Anderson R, Sieg K, Editors: *The Occupational Therapist as Consultant to Community Agencies: Conference Proceedings.* Gainesville, FL: University of Florida, College of Health Related Professions, 1975
15. Health: A look to the future. *Occup Ther Newspaper* 38(10):1, 15–16, 1984
16. Dataline: OT among twenty fastest growing occupations. *Occup Ther Newspaper* 38(3):6, 1984
17. Caplin G: *The Theory and Practice of Mental Health Consultation.* New York: Basic Books Inc, 1970
18. Bennis W, Benne K, Chin R, Editors: *The Planning of Change,* 2nd edition. New York: Holt Rinehart & Winston Inc, 1969
19. Lewin K: *Field Theory in Social Science.* New York: Harper, 1951
20. Leopold RL: Consultant and consultee: An extraordinary human relationship—Some thoughts for the occupational therapist. *Am J Occup Ther* 22:72–81, 1968
21. Gaupp P: Authority, influence and control in consultation. *Community Ment Health J* 2(3), 1966
22. West WL: 1967 Eleanor Clarke Slagle Lecture: Professional responsibility in times of change. *Am J Occup Ther* 22:9–15, 1968
23. Llorens LA: Occupational therapy in community child health. *Am J Occup Ther* 25:335–339, 1971
24. West WA: The growing importance of prevention. *Am J Occup Ther* 23:226–231, 1969
25. Wiemer RB: Some concepts of prevention as an aspect of community health. *Am J Occup Ther* 26:1–9, 1972
26. Finn GL: 1971 Eleanor Clarke Slagle Lecture: The occupational therapist in prevention programs. *Am J Occup Ther* 26:59–66, 1972
27. Grossman J: Nationally speaking: Preventive health care and community programming. *Am J Occup Ther* 31:351–354, 1977
28. Mazer JL: The occupational therapist as consultant. *Am J Occup Ther* 23:417–421, 1969
29. Jaffe E: The role of the occupational therapist as community consultant: Primary prevention in mental health programming. *Occup Ther Ment Health* 1(2):47–62, 1980
30. Rogers J: The study of human occupation. In *Health Through Occupation: Theory and Practice in Occupational Therapy,* G Kielhofner, Editor. Philadelphia: FA Davis, 1983, pp 93–121
31. Llorens LA: Preface. In *TOTEMS: A Competency-Based Educational Program,* EM Gilfoyle, Editor. Rockville, MD: American Occupational Therapy Association, 1980, vol 3, p v–vi
32. Gilfoyle EM: Eleanor Clarke Slagle Lectureship, 1984: Transformation of a profession. *Am J Occup Ther* 38:575–584, 1984
33. Gilfoyle EM, Editor: *TOTEMS: A Competency-Based Educational Program.* Rockville, MD: American Occupational Therapy Association 1980, vol 3, pp 19–20, 22–23
34. West W: The principles and process of consultation. In *Consultation in the Community: Occupational Therapy in Child Health,* L Llorens, Editor. Dubuque, IA: Kendall Hunt, 1973, pp 51–58
35. Livingston F, O'Sullivan N, Editors: *Occupational Therapy Consultancy.* Los Angeles: Occupational Therapy Consultants Group, 1978
36. White V: Sample rate per hour calculation. In *TOTEMS: A Competency-Based Educational Program,* E Gilfoyle, Editor. Rockville, MD: American Occupational Therapy Association, 1980, vol 3, p 76
37. American Occupational Therapy Association, Practice Division: Information Packet on *Private Practice.* Rockville, MD: American Occupational Therapy Association, 1982
38. Frazian BJW: Establishing and administrating a private practice in a hospital setting. *Am J Occup Ther* 32:296–300, 1978
39. Sorensen J: Nationally speaking: Occupational therapy in business: A new horizon. *Am J Occup Ther* 32:287–288, 1978
40. Hall K, Hickman L: Establishing a private practice. *Sensory Integration Specialty Section Newsletter* 3(4):1–2, 1980
41. Royee CB: Benefits from private practice in occupational therapy. *Sensory Integration Specialty Section Newsletter* 3(4):3, 1980
42. Caudwell-Klein E, Editor: [Special issue on private practice.] *Physical Disabilities Specialty Section Newsletter* 2(2):1–4, 1979

Section VIII

Payment, Regulatory, and Ethical Issues

This final section of the text treats major issues that affect the practice of occupational therapy. Chapter 18 discusses legislation and related administrative regulations pertaining to payment for occupational therapy services. The major provisions of three federal programs—Medicare, the Civilian Health and Medical Program of the Uniformed Services, and the Federal Employees Health Benefit Program—are summarized. So are the provisions of two federal-state programs, Medicaid and the Education for All Handicapped Children Act (Public Law 94-142), and a state-only program, workers' compensation. Private insurance plans, such as Blue Cross/Blue Shield, health maintenance organizations, and preferred provider organizations, are also covered.

Regulation is the unifying theme of Chapter 19, which, in separate sections, describes accreditation of health care organizations and certification and licensure of occupational therapy personnel. The chapter stresses the educational value of the accreditation process and the opportunity it can provide to develop quality programs. The background, the domain of regulation, the nature of the standards, and the procedures of four accrediting agencies that affect occupational therapy are summarized. *Certification, registration,* and *licensure* are defined, and certification and licensure are contrasted in a table. The chapter also answers some common questions about licensure.

In Chapter 20, "Ethics and Related Professional Liability," The American Occupational Therapy Association's "Principles of Occupational Therapy Ethics" are reproduced as text, and a commentary is offered on each set of principles. The commentary amplifies the principles as necessary, providing supplementary information and clarifying cloudy areas. Also, professional liability related to the principles is explained.

Chapter 18

Payment for Occupational Therapy Services

Susan Jane Scott, OTR

Payment for occupational therapy services is derived from a variety of sources, including federal, state, private, and commercial insurers and some individuals who pay out of pocket. Funds are available through two basic kinds of payment systems: insurance programs and grant programs. Insurance programs such as Medicare, Medicaid, workers' compensation, and private plans pay providers after the service is delivered. Grant programs such as the Education for All Handicapped Children Act (Public Law 94-142), Community Mental Health Centers, the Older Americans Act, and Social Security Title XX—Social Services include occupational therapy as part of an overall program for a specified population. These two types of payment systems are vastly different. Insurance programs are highly structured, with stringent guidelines regarding which services are covered, in what settings, by whom. Grant programs are more flexible, allowing state or local entities to provide specially designed programs as long as they meet broad national goals.

All payments systems regulate the provision of services. In some cases

---

Susan Jane Scott is the director of AOTA's Government and Legal Affairs Division. In that position she represents the views of the occupational therapy profession and segments of the rehabilitation community before the U.S. Congress and federal agencies.

the regulations are very strict. For example, Medicare defines everything from the nature of the service to the average number of service units expected to be provided to a patient with a particular diagnosis. Other systems, such as health maintenance organizations, are fairly heavily regulated regarding enrollment practices and eligibility requirements, but may, for the most part, provide services in the manner they choose.

The amount of regulation is related directly to the cost of the care and not necessarily to the quality. For example, Medicare may limit occupational therapy for a particular patient to nine visits in the home setting, deeming these all that are medically necessary. That limit is imposed to keep Medicare costs down. It has little to do with the number of treatments that would benefit the patient.

In advance of treatment, occupational therapy personnel are not liable for knowing whether a patient's/client's health plan will cover the service. In fairness, however, therapists should know and should inform the patient/client. Such candor can enhance the therapeutic relationship and also expedite payment. "This supports the need for occupational therapy personnel to determine as completely as possible the coverage of occupational therapy in all settings by all payers in [their] locality" (1, p 17). It also underscores the importance of occupational therapy managers knowing about the various payment systems.

This chapter examines the various forms of payment for occupational therapy services and the guidelines and the limitations that go along with them. Existing payment systems are divided into federal, state, and private.[1] Government payment systems in particular are greatly influenced by forces in the larger society, and thus their characteristics are subject to change.

FEDERAL PAYMENT SYSTEMS

Medicare

Established by Congress in 1965 as Title XVIII of the Social Security Act, Medicare is by far the largest single payer for occupational therapy services. Beneficiaries of the program are the nation's elderly, sixty-five years of age and older, people who are disabled, and some people with end stage renal disease. In 1985 an estimated 20 percent of the occupational therapy profession served Medicare beneficiaries in hospital inpatient and outpatient settings, physicians' offices, skilled nursing facilities, comprehensive outpatient rehabilitation facilities, hospices, and through home health agencies (2). The program consists of two parts: Part A—Hospital Insurance Program, which pays for hospital, skilled nursing facility, home, and hospice care; and Part B—Supplementary Medical Insurance Program, which covers hospital outpatient, physician, and other professional services. The coverage requirements for occupational therapy services under these two parts are summarized in Table 1 and discussed below.

---

[1]Some sections of this chapter dealing with federal, state, and private payment systems are adapted in part from the *Federal Report*, No. 83-2, March 1983, and the *Occupational Therapy Medicare Handbook*, 1982, both written by staff of The American Occupational Therapy Association's Government and Legal Affairs Division and published by AOTA.

TABLE 18–1
Coverage for Occupational Therapy Services Under Medicare Parts A and B

Setting	Part A	Part B
Hospital inpatient	Occupational therapy covered at hospital's option	—
Skilled nursing facility	Occupational therapy covered	—
Home health care	Occupational therapy covered; need for occupational therapy alone not sufficient to qualify patient for benefit, but occupational therapy may continue after other services end	Occupational therapy covered; need for occupational therapy alone not sufficient to qualify patient for benefit, but occupational therapy may continue after other services end
Hospice	Occupational therapy covered	—
Hospital outpatient	—	Occupational therapy covered if rendered by hospital personnel, under supervision of attending physician
Other outpatient	—	Occupational therapy covered if rendered as incident to physician's services in physician's office or physician-directed clinic, by clinic's or physician's employee, under physician's supervision; must be directly related to condition for which physician is treating patient, must be billed for by physician
Comprehensive outpatient rehabilitation facility	—	Occupational therapy covered

Note: All services must be prescribed by a physician and furnished according to a written plan of care approved by the physician.

Part A—Hospital Insurance Program. Nonpsychiatric occupational therapy services are covered under Part A when provided to eligible beneficiaries who are inpatients of hospitals and skilled nursing facilities, patients receiving posthospital home health services from a home health agency participating in Medicare, or patients receiving hospice care.

Until October 1983, Medicare paid hospitals on a retrospective basis for reasonable costs incurred in providing specific services (such as occupational therapy) to inpatients. Since that time, under the Prospective Payment System (PPS), hospitals have received a predetermined fixed sum for each discharged patient. This sum is set according to a schedule of 470 Diagnosis Related Groups (DRGs). Hospitals now choose which services to provide to inpatients, and occupational therapy is one of the services that may be provided to certain patients. Some hospitals—psychiatric, rehabilitation, pediatric, and long-term care—are temporarily exempt from the PPS, as are psychiatric and rehabilitation units of acute care general hospitals. These facilities and units continue to be paid retrospectively on a reasonable cost basis, and occupational therapy is a reimbursable service. In addition, four states—Maryland, Massachusetts, New Jersey, and New York—are exempt.[2]

The Medicare law specifically identifies occupational therapy as a covered skilled nursing and home health service under Part A. However, when inpatients of a skilled nursing facility are switched to Part B because they have exhausted their inpatient days of coverage under Part A, occupational therapy services are no longer covered. In a home care setting, the need for intermittent skilled nursing care, physical therapy, or speech therapy alone, qualifies a homebound patient for home health benefits, but the need for occupational therapy alone does not. However, Medicare patients may continue to receive occupational therapy services under the home health benefit after their need for skilled nursing, physical therapy, or speech therapy ends.

Some limitations and qualifying conditions apply in the Part A program:

1. All services must be prescribed by a physician and furnished according to a written plan of care approved by the physician.
2. To qualify for skilled nursing inpatient benefits, patients must need skilled nursing care or skilled rehabilitation services on a daily basis.
3. For posthospital home health services a plan of care for the patient must be established within fourteen days after the patient's discharge from a hospital or skilled nursing facility. This plan must be reviewed periodically by the physician who is responsible for the patient. A plan for occupational therapy would be a part of the overall plan.

Part A covers hospice care for eligible Medicare beneficiaries who have been certified by a physician as "terminally ill," defined in the regulations as a medical prognosis of less than six months to live. The benefit consists of three "election periods"—two of ninety days and a subsequent one of thirty days—that a beneficiary may use during his or her lifetime. A patient who elects to receive hospice benefits must waive inpatient Medicare benefits during the election period.

Medicare defines a hospice as a public agency or a private organization that is primarily engaged in providing care to terminally ill people and that meets Medicare's conditions of participation for hospices. Included are hospice centers, hospitals, special units of hospitals, skilled nursing facilities, home health agencies, and comprehensive outpatient rehabilitation facilities.

Medicare regulations for hospices mandate that four core services be available to patients twenty-four hours a day: counseling, nursing, physician services, and social services. Also, the hospice is required to provide, on an as needed basis, occupational therapy, physical therapy, speech-language therapy, home health aids, homemaker services, and medical supplies, either directly or under a contractual arrangement.

The regulations describe the purposes of occupational therapy services as controlling a patient's symptoms or enabling a patient to maintain activities of daily living and basic functional skills. All hospice employees and additional service providers, such as occupational therapists, must

---

[2]These exemptions are subject to change.

be licensed, certified, or registered in accordance with applicable state laws.

Hospice benefits are paid on a prospective basis. The rates are based on four primary levels of care corresponding to the degree of illness and the amount of care required.

Psychiatric occupational therapy services are covered on a hospital inpatient basis, under a provision of Part A that requires hospitals to have a sufficient number of qualified therapists to provide comprehensive therapeutic activities for psychiatric inpatients. The beneficiary must have a diagnosis of "mental illness," and the services must stay within a limit on all psychiatric services of 190 days over the life of a beneficiary (3).

Part B—Supplementary Medical Insurance Program. Nonpsychiatric occupational therapy services are covered under Part B when furnished in the home; as incident to a physician's services in a private office or a physician-directed clinic; as incident to a physician's services in the outpatient department of a hospital; or in a comprehensive outpatient rehabilitation facility.

As with posthospital home health benefits under Part A, the need for occupational therapy alone does not qualify a beneficiary for home health care, but patients may continue to receive occupational therapy services under the home health benefit after their need for skilled nursing, physical therapy, or speech therapy ends. As a practical matter, home health benefits under Parts A and B have been the same since 1980, when Congress removed the one-hundred-visit limit on Part A.

Occupational therapy services furnished to patients in a physician's office or a physician-directed clinic are covered under the Medicare law's provision that they be incident to a physician's professional service. The therapist providing the services must be employed (either full- or part-time or under contract) by the physician or the clinic and perform the therapy under the physician's direct supervision. The physician's presence in the office or the clinic satisfies the latter requirement. Other requirements are that the provision of the services be directly related to the condition for which the physician is treating the patient, and that the physician bill Medicare for the services.

Medicare covers occupational therapy services furnished to hospital outpatients incident to a physician's services, if the services are provided on a physician's orders by hospital personnel under the supervision of hospital medical staff. Medicare still pays for outpatient services on a retrospective, reasonable-cost basis.

Psychiatric occupational therapy services are covered under Part B in only one outpatient setting, comprehensive outpatient rehabilitation facilities. Medicare places a ceiling of $250 on the total cost of psychiatric services reimbursed under this provision (3).

Medicare conditions of participation. To be paid by Medicare, a service provider must meet all state and local requirements and comply with Medicare's own conditions of participation. The conditions are monitored and periodically revised by the Health Care Financing Administration (HCFA), the agency that administers Medicare.

Hospitals accredited by the Joint Commission on Accreditation of Hospitals or the American Osteopathic Association are deemed to have met the conditions of participation. Nonaccredited hospitals, skilled nursing facilities, home health agencies, and comprehensive outpatient rehabilitation facilities are surveyed by state health agencies using HCFA guidelines.

In hospitals, occupational therapy services must be provided by therapists certified by the American Occupational Therapy Association (AOTA). Certified occupational therapy assistants (COTAs) may provide services under the general supervision of a registered occupational therapist (OTR). General supervision has been defined in Medicare guidelines as "initial direction and periodic inspection of the activity" of a COTA, "but not necessarily on site" (4, p B-3). In skilled nursing facilities, home health agencies, and comprehensive outpatient rehabilitation facilities, occupational therapy services must be provided by occupational therapists who are eligible to take the AOTA certification examination, and occupational therapy assistants must be eligible for certification by AOTA. In all Medicare settings, personnel must be state licensed where applicable.

Durable medical equipment. Expenses incurred by a beneficiary for the rental or the purchase of durable medical equipment are reimbursable if the equipment is used in the patient's home and if it is necessary and reasonable to treat an illness or an injury or to improve the functioning of a malformed body member. Medicare defines durable medical equipment as that which can withstand repeated use, is primarily and customarily used to serve a medical purpose, and generally is not useful to a person in the absence of illness or injury. An example is oxygen-assistance breathing equipment. Raised toilet seats and bathtub grab bars are not covered because they are not considered medically necessary.

Medicare payment for occupational therapy services. In 1975, HCFA (then the Bureau of Health Insurance) issued guidelines for Medicare payment of occupational therapy services. These guidelines, which appear in Appendix F, apply to all settings in which occupational therapy is a covered service. Claims for and documentation of occupational therapy services should clearly reflect the elements of the guidelines, or payment may be delayed or denied. Intermediaries and carriers (insurance companies that administer Medicare claims) are bound by these guidelines, so denials that conflict with them should be strongly challenged. Appendix G offers advice on what to do if Medicare payment is denied.

Civilian Health and Medical Program of the Uniformed Services

The Civilian Health and Medical Program of the Uniformed Services (CHAMPUS) is a U. S. Department of Defense program of health care for the dependents of active duty members of the armed forces, and for retired members. It shares the cost of medical and other health care that eligible beneficiaries receive from civilian sources. For dependents, CHAMPUS is considered the last payer, so if other coverage exists, it must be used first. The CHAMPUS program pays for services through fiscal intermediaries such as Blue Cross/Blue Shield. The amount of payment is based on reasonable charges. CHAMPUS coverage is provided under a basic program and a special program of rehabilitative benefits.

The basic program. Under the basic program CHAMPUS beneficiaries can obtain both inpatient and outpatient medical and mental health care from civilian sources. Until fall 1984 the basic program covered occupational therapy only on a hospital inpatient basis, specifically excluding coverage in any other settings. However, federal regulations published September 14, 1984, expanded medical and mental health coverage for occupational therapy to hospital outpatient settings.

To qualify for payment, occupational therapy services must be judged medically necessary by a supervising physician, and must be intended to help the patient overcome or compensate for disability resulting from illness, injury, or the effects of a CHAMPUS-covered condition. The occupational therapist must be an employee of a CHAMPUS-authorized provider and must render the services in connection with CHAMPUS-authorized care in an organized inpatient or outpatient rehabilitation program. The employing institution must bill for the services (5).

The special program of rehabilitative benefits. The special program offers rehabilitative benefits for seriously physically handicapped and moderately or severely mentally retarded spouses and children of active duty members. Coverage is provided on an inpatient and outpatient basis, but the requirements for a beneficiary to qualify for the benefits are extremely stringent. Under this program the beneficiary pays only a small deductible. A handbook distributed by CHAMPUS (6) provides details about coverage and payments.

Federal Employees Health Benefit Program

The Federal Employees Health Benefit Program covers federal government employees and retirees. The program is implemented by over two hundred private plans, including two that are governmentwide, several that are sponsored by employee organizations, and many that are local, comprehensive plans (such as health maintenance organizations). The federal law and regulations governing the scope of the services that must be provided do not specify particular services, only general ones such as hospital, surgical, medical, and others. The coverage of specific services such as occupational therapy, and the settings in which they may be provided, is determined by each plan. As a general rule, the plans cover nonpsychiatric occupational therapy services in hospital inpatient settings, and, to some extent and indirectly, psychiatric services (3). The plans vary in their coverage of occupational therapy in other settings.

STATE PAYMENT SYSTEMS

Medicaid

Medicaid, Title XIX of the Social Security Act, is a joint federal-state program that provides health care to the poor and the medically indigent. States have great flexibility in the definition of *medically indigent* and in the makeup and the administration of the program, so benefits vary significantly from state to state. States must include all recipients of Aid to Families with Dependent Children (AFDC) and most beneficiaries of

Supplementary Security Income (SSI). Not all states provide Medicaid coverage for the medically needy. "Some states have a spend-down provision under which families with moderately high incomes may become eligible for Medicaid when their medical expenses reduce their income below the state standard" (7, p 20).

Medicaid services fall into two categories: mandatory and optional. Mandatory services include hospital services; laboratory work and X-rays; skilled nursing facility services; physician services; early and periodic screening, diagnosis, and treatment for those under twenty-one; and family planning. Optional services are those that the states may choose to provide. Occupational therapy is one, along with physical therapy, speech therapy, drugs, psychiatric care, and others. The option includes psychiatric occupational therapy services. Some states have opted to cover occupational therapy services in various settings, and others have not. Information on Medicaid coverage of occupational therapy may be obtained from a state's Office of Medical Assistance (Medicaid).

The Education for All Handicapped Children Act

Enacted by Congress in 1975, the Education for All Handicapped Children Act (Public Law 94-142) requires that any public school system receiving federal assistance provide handicapped children with a free, appropriate education in the least restrictive environment. Federal grants assist state and local education agencies in fulfilling this mandate. The law entitles handicapped children not only to special education services, but to the related services they need to benefit from special education. Occupational, physical, and speech therapy are defined as related services, among others (8). Occupational therapy services must be provided by qualified therapists as defined in each state, and must be directed toward helping the child benefit from special education services. Over five thousand OTRs and COTAs provide services to children in school settings (2). About half of the OTRs receiving payment for services under this program are salaried employees of the school system. The remainder have contractual arrangements to serve children in one or more school system.

For a child to receive occupational therapy it must be included as a related service in the child's individualized education program (IEP). The IEP, which is mandated by law, is developed by a team of professionals and the child's family or guardian. Although the occupational therapy treatment plan may include various modalities and treatment approaches, the service must be clearly identified as occupational therapy because that is the legally mandated service. If school personnel or parents believe that a child needs occupational therapy as a related service and it is not included in the IEP, a due process hearing can be requested. Appendix H explains the procedure.

Although federal law mandates the provision of services to handicapped children and provides some monies for states to meet the mandate, the vast majority of decisions under Public Law 94-142 are made by state and local officials, and most of the funding is derived from state and local sources. Occupational therapy personnel in school settings need to work closely with local and state education officials on issues related to funding, human resources, and regulation of services.

Workers' Compensation

Workers' compensation is a state-sponsored program supported by employer contributions and administered by insurance carriers. A beneficiary receives services identified by the workers' compensation law in his or her state. As with Medicaid, the coverage of health services, including occupational therapy, varies substantially across the states. The amounts of deductibles and copayments also vary, as do the duration and scope of services. Occupational therapy personnel providing services to people covered by workers' compensation should investigate the coverage of occupational therapy under their particular state's law. They should also check whether services are paid for according to prevailing charge, reasonable cost, or predetermined fee.

In several states, workers' compensation programs have established maximum allowable fees for individual modalities or procedures, using a uniform description and coding system. Sometimes the allowable fee is not comparable with a reasonable charge. If this is the case, local practitioners should work with the state workers' compensation governing board to obtain adjustments in the fee schedules (9).

PRIVATE PAYMENT SYSTEMS

Together the several thousand health insurance plans operating in the United States represent the largest source of payment for health care. No single form of private insurance prevails, nor are coverage requirements necessarily similar across the plans. Three points about them may help managers and practitioners understand their operation:

1. There are profit and nonprofit health plans in this sector. For example, Blue Cross/Blue Shield plans are nonprofit, but Aetna and Prudential are operated for profit. Both types are private, however, and must adhere to state insurance codes, which establish coverage requirements.
2. According to a July 1984 issue of *Pension World*, "nearly half of all employers providing health insurance to their work forces now self-insure at least part of their medical benefits package" (10, p 12). Courts have ruled that these self-funded plans are governed not by state insurance codes, but by federal standards set forth in the Employee Retirement Income Security Act (ERISA). These are very general, minimum standards and do not mention occupational therapy.
3. The many plans of Blue Cross/Blue Shield across the country are quasi-independent. No master contract governs their coverage requirements. Thus, a Blue Cross/Blue Shield plan in one state or city may have completely different coverage requirements for occupational therapy than a plan in another state or city.

Occupational therapy personnel should investigate how their services are covered by the private insurance plans operating in their local area. Usually one or more plans tend to dominate in an area, so this information should not be difficult to obtain. Most types of private insurance plans still pay for services on a retrospective basis. This could change in the years ahead, however, influenced by the Medicare Prospective Payment System.

Prepaid Health Plans

Many prepaid health plans are available now, and their number is increasing. A popular type is the health maintenance organization (HMO). HMOs provide comprehensive, coordinated medical services in a limited geographic area to a group of voluntarily enrolled members. For access to these services the members pay a fixed premium at regular intervals and receive services at no extra or very little cost.

Health Maintenance Organizations are of three basic types: group/staff HMOs, individual practice associations (IPAs), and network HMOs. In a group/staff HMO, care is provided in one or more locations either by a group of physicians who contract with the HMO or by physicians whom the HMO employs directly. In an IPA, the HMO contracts individually with physicians, who provide services to HMO members out of their own offices. In a network HMO, services are provided by two or more group practices with which the HMO has a contractual arrangement (11).

A new form of HMO is known as the social/health maintenance organization (SHMO). Designed to address the needs of the elderly as this proportion of the population grows, the SHMO offers health and social services to enrollees on a prepaid basis. The services provided include those covered under Medicare Parts A and B, some long-term-care services, and other benefits such as eyeglasses, prescription drugs, and hearing aids. All of the services are coordinated through a single system, using a combination of public and private funding. To the extent that occupational therapy is covered under Medicare Parts A and B, it is included in the services provided by the SHMO (12).

In all these kinds of plans the incentive to health care organizations and practitioners is to provide only necessary health care. Occupational therapy services may be included in one or more of the plans operating in an area, but that has to be determined. If the service is not included, its addition to a plan could be negotiated.

Recent changes in federal regulations governing HMOs make it easier and more attractive for them to enroll Medicare beneficiaries. HMOs serving Medicare beneficiaries must provide all of the benefits that the Medicare law stipulates, including occupational therapy (see the earlier section on Medicare coverage, under Federal Payment Systems). The new regulations offer an opportunity for occupational therapy personnel to expand their services and programming through these new types of organizations.

A recent phenomenon related to the HMO is the preferred provider organization (PPO). The PPO, which first appeared in 1980, has emerged primarily as a result of two factors: the interest of business coalitions in reducing health care costs and an oversupply of physicians or hospital beds in certain areas of the country. The PPO is not an entity, but an arrangement that gives preference to certain "preferred" providers. These are providers with whom fees have been negotiated, often at discounted rates. PPOs cover the services of nonpreferred providers as well, but not at particularly competitive rates, and often they give consumers further incentives to use preferred providers by offering reduced deductibles, no copayments, or special benefits. Preferred providers are usually hospitals and physicians, but may also be skilled nursing facilities or home health agencies (13).

Self-Pay

In many cases a patient/client needs and receives occupational therapy, but has insufficient coverage or none at all and thus must pay for the services out of pocket. This can be a major problem when a patient/client assumes that his or her plan covers all necessary medical care. The problem occurs most often in outpatient settings, because occupational therapy is frequently not covered in them, or the coverage is vague. These possibilities underscore the importance of occupational therapy personnel understanding the provisions of health plans in their area and talking openly about payment with a patient/client before any services are rendered.

DOCUMENTATION

Critical to timely payment for occupational therapy services under any system is proper documentation. Most systems require a plan of treatment which has to be approved by a physician. The plan must clearly indicate the specific occupational therapy intervention proposed for the patient. Care should be taken to show the occupational therapy services as different from other services that the patient may be receiving, such as nursing or physical therapy. Progress notes should chart specific measurable patient progress, record alterations in the treatment plan, and summarize the patient's status when treatment is discontinued. The medical record may become a legal document if placed in evidence during a court proceeding, so all entries should be strictly correct and carefully thought out. The medical record also documents that services were provided, and this could be linked directly to payment in many cases. A good rule of thumb to remember is, "If it isn't written in the record, it didn't happen."

The goals and philosophy of the payment program should be reflected in documentation. For example, Medicare is an acute medical insurance program. Notes on Medicare patients should address occupational therapy intervention for acute medical problems such as pain, limited range of movement, and so forth. Similarly the occupational therapy portion of the IEP for a child receiving services under Public Law 94-142 should indicate how occupational therapy will address a child's functional problems so that he or she can benefit from special education services.

Good documentation is also important for describing occupational therapy programs and services. Education of physicians, nurses, facility administrators, and insurance claims reviewers may require the development of good fact sheets, protocols, case examples, and payment guidelines. Chapter 16 discusses such internal and external communications at length. The Medicare occupational therapy guidelines and the AOTA Uniform Terminology (14) may be useful as well.

It may also be necessary to supply written documents supporting the efficiency and cost effectiveness of occupational therapy. The AOTA has identified a number of studies related to these subjects that might prove helpful (15). Again, in any documentation, occupational therapy must come through as distinct from other services and reasonable and necessary for the patient/client.

CODING OF SERVICES FOR BILLING

A subject related to documentation is the coding of occupational therapy services for billing purposes. Various payers require different systems. For Part A inpatient hospital services the Medicare program uses the Uniform Bill #82 (UB-82, formerly HCFA 1450), which includes information about the patient's age, sex, principal diagnosis, any surgical procedures, complications or accompanying conditions, and services received. Information from the UB-82 is used by Medicare intermediaries to establish a specific DRG number (from 1 through 470) for each patient at discharge. The hospital then receives a predetermined payment rate relating to the DRG number. As of July 1985, skilled nursing facilities, home health agencies, and comprehensive outpatient rehabilitation facilities must also use this system, and an increasing number of commercial insurers and state Medicaid programs are adopting it (16).

Occupational therapists in private practice or in physicians' offices have sometimes used CPT codes for billing purposes. CPT, short for *Physicians' Current Procedural Terminology* (17), is a listing of descriptive terms and identifying codes for reporting medical services and procedures performed by physicians. The purpose of the terminology is to provide a uniform language that accurately designates medical, surgical, and diagnostic services and provides an effective means of reliable, nationwide communication among physicians, patients/clients, and third parties. The CPT is prepared by an editorial committee and the staff of the American Medical Association with the assistance of physicians representing all specialties of medicine. The present version, CPT-4, is the fourth edition of a work that first appeared in 1966.

The CPT-4 codes form a part of another, more widely used system, the HCFA Common Procedure Coding System (HCPCS). This was developed by HCFA to satisfy the operational needs of Medicare Part B and Medicaid fee-for-service reimbursement programs. To the CPT-4 codes, HCPCS adds additional codes and modifiers developed by other professionals and insurers to meet their reporting needs. Also included are codes developed by HCFA, state agencies, and commercial carriers to meet the claims-processing needs of Medicare and Medicaid.

The HCPCS is fast becoming a national system. Blue Cross/Blue Shield Association requires all of its participating plans to use the system, and the Health Insurance Association of America has endorsed its use by commercial insurance companies (16). State Medicaid programs are expected to adopt it in the near future.

EXPANDING PAYMENT FOR OCCUPATIONAL THERAPY SERVICES

Much progress has been made in recent years in expanding payment for occupational therapy services. National efforts have been successful in broadening Medicare coverage to home health, comprehensive outpatient rehabilitation facilities, hospice programs, and HMOs. Local and state efforts have resulted in better coverage under Medicaid, the Federal Employees Health Benefit Program, and private insurance plans. In 1984 the Health Insurance Association of America reaffirmed its support for inclusion of occupational therapy in insurance plans, stating in its *Report on Consumer and Professional Relations* "that *Occupational Therapy* is a professional health care service which, when properly used, can be instrumental in decreasing hospital confinement, disability, and the ultimate cost of health care" (18, p 3).

Further expansion of payment for occupational therapy services is a national, state, and local—but collective—effort. Critical to success is good documentation of the medical necessity and the cost effectiveness of occupational therapy services. The efficacy data studies that AOTA has identified (15) support these conclusions. A research study underway at AOTA seeks more evidence. Also available from AOTA is an extensive package of audiovisual materials that may be used to educate potential payers about occupational therapy (19).

Consumer demand for occupational therapy services to be included in insurance plans available to them can be extremely helpful, as can physician and other professional support. New payment sources are developing for occupational therapy personnel, such as shopping center clinics, health maintenance organizations, and industry wellness programs. Treating patients/clients and testifying as expert witnesses in disability cases is an area of occupational therapy involvement that is growing dramatically. As the health care industry changes in response to public demand for lower health care costs, occupational therapy personnel should have many more chances to demonstrate the value and cost effectiveness of their services.

SUMMARY

Payment for occupational therapy services is derived from a variety of sources, including federal, state, private, and commercial insurers and some individuals who pay out of pocket. Funds are available through two basic kinds of payment systems: insurance programs (e.g., Medicare) and grant programs (e.g., the Education for All Handicapped Children Act). The former are highly structured, the latter more flexible.

Federal payment systems include Medicare, the Civilian Health and Medical Program of the United States (CHAMPUS), and the Federal Employees Health Benefit Program. Medicare beneficiaries are the nation's elderly sixty-five years of age and older, people who are disabled, and some people with end stage renal disease. Benefits are paid under two parts: Part A, which provides hospital insurance, and Part B, which offers supplementary medical insurance. Under Part A, nonpsychiatric occupational therapy services are covered when provided to eligible beneficiaries who are inpatients of hospitals and skilled nursing facilities, patients/clients receiving posthospital home health services from a home health agency participating in Medicare, or patients/clients receiving hospice care. Psychiatric services are covered on a hospital inpatient basis.

Part B covers nonpsychiatric occupational therapy services when they are furnished in the home; as incident to a physician's services in a private office or a physician-directed clinic; as incident to a physician's services in the outpatient department of a hospital; or in a comprehensive outpatient rehabilitation facility. Psychiatric services are covered only in the latter type of facility.

Nonpsychiatric and psychiatric services under Part A or Part B must be prescribed by a physician and furnished according to a written plan of care approved by the physician. Some additional conditions and limitations apply in particular settings.

Since October 1983, under the Prospective Payment System, hospitals have received a predetermined fixed sum for each discharged patient/client. Some types of hospitals and some units of hospitals are temporarily exempt from this system and continue to be paid for their services on a retrospective, reasonable-cost basis. Outpatient services are also still paid on the latter basis.

The CHAMPUS is a U. S. Department of Defense program of health care for the dependents of active duty members of the armed forces, and for retired members. For dependents, CHAMPUS is considered the last payer, so if other coverage exists, it must be used first. Under the basic program CHAMPUS beneficiaries can obtain both inpatient and outpatient medical and mental health care from civilian sources. To qualify for payment, occupational therapy services must be judged medically necessary by a supervising physician. Other conditions apply. A special program offers rehabilitative benefits for seriously physically handicapped and moderately or severely mentally retarded spouses and children of active duty members. Qualifying requirements are extremely stringent, however.

The Federal Employees Health Benefit Program, which covers federal government employees and retirees, is implemented by over two hundred private plans. Coverage of occupational therapy services is determined by each plan.

State payment systems include Medicaid, the Education for All Handicapped Children Act, and workers' compensation. Medicaid is a joint federal-state program that provides health care to the poor and the medically indigent. Benefits vary from state to state. Occupational therapy is an optional service that states may choose to cover.

The Education for All Handicapped Children Act entitles handicapped children to a free appropriate education in the least restrictive environment and to the related services they need to benefit from that education. Occupational therapy is defined as a related service. For a child to receive it, it must be included in the child's individualized education program.

Workers' compensation is supported by employer contributions and administered by insurance carriers. A beneficiary receives services identified by the particular law in his or her state. Coverage of occupational therapy varies across states.

Private payment systems represent the largest source of payment for health care. No single form prevails, and coverage requirements are not uniform. Most types of private plans still pay for services on a retrospective, reasonable-cost basis, but prepaid health plans are proliferating, among them, health maintenance organizations. Under these kinds of plans, based on payment of a fixed sum at regular intervals, the incentive to health care organizations and practitioners is to provide only necessary health care.

In many cases a patient/client must pay for occupational therapy services out of pocket. This underscores the need for occupational therapy personnel to understand payment systems and talk openly with patients/clients about their coverage.

Critical to timely payment for services is proper documentation. Care should be taken to show occupational therapy services as different from others. The goals and philosophy of the payment program should be reflected in the documentation.

Several systems exist for coding services. Various payers require different systems. Two widely used ones are Uniform Bill 82 and the U. S. Health Care Financing Administration's Common Procedure Coding System.

Much progress has been made in recent years in expanding payment for occupational therapy services. Further expansion is a national, state, and local—but collective—effort. As the health care industry changes, occupational therapy personnel should have many more chances to demonstrate the value and cost effectiveness of their services.

References

1. American Occupational Therapy Association, Government and Legal Affairs Division: *Federal Report*, No 83-2, March 1983.
2. American Occupational Therapy Association, Membership Services: *Member Data Survey*. Rockville, MD: American Occupational Therapy Association, 1982
3. Peters ME: Reimbursement for psychiatric occupational therapy services. *Am J Occup Ther* 38:307–312, 1984
4. Article 3101.9, Medicare coverage of occupational therapy services. In *Occupational Therapy Medicare Handbook*, American Occupational Therapy Association, Government and Legal Affairs Division. Rockville, MD: American Occupational Therapy Association, 1982
5. 32 *Code of Federal Regulations* §199.10.
6. *CHAMPUS Handbook*. Aurora, CO: CHAMPUS, 1983 (Address: CHAMPUS Information Office, Aurora, CO 80045-6900)
7. *Medicare/Medicaid Fact Finder*. Washington, DC: McGraw-Hill, Washington Health Letters, 1984 (Address: 1120 Vermont Avenue, N.W., Washington, DC 20005)
8. Rourk JD: Funding health services for children. *Am J Occup Ther* 38:313–319, 1984
9. Hershman AG: Reimbursement in private practice. *Am J Occup Ther* 38:299–306, 1984
10. Self-insurance: Key to health costs? *Pension World*, July 1984, p 12
11. *HMO Fact Sheet*. U. S. Department of Health and Human Services, Public Health Service, Office of Health Maintenance Organizations, April 1985
12. American Occupational Therapy Association, Government and Legal Affairs Division: *Federal Report*. No 84-5, September 1984, pp 8–10
13. Davy JD: Preferred provider organizations. *Am J Occup Ther* 38:327–329, 1984
14. American Occupational Therapy Association: Uniform terminology for reporting occupational therapy services and occupational therapy product output reporting system. In *Reference Manual of the*

Official Documents of the American Occupational Therapy Association. Rockville, MD: American Occupational Therapy Association, 1983

15. American Occupational Therapy Association, Quality Assurance Division: *Efficacy Data Briefs: Outpatient Stroke Therapy Reduces Functional Deterioration*, No 1, March 1983; *Stroke Rehabilitation, Including Occupational Therapy as Part of Team, Shows Statistically Significant Long-Term Functional Gains*, No. 2, July 1983; *Research Shows Shorter Hospitalization Related to Occupational Therapy*, No 3, March 1983; *Rehabilitation Can Be Cost-Effective in Treatment of Multiple Sclerosis*, No 4, November 1983; *Research Shows Day Treatment, Including Occupational Therapy, Adds Significantly to Benefits of Antipsychotic Drugs in Care of Schizophrenic Patients*, No 5, October 1984. Rockville, MD: American Occupational Therapy Association, Quality Assurance Division
16. Health Care Financing Administration develops uniform coding systems. *Occup Ther News* 39(4):6, 1985
17. Finkel AJ, Editor: *Physicians' Current Procedural Terminology*, 4th edition. Chicago: American Medical Association, 1981
18. Health Insurance Association of America: Update on occupational therapy. *Report on Consumer and Professional Relations*, January 31, 1984
19. *Occupational Therapy Promotion Kit*. Rockville, MD: American Occupational Therapy Association, 1984

Additional Resource

Reimbursement. *Am J Occup Ther* (special issue) 38:293–343, 1984

Chapter 19

Regulation and Standard Setting

Susan B. Fine, MA, OTR, FAOTA
Jeanette Bair, MBA, OTR, FAOTA
Stephanie Presseller Hoover, EdD, OTR
Jane Davy Acquaviva, OTR

In health care, as in other fields, mechanisms exist for setting standards and applying them to organizations and individuals delivering professional services. These mechanisms—accreditation, certification, licensure and standards of practice—serve both the public and the

---

Susan B. Fine has 25 years of experience as an administrator of psychosocial rehabilitation programs and as an educator in management methods. Currently the director of the department of therapeutic activities at New York's Payne Whitney Clinic, she is AOTA's representative on the Joint Commission on Accreditation of Hospitals' Professional Technical Advisory Committee for Psychiatric Facilities and its Task Force on Rehabilitation Standards.

Jeanette Bair is the director of AOTA's Practice Division, in which capacity she is the staff liaison to the Commission on Practice and to the four accrediting agencies discussed in this chapter. Before joining the AOTA staff, she held various management positions in clinical settings.

Stephanie Presseller Hoover is the director of AOTA's Education Division. Her career has included experiences as a practitioner in pediatrics, an administrator in a rehabilitation department, an instructor in higher education, and a consultant.

As assistant director of the Government and Legal Affairs Division of the American Occupational Therapy Association, Jane Davy Acquaviva has been actively involved for the past six years in the issues surrounding state regulation of occupational therapy personnel.

profession. They assure the public of qualified professionals and adequately equipped, competently staffed organizations. For the profession they publicly confirm the quality of individual organizations and the competence of individual practitioners. Both organizations and individuals gain in status from such recognition. Accreditation also establishes the eligibility of organizations to receive government grants and contracts, and an official seal of approval qualifies both establishments and individuals for third-party reimbursement.

The application of standards at the state level often has the force of law because legislatures have created professional boards and commissions to accredit programs of preparation and to license individual practitioners. At the national level, accreditation, certification, licensure, and standards of practice, where they exist, are ostensibly voluntary. This voluntary regulation is usually accepted by the public because the professions involved have demonstrated a commitment to maintain standards themselves. The voluntary nature of this regulation is questionable, however. Because the federal government and insurance companies depend on national accreditation to determine eligibility for grants and contracts and third-party reimbursement, national accreditation is essentially mandatory.

VOLUNTARY ACCREDITATION OF ORGANIZATIONS

Voluntary regulation of health care organizations began in 1917 with hospital regulation, the development of which is well documented in the literature (1–6). Prompted by the revelations of the landmark Flexner Report (5) and the medical profession's desire to avoid government regulation of hospital practice (6), the American College of Surgeons formulated "Minimum Standards for Hospitals" in 1917. The success of this voluntary effort to improve the quality of health care is reflected in the change from a 13 percent rate of accreditation that first year to a 94 percent rate by 1945 (4). The marked growth of the regulatory process over the years is illustrated by the increase in the length of the standards for general hospitals, from 1 page in 1917 to 226 pages in 1982 (2).

"As they've evolved, standards . . . have shifted from being the 'minimum essential' to the 'optimal achievable'" (7, p 299). This expansion has been met by enthusiastic praise as well as rigorous criticism (2, 8, 9). Pointing to the variety of agencies as well as the mass of regulations and required documentation, many view the regulatory process as having grown "from a paper tiger into a man eating beast" (3, p 113). Intense concerns about whether or not accreditation is really the key to quality care have been matched by concerns for cost containment and a variety of ethical and interdisciplinary issues related to regulation (1, 8).

The practice of occupational therapy is affected by regulation of a variety of health care settings: hospitals, rehabilitation facilities, agencies and facilities for developmentally disabled people, and home and community health agencies. Table 1 identifies the agencies operating in these domains and presents information about pertinent characteristics. Each agency is discussed in further detail on the following pages. Accreditation/approval of education in occupational therapy is also explained.

The Accreditation Process

Typically, an organization seeking accreditation initiates the accreditation process by submitting an application for a review or a survey. Several of the accrediting agencies then require a self-study on the basis of their standards. The next step is a site survey, in which a team of surveyors visits the organization. The organization is notified in advance of the designated time for the visit. Depending on an organization's size and the scope of its services, the visit may last from one to four days, and the survey team may involve from one to four professionals from various fields of health care. The cost of the survey is borne by the organization seeking accreditation. Once an organization is accredited, to maintain its accreditation, it must undergo periodic review, normally every three years.

The final decision regarding accreditation is made by different bodies within the various accrediting agencies, depending on an agency's structure and purpose. In agencies whose major purpose is accreditation, such as the Joint Commission on Accreditation of Hospitals, the agency's governing board usually makes the final decision. When a professional association operates the accrediting program, the decision frequently rests with an internal commission or committee. If accreditation or reaccreditation is denied, an appeals process normally exists for challenging the decision. A common practice of accrediting agencies is to publish a list of the organizations they have accredited.

Across agencies there is variability in the process for developing and revising accreditation standards. Table 1 summarizes the processes followed in the four agencies discussed in this chapter.

Importance of Accreditation for Occupational Therapy

An occupational therapy manager whose organization is being surveyed should expect to participate in the process through advanced planning with other members of the organization's administration, submission of policies and procedures manuals and other documents representing compliance with the standards, hosting an inspection of the physical plant, and interviews with the survey team. The latter frequently involve discussion of personnel (their formal preparation, credentials, qualifications, and experience, and provisions for continuing assessment of their competency), staff continuing education and supervision, methods of documentation, referrals, and quality assurance activities. If the occupational therapy manager handles these interviews skillfully, he or she is able not only to demonstrate compliance but to educate surveyors about the purpose and value of occupational therapy services.

Despite the inadequacies of some standards, the difficulties that frequently plague the survey visit, and the variability in surveyors' knowledge and understanding of all aspects of an organization's services, the accreditation process can provide important opportunities for occupational therapy managers to clarify program goals and develop effective strategies for implementation of clinical, research, and educational components. Instead of managers and practitioners viewing accreditation as an intrusive inspection visit for which they must spend time and effort

(*text continued on page 345*)

TABLE 19–1
Accreditation Agency Characteristics

Agency	Domain of Accreditation	Sponsored By	Standards Developed By	Accreditation Decided By
Joint Commission on Accreditation of Hospitals (JCAH)	General hospitals, psychiatric and substance abuse programs, hospice programs, ambulatory health care organizations, long-term-care facilities, mental retardation and developmental disabilities programs, and community mental health centers	American College of Physicians, American College of Surgeons, American Dental Association, American Hospital Association, American Medical Association	JCAH staff with input from task forces on particular chapters, Professional and Technical Advisory Committees, field reviews; final approval by JCAH Board of Commissioners	JCAH Board of Commissioners
Commission on Accreditation of Rehabilitation Facilities (CARF)	Free-standing rehabilitation organizations or rehabilitation programs operated as units within larger institutions; private nonprofit, proprietary, and public agency operated facilities	American Academy of Physical Medicine and Rehabilitation, American Hospital Association, American Occupational Therapy Association, American Physical Therapy Association. Goodwill Industries of America, National Association of Jewish Vocational Services, National Association of Private Residential Facilities for the Mentally Retarded, National Easter Seal Society, United Cerebral Palsy Association	Ad hoc committees reaching consensus regarding practice in the field; final approval by CARF Board of Trustees	CARF Board of Trustees

Accreditation Council (for services for mentally retarded and other developmentally disabled persons—AC MRDD)	Any agency serving developmentally disabled people	American Association of Mental Deficiency, American Occupational Therapy Association, American Psychological Association, Association for Retarded Citizens of the U. S., Epilepsy Foundation of America, National Association of Private Residential Facilities for the Mentally Retarded, National Association of Service Workers, National Society for Children and Adults with Autism, United Cerebral Palsy Association	Service providers and consumers; final approval by AC MRDD Board of Directors	AC MRDD Board of Review
NLN/APHA Program for Home Health Agencies and Community Nursing Services	Agencies that offer nursing and other health services outside hospitals, extended care facilities, and nursing homes	National League for Nursing, American Public Health Association	Accreditation Standards Committee of NLN's Council of Home Health Agencies and Community Health Services	Board of Review

writing up what they suspect the surveyors want, they should learn how to make standards work for them and their programs on a continuing basis. Standards provide occupational therapy personnel with a mandate to define and document their work, an opportunity the profession can ill afford to ignore. Standards can foster effectiveness and efficiency by helping managers monitor and improve the use and the quality of occupational therapy services and heighten the visibility and credibility of occupational therapy within an organization. Further, standards can support managers in promoting the needs of their department or program with the administration.

Understanding and interpreting standards skillfully and logically, in keeping with patients'/clients' needs and an organization's objectives and resources, is the responsibility of the occupational therapy manager. Resource materials prepared by accrediting agencies are helpful in developing a fuller understanding of the intent and the potential of their standards. Information about these resources can be obtained directly from the agencies [see (11, 13–15) for addresses].

Hospital Accreditation

At the forefront of the regulatory process is the Joint Commission on Accreditation of Hospitals (JCAH), the largest and most influential private organization involved in voluntary accreditation in health care. The JCAH strives to "enhance, through a voluntary accreditation process, the quality of care and services provided in organized health care settings" (10, p 1211). The impact of JCAH standards has spread considerably since the 1960s when JCAH accreditation became the "preferred route" for hospitals to demonstrate eligibility for Medicare and Medicaid reimbursement (2). "More than 7,400 facilities and programs, including 75% of the nation's acute care general hospitals, participate in JCAH activities" (11).

To achieve its stated goals, the JCAH develops and refines standards, surveys, and evaluates organizations at their request to measure compliance with standards; awards accreditation when it is merited; and recommends methods to improve the quality of patient care. The Commission's ability to keep up-to-date with developments in the many specialties that make up the health care industry depends, to a large extent, on the diversity and number of experts who serve on advisory committees and participate in field reviews of standards. These committees include the Policy Advisory Committee, the Professional and Technical Advisory Committees (PTAC), the Advisory Committee on Education and Publications, and the Committee on Health Care Safety. American Occupational Therapy Association (AOTA) members, along with representatives of other professional organizations and service providers, have participated actively on PTAC for psychiatric facilities since 1980 and on the Rehabilitation Standards Chapter Task Force as well. Both areas of involvement have provided opportunities to increase the visibility and the influence of occupational therapy in patient advocacy and health care policy making.

The format and content of JCAH standards have varied over the years. The most recent revisions, published in 1985, reflect a trend toward a single set of standards for all hospitals. The incorporation of psychiatric and substance abuse standards into the *Accreditation Manual for Hospitals* is particularly significant. For mental health practitioners the shift away from the Consolidated Standards formerly used for psychiatric and substance abuse programs with over one hundred beds, has resulted in a diminished commitment to a multidisciplinary team approach. A reading of the Medical Staff Chapter of the manual reveals a stronger focus on the medical model, with more discretion left to each institution and members of the medical staff. Revisions in the chapter that relate to staff composition and organization, staff responsibilities, and clinical privileging are of special interest in this regard (12).

The new standards represent a welcome departure from their overly detailed and prescriptive predecessors, although the degree of specificity needed to appropriately guide and educate hospital administrators, staff, and surveyors continues to be a central issue. "On the one hand, they must be specific enough to allow meaningful application without chaotic disagreements over their interpretation. On the other hand, they must be general enough to permit reasonable differences between hospitals and services and to permit feasible implementation" (1, p 1209).

For all areas of patient care, quality assurance guidelines have been strengthened. Time pressures and a tendency "to avoid formal assessment of patient outcomes" (2, p 26) may often deter full involvement of occupational therapy personnel in innovative quality assurance activities. The life of many treatment programs in today's cost-cutting era, however, may well hinge on favorable evidence from productivity analyses, patient care audits, and outcome studies.

Also in the new manual, standards for appropriate treatment environments have been raised, and some gains for the biopsychosocial needs of patients are evident in the expectation that assessments include social, emotional, and behavioral status. A summary of all changes made since 1984 can be found in Appendix B of the 1985 *Accreditation Manual for Hospitals* (12).

Accreditation of Rehabilitation Facilities

Accreditation of rehabilitation facilities is primarily the domain of the Commission on Accreditation of Rehabilitation Facilities (CARF). CARF was created in 1966, merging the functions of the Association of Rehabilitation Centers and the National Association of Sheltered Workshops and Homebound Programs. CARF is an "organization independent from those it accredits which establishes and maintains a nationwide set of standards of quality developed in a participatory fashion, and designed to address the needs of people with disability" (13, p v). A number of public agencies and insurance providers require organizations to have CARF accreditation to be eligible for reimbursement.

During CARF's first seven years its standards focused on administrative issues in rehabilitation organizations, number and levels of staff, types and levels of services provided, and physical plant. In 1973, while continuing to develop standards for evaluating the various component programs of rehabilitation, CARF began to develop qualitative standards to evaluate the outcomes of rehabilitation.

CARF's *Standards Manual for Facilities Serving People with Disabilities* is organized into two main sections, Standards for All Programs and Standards for Individual Programs and Services. From these latter standards an organization may choose the set on which it wants to be surveyed. They cover hospital-based rehabilitation, spinal cord injury programs, chronic pain management programs, outpatient medical rehabilitation, infant and early childhood development programs, vocational evaluation, work adjustment, occupational skill training, job placement, work services, activity services, residential services, independent living programs, and psychosocial programs. In the survey an organization's practices are compared with the manual's standards for that type of facility.

The CARF standards are very specific to the functioning of occupational therapy in rehabilitation. Many of the standards for individual programs require that occupational therapy be provided and delineate the services that should be offered. As with the JCAH standards, the CARF standards are a tool to measure the quality of services.

Accreditation of Services for Developmentally Disabled People

The agency chiefly responsible for accreditation of services for developmentally disabled people is the Accreditation Council for services for mentally retarded and other developmentally disabled persons (AC MRDD). The development of standards in this area began in 1952 when the American Association of Mental Deficiency (AAMD) issued the report of a special committee recommending standards for institutions serving the mentally retarded. Twelve years later, the AAMD published *Standards for State Residential Institutions for the Mentally Retarded.* At the same time it established a committee to continue revising the standards and plan for formal accreditation activities. In 1966, supported by a grant from the U.S. Department of Health, Education, and Welfare, AAMD created a national planning committee to develop a structure for an accrediting agency. The result was the establishment of an accreditation council under the JCAH. In 1979, during a reorganization of the JCAH structure, AC MRDD established an accreditation program independent of JCAH.

AC MRDD's objective is "to promote the delivery of comprehensive and coordinated services within a service delivery system that meets all the needs of every developmentally disabled individual" (14, p ix). Its accreditation process is intended to be both "educational and evaluative" (14, p vii).

Each section of the standards deals with definitions and principles of implementation. Standards cover the following areas: Individual Program Planning and Implementation, Alternative Living Arrangements, Achieving and Protecting Rights, Individual Program Support, Safety and Sanitation, Research and Research Utilization, and the Agency in the Service Delivery System. The focus of the standards is on implementing individual programs in accordance with "the developmental model, the principle of normalization, and the interdisciplinary approach" (14, p vi).

As a sponsoring organization of AC MRDD, the AOTA has two representatives on the Board of Directors. The standards set by the agency affect a large population of occupational therapy patients/clients and provide a framework for quality service delivery in this area of practice.

Regulation of Home Health Agencies and Community Nursing Services

Accreditation of home health agencies and community nursing services occurs under a program jointly sponsored by the National League for Nursing (NLN) and the American Public Health Association (APHA). The program is administered within the NLN, by the Council of Home Health Agencies and Community Health Services. The framework of an organization is evaluated because it is felt that a relationship exists between the quality of administrative practices and the services that are delivered.

Accreditation decisions are based on the degree to which an agency meets the standards "in relationship to its own stated purposes and the attempts it makes to meet the health needs of the community it serves" (15, p 1).

The number of occupational therapy personnel working in home care agencies is growing daily. They are guided by the *Standards of Practice: Home Health,* approved by the AOTA Representative Assembly in 1978. The AOTA's involvement in the Accreditation Committee provides an opportunity to advise NLN regarding the standards necessary to ensure quality in the delivery of services. Several occupational therapists serve on the Professional Review Panel of the accreditation program.

Regulation of Educational Programs

Educational programs in occupational therapy are regulated by the AOTA using two sets of standards: *Essentials of an Approved Program for the Occupational Therapy Assistant* (16) and *Essentials of an Accredited Program for the Occupational Therapist* (17). The former are handled independently; the latter are administered in collaboration with the Committee on Allied Health Accreditation of the American Medical Association (AMA). The standards address both academic and fieldwork education and are used as minimum requirements for program development and evaluation.

The Educational Standards Review Committee of the AOTA's Commission on Education (COE) is responsible for the periodic revision of both sets of standards. Once this process is completed, most recently in 1983, the standards must be approved by the COE, the AOTA Representative Assembly, and, for professional-level programs only, the AMA.

Approximately every five years, on a staggered basis, all occupational therapy programs in U.S., District of Columbia, and Puerto Rican colleges and universities are visited to determine whether they continue to meet the educational standards. This process is managed by the Accreditation Committee of the AOTA Standards and Ethics Commission. Any questions about interpretation of *Essentials* are referred to the Educational Standards Review Committee.

Educational programs in occupational therapy are the profession's source of supply of human resources. *Essentials* provides a mechanism for the profession indirectly to ensure that new practitioners have the necessary skills and knowledge to enter the practice arena. Only graduates of approved/accredited programs are able to take the AOTA's national certification examination.

VOLUNTARY AND MANDATORY REGULATION OF INDIVIDUALS

Historically, the public has expected health practitioners to have certain credentials demonstrating professional or technical competence in their chosen field. Some members of the public even ask health care providers where and when they received their training. More often the public relies on a credentialing process run by state governments to ensure that health professionals are qualified to practice.

For over fifty years occupational therapy personnel have been certified by the AOTA, their national professional association. More recently, state laws also began to provide for certification or licensure of occupational therapy personnel.

Certification and Registration

Certification may be voluntary or mandatory.

Voluntary certification. In voluntary certification, also known as non-governmental title control, usually a professional organization establishes its own program to recognize those who have attained entry-level competence in the broad areas of responsibility of a given occupation (18). A person completing the certification process is granted a certificate and may use a special designation with his or her name. For instance, the American College of Life Underwriters grants the use of the title *chartered life underwriter* (CLU) after an insurance agent has successfully passed certain tests (18). Likewise, the AOTA grants the use of *occupational therapist, registered* (OTR) and *certified occupational therapy assistant* (COTA) after a person has met certain requirements.

The AOTA's voluntary certification program has been in existence since 1932. The three essential elements in the AOTA's certification process include graduation from an accredited/approved occupational therapy program, successful completion of supervised fieldwork experience, and passing the national occupational therapy certification examination for registered occupational therapists and certified occupational therapy assistants.

Mandatory certification. In mandatory certification, or title control, state law prohibits a person from using a certain title or from holding himself or herself out to the public as "certified" or "registered." People allowed to use the title must meet certain entry-level requirements. For example, in Hawaii, the titles *occupational therapist* and *occupational therapy assistant* and the words *registered* and *certified* used respectively in conjunction with the titles are protected by law. People may, however, practice or provide "occupational-therapy-type" services, as long as they do not refer to their business as occupational therapy or themselves as occupational therapists. According to Hawaii law, occupational therapy personnel must complete the same requirements as those of the AOTA for certification.

Mandatory certification does not govern the practice of a professional group. It only protects a title.

Registration. The term *registration* has a number of different meanings. It usually means that an association or a government agency maintains an official roster of people who have met its certification requirements. Registration can be voluntary, as with a professional association, or mandated by law with a government agency. Title acts are sometimes called registration acts. When this occurs, a registration act is the same as mandatory certification or title control.

Licensure

Licensure, or practice control, is "the process by which an agency of government grants permission to an individual to engage in a given occupation upon finding that the applicant has attained the minimal degree of competence necessary to ensure that the public health, safety, and welfare will be reasonably well protected" (19, p 17). Licensure differs from certification in that it protects not only the title of a profession, but also the scope of practice as defined in the licensure law. A licensure law is therefore often referred to as a practice act. Table 2 contrasts the essential elements of a licensure law and a certification law for occupational therapy personnel.

Some certification laws include all the elements of a licensure law with the exception of the practice language underlined in the licensure column in Table 2. This type of certification law is usually viewed as stronger than that typified in Table 2 because of the provision for an occupational therapy board, which can write rules, deal directly with complaints, and sanction occupational therapy personnel. Without a board, all problems are referred to the attorney general's office, which handles a broad range of issues, most of them probably more pressing than occupational therapy concerns. This procedure also takes decisions outside the profession and seeks judgments on professional problems from people who are not expert in the matters to be adjudicated. Provisions for a board, an application, and the issuance of a state certificate necessitate a fee, but enforcement and thus consumer protection are strengthened through these additional sections in a law.

Powers and duties of licensure boards. The powers and the duties of licensure boards vary according to the administrative structure imposed by a state. Boards range from autonomous bodies to advisory councils (see Table 3).

An example of an autonomous board is the North Dakota occupational therapy licensure board. The board is fully responsible for implementing the licensure law. Board members write regulations, send out applications, collect fees, issue licenses, and hear complaints. They purchase clerical, printing, legal, or investigative services as needed, usually from other state agencies.

Most states have licensure boards or advisory councils that are essentially autonomous but receive administrative services, review, and funding from a central agency. In a few states a central agency administering licensure laws maintains complete licensure authority. This is true in New York, where the occupational therapy board only advises the Board

TABLE 19–2
A Comparison of State Licensure and Certification in Occupational Therapy

	Licensure/Practice Act	Certification/Title Act
Definitions	Occupational therapy, occupational therapist, and occupational therapy assistant	None
Prohibition language	"No person shall *practice occupational therapy or* hold himself or herself out as an occupational therapist, or as being able to practice occupational therapy, or to render occupational therapy services in this State unless he or she is licensed under the provisions of this Act."	"No person shall hold himself or herself out as an occupational therapist, or as being able to practice occupational therapy, or to render occupational therapy services in this State unless he or she is certified under the provisions of this Act."
Exemption language	"This exempts other licensed professionals, occupational therapy students, occupational therapy fieldwork interns, and federal government employees from being licensed.	None
Requirements	Entry level	Entry level
Fees	Yes	None
Enforcement	Delegated to an occupational therapy board, usually consisting of occupational therapy personnel and a consumer, occasionally including another health professional	Usually delegated to the state attorney general's office
Examples of this type of legislation	Maryland	California, Hawaii

of Regents within the Department of Education. Similarly, in Connecticut the Department of Health Services has the sole responsibility for administering the occupational therapy licensure program.

Regardless of structure, the most broad-reaching power licensure boards have is that of writing regulations, which have the force of law. Boards establish rules for issuance of a license, for supervision of assistants and unlicensed occupational therapy personnel, and for continuing competency requirements when specified by law. These rules affect everyone wishing to practice in a given state.

Boards protect the public by providing consumer information, monitoring licensees, and investigating complaints. They have the power to

TABLE 19–3
Variations in the Powers of Licensure Boards

Autonomous ←		→ **Advisory**
Independent board that makes all decisions and performs all administrative functions	Autonomous board, located in a central agency that performs administrative functions such as staffing and budget	Advisory board, attached to a central agency with complete licensure authority

discipline licensees using a broad range of sanctions ranging from a reprimand to loss of a license. The latter removes the licensee's right to practice in that state and is thus used only in extreme cases. Discipline may include such actions as peer review of records, supervision, continuing education, and temporary loss of a license.

The Future of Licensure and Certification

Although government regulation of health professionals has been viewed critically by many in the 1970s and 1980s, the public has become accustomed to mandatory licensure or certification. Critics of licensure propose a system that would encourage consumers to rely on information and their own judgment regarding the preparation of health professionals. Although programs to modify the state licensure structure have been proposed, public policy has not shifted sufficiently for adoption of such changes. Therefore, voluntary and mandatory certification and licensure are likely to continue for some time in the future.

Standards of Practice

The AOTA has developed guidelines to assist its members in the management of occupational therapy services and to serve as minimum standards for occupational therapy practice. There are six different sets of standards. One set (reproduced in Appendix I) is applicable to all client populations and the programs in which clients are served. The other five sets apply to clients with physical disabilities, developmentally disabled clients, mental health programs, home health programs, and schools.

SUMMARY

In health care, as in other fields, mechanisms exist for setting standards and applying them to organizations and individuals delivering professional services. These mechanisms—accreditation, certification, licensure, and standards of practice—serve both the public and the profession.

Health care organizations have a well-established tradition of voluntarily regulating themselves, beginning with hospital regulation in 1917. The regulation itself is controversial, however. Concerns are expressed about the sheer massiveness of regulations and the required documen-

Common Questions Regarding Licensure

- *How does a licensure law affect the practice of occupational therapy? Will it limit what I can do?*

A licensure law requires a person to hold a valid license to practice as an occupational therapist or an occupational therapy assistant. Regulations implementing the law might address the supervision of occupational therapy assistants and aides and thus affect the management of staff. Regulations might also require continuing education and thus influence continuing education choices.

A licensure act defines practice in entry-level terms because its primary purpose is to establish a competency level to enter a field. Some occupational therapy personnel, through appropriate education and experience, may acquire advanced skills not addressed in the licensure act's definition of occupational therapy. Licensure does not prohibit occupational therapy personnel from obtaining advanced skills, just as it does not prohibit physicians from doing so. Physicians are licensed as general practitioners, but most physicians specialize in one area of medicine not identified through the licensure process. Likewise, an occupational therapist or an occupational therapy assistant may specialize. Specialty areas are currently not addressed in any occupational therapy licensure law.

Occupational therapy licensure laws have reportedly weeded out unqualified people and provided a state standard for occupational therapy personnel to which all state programs involving occupational therapy turn for guidance. At this time, there is no evidence to indicate any adverse effect of occupational therapy licensure laws.

- *What are the requirements for licensure? Do I have to take the AOTA examination again?*

As of the end of 1984, there were twenty-nine jurisdictions licensing occupational therapy personnel. Thus far, the examination used for the AOTA certification has been adopted by all jurisdictions as the licensing examination. Therefore, passing the AOTA certification examination also meets the licensure examination requirement in the twenty-nine licensure laws.

- *Beyond getting a license to practice, what is the role of the occupational therapist and the occupational therapy assistant in states with licensure laws?*

Individual occupational therapy personnel are in a position to identify unqualified practitioners and licensed practitioners violating practice or ethical standards. When such violations are observed, they should be referred to the licensure board and to the AOTA Standards and Ethics Commission.

tation. Questions are raised about accreditation's effect on cost containment and its contribution to quality care. There are also a variety of ethical and interdisciplinary issues.

Typically, an organization seeking accreditation initiates the accreditation process by submitting an application for a review. With some agencies the next step is self-evaluation. A site visit to the organization by a team of professionals follows. Once an organization is accredited, it must undergo periodic review to maintain its accreditation.

An occupational therapy manager whose organization is being surveyed should expect to participate in the process through advanced planning, submission of documents, hosting an inspection of the plant, and interviews with the visitors. The visit, and the larger accreditation process, can provide important opportunities for managers to clarify program goals and develop effective strategies for implementation of clinical, research, and educational components.

The organization that sets standards for hospitals is the Joint Commission on Accreditation of Hospitals. It strives to "enhance . . . the quality of care and services provided in organized health care settings." To achieve this and other goals, it develops and refines standards, surveys and evaluates organizations to measure compliance with standards, awards accreditation when merited, and recommends methods to improve the quality of patient/client care.

The format and content of JCAH standards have varied over the years. The current ones reflect a trend toward a single set for all hospitals. They also depart noticeably from their overly detailed and prescriptive predecessors.

Several organizations set standards in the rehabilitation field: the Commission on Accreditation of Rehabilitation Facilities (CARF), the Accreditation Council for services for mentally retarded and other developmentally disabled persons (AC MRDD), and, jointly, the National League for Nursing and the American Public Health Association (NLN/APHA). CARF's standards are qualitative, focusing on the outcomes of rehabilitation. They cover a broad range of programs, from hospital-based rehabilitation to independent living. AC MRDD promotes "the delivery of comprehensive and coordinated services within . . . a system that meets all the needs of every developmentally disabled individual." Its standards encourage the implementation of individual programs in accordance with "the developmental model, the principle of normalization, and the interdisciplinary approach." NLN/APHA together operate a program to accredit home and community health agencies. The framework of an organization is evaluated because it is felt that a relationship exists between the quality of administrative practices and the services that are delivered.

Educational programs in occupational therapy are regulated by the AOTA. Programs for occupational therapy assistants are handled independently; programs for occupational therapists are administered in collaboration with the American Medical Association.

Regulation of individual service providers in occupational therapy occurs under both voluntary and mandatory processes. Certification may be voluntary or mandatory. In voluntary certification, usually a professional organization establishes its own program to recognize, by permitting the use of certain titles, those who have attained entry-level competence in the broad areas of responsibility of a given occupation. In mandatory certification, state law controls who may use certain titles. Registration, which may also be voluntary or mandatory, usually means that an association or a government agency maintains an official roster of people who have met its certification requirements.

Licensure differs from certification in that it protects not only the title of a profession, but also the scope of practice as defined in the licensure law. Licensure laws also provide for boards, usually consisting of occupational therapy personnel and a consumer, occasionally including another health professional. The powers and duties of licensure boards vary according to the administrative structure imposed by a state. Boards range from autonomous bodies to advisory councils. The most broad-reaching power they have is that of writing regulations which govern the issuance of licenses, the supervision of other occupational therapy personnel, and the requirements for continuing competence. Boards protect the public by providing consumer information, monitoring licensees, and investigating complaints.

The AOTA has developed six sets of standards of practice to guide practitioners. One set is general and the other five apply to client groups or settings.

References

1. Lieberman PB, Astrachan BM: The JCAH and psychiatry: Current issues and implications for practice. *Hosp Community Psychiatry* 35:1205–1210, 1984
2. Ostrow PC: The historical precedents for quality assurance in health care. *Am J Occup Ther* 37:23–26, 1983
3. Johnson EA, Johnson RL: *Hospitals in Transition.* Rockville, MD: Aspen Systems Corp, 1982
4. Somers AR: *Hospital Regulation: The Dilemma of Public Policy.* Princeton, NJ: Princeton University, 1969
5. Flexner A: *Medical Education in the United States and Canada.* New York: Carnegie Foundation, Merrymount Press, 1910
6. Starr P: *The Social Transformation of American Medicine.* New York: Basic Books Inc, 1982
7. Bonn EM: Accreditation and regulation of psychiatric facilities. In *Psychiatric Administration: A Comprehensive Text for the Clinician-Executive,* JA Talbott, SR Kaplan, Editors. New York: Grune & Stratton, 1983
8. Houck JH: Regulation and accreditation: The pros and cons for psychiatric facilities. *Hosp Community Psychiatry* 35:1201–1204, 1984
9. Michels R: Commentary: Assessing the quality of quality assessment. *Hosp Community Psychiatry* 35:1179, 1984
10. Widmann DE: Recent changes in JCAH standards affecting the accreditation of psychiatric facilities. *Hosp Community Psychiatry* 35:1211–1214, 1984
11. Joint Commission on Accreditation of Hospitals: *Facts About JCAH.* Chicago: Joint Commission on Accreditation of Hospitals. (Address: 875 North Michigan Avenue, Chicago, IL 60611)
12. Joint Commission on Accreditation of Hospitals: *Accreditation Manual for Hospitals.* Chicago: Joint Commission on Accreditation of Hospitals, 1985, pp 73–88, 203–205
13. *Standards Manual for Facilities Serving People with Disabilities.* Tucson, AZ: Commission on Accreditation of Rehabilitation Facilities, 1985 (Address: 2500 North Pantano Road, Tucson, AZ 85715)
14. *Standards for Services for Developmentally Disabled Individuals.* Washington, DC: Accreditation Council for Services for Mentally Retarded and Other Developmentally Disabled Persons, 1983 (Address: 5101 Wisconsin Avenue, N. W., Washington, DC, 20016)
15. *Criteria and Standards Manual for NLN/APHA Accreditation of Home Health Agencies and Community Nursing Services,* publication No. 21-1306. New York: National League for Nursing, 1980 (Address: 10 Columbus Circle, New York, NY 10019)
16. American Occupational Therapy Association: Essentials of an approved program for the occupa-

tional therapy assistant. In *Reference Manual of the Official Documents of the American Occupational Therapy Association*. Rockville, MD: AOTA, 1983

17. American Occupational Therapy Association: Essentials of an accredited program for the occupational therapist. In *Reference Manual of the Official Documents of the American Occupational Therapy Association*. Rockville, MD: AOTA, 1983
18. Shimberg B: *Occupational Licensing: A Public Perspective*. Princeton, NJ: Educational Testing Service, 1982
19. US Department of Health, Education, and Welfare: *Credentialing Health Manpower*, publication No. (05)77-50057. Public Health Service, July 1977

Chapter 20

Ethics and Related Professional Liability

Carlotta Welles, MA, OTR, FAOTA

This chapter uses the "Principles of Occupational Therapy Ethics" of the American Occupational Therapy Association (AOTA) (1) as an organizational structure for a discussion of ethics and related professional liability in occupational therapy. (Excerpts from the Principles are presented in italics to differentiate them from the rest of the chapter text.) The Principles were approved by the AOTA Representative Assembly in 1977 and revised by it in 1979. Each section of the Principles is amplified by a commentary that supplements, clarifies, or illustrates points made in the section. The commentary also discusses implications for professional liability. The text of the Principles is an integral part of the text of this chapter. That is, the commentary does not reiterate the ethical principles and the guidelines contained in each section, nor does it explain any that are self-evident; rather it elaborates on those that are not clear on their face or have been difficult to interpret. The intent of the chapter is to make ethics and professional liability easily understood, widely taught, and universally applied within the profession.

A recipient of the AOTA Award of Merit, Carlotta Welles is now semiretired but teaches and writes about ethics and professional liability, and serves as a consultant on financial matters. She formerly chaired the Occupational Therapy Assistant Program at Los Angeles City College.

PREAMBLE

The American Occupational Therapy Association (AOTA) and its component members are committed to furthering man's ability to function fully within his total environment. To this end the occupational therapist renders service to clients in all stages of health and illness, to institutions, other professionals, colleagues, students and to the general public.

In furthering this commitment the American Occupational Therapy Association has established the Principles of Occupational Therapy Ethics. The Principles are intended for use by all occupational therapy personnel, including practitioners in all settings, administrators, educators, and students. Licensure laws and regulations should reflect and support these Principles which are intended to be action oriented, guiding and preventive rather than negative or merely disciplinary. The Principles, likewise, should influence the consulting, planning, and teaching of occupational therapists.

It should be noted that these Principles are intended only for internal use by the American Occupational Therapy Association as a guide to appropriate conduct of its members. The Principles are not intended to define a standard of care for patients or clients of a particular community.

Professional maturity will be demonstrated in applying these basic Principles while exercising the large measure of freedom which they provide and which is essential to responsible and creative occupational therapy service.

For the purpose of continuity the following definitions will support information in this document: Occupational therapist includes registered occupational therapists, certified occupational therapy assistants, occupational therapy students; clients include patients, students, and those to whom occupational therapy services are delivered.[1]

Commentary

Ethics concern behavior that is moral and considerate of the rights of others. Ethics set a standard of behavior for individuals and groups. Ethics are particularly important to professions. In fact, ethical conduct is a hallmark of professional behavior. One of the reasons the public trusts professionals is that professions promulgate, monitor, and enforce ethical standards.

Most ethical standards are supported by law in some form. If a person can prove he or she was damaged by the unethical practices of another (i.e., breach of duty), the person may initiate a tort action (a civil law suit) and, if the action is successful, collect damages, usually money, as compensation for the injury. Therefore, ethics should not be considered separately from law, although in ethics there may be an ethical violation where there is no actual damage.

The ethical standards of a profession apply to all its members. They are mandatory. Adherence to them is not a voluntary matter, nor are they to be followed only when it is easy or convenient to do so. Moreover, a professional person cannot be released from conformance to a standard

---

[1]This definition of *occupational therapist* applies to the principles only. The commentary, like the rest of the text, uses *occupational therapist* in the narrower sense and employs the broader term *occupational therapy personnel* when it applies.

by arguing that others are violating it or by securing permission from a supervisor, a physician, or an administrator to perform an unethical act. In other words, the Principles established by the AOTA cannot be negated by an individual member or by someone outside the profession. Such is the strength of the ethical standards of a profession, an invaluable asset to that profession, each of its members, and the public.

The Principles include the major aspects of ethical standards and practices, but they also represent principles to be applied universally to the practice of occupational therapy. That is, there may be additional ways in which occupational therapy personnel should be ethical that are not specifically outlined. Also, the principles are applicable even if the details of a given situation are different.

In ethics the concern is with actual behaviors and relationships and their outcomes, rather than with the *intent* of what is done. Substandard practices, even with good intent, may damage another. Careful study of this chapter and the resources listed at the end of it, mature thinking, and consultation with others as needed should serve occupational therapy personnel well in functioning as ethical health professionals.

I. [PRINCIPLES] RELATED TO THE RECIPIENT OF SERVICE

The occupational therapist demonstrates a beneficent concern for the recipient of services and maintains a goal-directed relationship with the recipient which furthers the objectives for which it is established. Services are evaluated against objectives and accountability is maintained therefore. Respect shall be shown for the recipients' rights and the occupational therapist will preserve the confidence of the client relationship.

Guidelines: *Recipients of occupational therapy services refer to clients, patients, students and the employers of occupational therapists, i.e., agencies, facilities, institutions, etc.*

It is the professional responsibility of occupational therapists to provide services for clients without regard to race, creed, national origin, sex, handicap or religious affiliation. Occupational therapists recognize each client's individuality and worth as a unique person.

Services provided should be planned in concert with clients' involvement in goal-directed activities, in accordance with the overall habilitation or rehabilitation plan. Treatment objectives and the therapeutic process must be measurable to insure professional accountability.

Clients' and students' rights are to be protected as stipulated in the Federal Privacy Act of 1974, in addition to any specified rules, regulations or procedures as may be required by the employer.

The financial gain of occupational therapists should never be paramount to the delivery of services. Those occupational therapists who are compensated by virtue of being a direct service provider or vendor have the right to assess reasonable fees for profit.

Occupational therapists are obligated to provide the highest quality of service to the recipient. If further services would be beneficial to the client, the referring practitioner should be informed. It is also incumbent upon occupational therapists to recommend termination of services when established goals have been met, or when further services would not produce improved recipient performance.

Occupational therapy educators are obligated to provide the highest quality educational services supporting the AOTA "Essentials" and the current theory that supports service delivery.

Commentary

Patients/clients. Occupational therapy personnel provide restorative services to patients/clients. Sometimes there are too many patients/clients to be served effectively with existing personnel and resources. Those best served by occupational therapy should be seen. Those who cannot be helped should not be accepted. Objective criteria and methods should be devised to discharge those who can no longer profit from occupational therapy. This process may be called triage.

Students. Occupational therapy personnel also educate students, their own and others'. The section of this chapter on Principles Related to Education discusses the admission of students to educational programs, as well as other ethical aspects of educational programs.

Rights of individuals. The law gives certain rights or freedoms to all citizens. The first right is *freedom from bodily harm.* Assault, which may be physical or verbal, is attempted battery without physical contact, and battery is "any unlawful touching which is without justification or excuse" (2, p 105) or which is unwanted. Legally an adult patient/client (of sound mind) must consent to treatment from anyone and can refuse any touching, including that from occupational therapy personnel. A patient/client is required to give written consent for surgery, participation in research, being photographed, and other forms of medical care. The same patient/client gives "implied consent" by engaging in occupational therapy activity. The skillful therapist secures this all-important implied consent by many means—for example, conforming to the treatment schedule, showing competence in giving patient/client services, maintaining a pleasant uncluttered treatment setting, and carrying on cordial relationships with patients/clients.

Although occupational therapy personnel do not injure their patients/clients purposely, a patient/client may be accidentally injured in many ways. They may fall, or be hurt by tools, equipment, or falling objects. A therapist may inadvertently cause emotional distress. It is well to make an inventory of all such possibilities and provide for avoiding them.

The second right of all citizens is *the right to privacy,* which is easily abrogated in the health care setting. Privacy is interpreted to have two meanings: information about oneself and privacy for one's physical person. Patients/clients have the right to have no one outside the organization know that they are present in a facility for care, or what their diagnosis and problems are. Records containing such information may not be taken outside the facility. Moreover, information about patients/clients cannot be used as social conversation. The section of this chapter on Principles Related to Records, Reports, Grades and Recommendations covers appropriate uses of patient/client records.

Traditionally patients/clients have been very accepting of (i.e., have consented to) the many invasions of their physical privacy. In the name of teaching they have been presented at grand rounds, examined before classes of students, and had their history described at length to everyone present. Although patients/clients have the right to refuse all of this, they seldom do for fear of not receiving the care they very much need. Their permission must be secured before they are used for teaching, and care must be taken to minimize the trauma that their use in teaching may cause.

Photography in the occupational therapy clinic may be damaging to patients/clients, or it may be helpful. Appropriate publicity about the profession can do much to create public understanding and support of its programs. Proper written consent to be photographed must be secured beforehand from each adult patient/client and from the parent or the guardian of each child patient/client. Consent forms are not devised by therapists but are prepared for institutions by their attorneys or by the attorneys of the hospital association in the state. Therapists in private practice should seek help from an attorney in this matter.

The purpose of these precautions is to protect the privacy of the individual. Photographs of hands, feet, braces, and so forth that do not identify an individual by name are probably safe to take with only oral consent. If a therapist has any doubt, written consent should be obtained.

As stated in the guidelines, occupational therapy personnel have a right to be paid for their services, as do other health care professionals. Neither ethical standards nor the law makes a distinction, however, as to whether occupational therapy personnel are paid or unpaid. If a therapist has created a professional relationship with a patient/client by giving him or her any sort of occupational therapy service or advice, that therapist is expected to conform to the highest standards of care and treatment (3). Therefore, it is unwise to enter into informal relationships in which one cannot maintain such standards—for example, casually giving occupational therapy services or advice to a neighbor or a friend.

Different relationships of therapists to patients/clients. Therapists have different relationships to the recipient of service depending on their role and job description. Most of this chapter concerns the role of the treating therapist, but there are also the roles of supervisor and consultant.

The primary role of a *supervisor* is to assign people to duties within their known competence. Therefore, supervisors must have a clear understanding of the duties to be performed (although they do not necessarily have to know how to perform the duties well themselves, just as the captain of a ship is not expected to be able to perform all of the functions involved in running the ship). Supervisors must also have an objective assessment of the skills and the abilities of each supervisee so that duties can be matched with people fully qualified to perform them. The assessments of duties and qualifications should be conducted objectively and recorded. Once a supervisor has evaluated the success of an assignment and found it to be working well, the law does not expect the supervisor to be constantly on site, provided he or she is available from time to time if needed for help or consultation.

The closeness of supervision is governed by (a) the degree of difference (that is, the amount of discretion) permissible in the supervisee's function, (b) the possible risks and hazards involved, and (c) the supervisee's areas of competence and possible deficiencies. Once a supervisor has properly attended to assessments of duties and qualifications and an evaluation of the assignment, he or she is not required actually to control the work of the therapist. Occupational therapy personnel are expected by law to be fully competent for the duties undertaken. If not, help should be sought, or the duties refused. If there is an untoward medical event [that is, "one occurring unexpectedly and not naturally or not in the ordinary course of events" (2, p 1378)] the courts will find the supervisee at fault rather than the supervisor (provided that adequate performance of the supervisor's duties is well documented).

A *consultant* is legally in a different position. The correctness of the advice, the teaching, and the recommendations offered should be documented, as well as exactly what consultation was given to whom. It is a good idea to formalize consultation with a memorandum to all concerned covering the date, the content, and the name of the consultee(s). Beyond this, the consultant usually has no legal responsibility for the actual performance of those involved. He or she is not in a line relationship to them, did not employ them, does not assign them, and cannot discharge them.

II. [PRINCIPLES] RELATED TO COMPETENCE

The occupational therapist shall actively maintain and improve one's professional competence, represent it accurately, and function within its parameters.

Guidelines: *Occupational therapists recognize the need for continuing education and where relevant, they obtain training, experience, self-study or counsel to assure competent occupational therapy services.*

Occupational therapists accurately represent their competence, education, training, and experience. Occupational therapists must accurately represent their skills and should not provide services or instructions, either for pay or in a voluntary capacity, that are not within their demonstrated competencies.

Occupational therapists must recognize the skills necessary to manage a client or a position. If client needs exist that the therapist cannot effectively manage, the therapist should seek consultation or refer the client to an occupational therapist or another professional who can provide the required service.

Commentary

The three standard designations of occupational therapy personnel used in this country today—registered, certified, and licensed—*indicate* a general competence in occupational therapy. Various college and university degrees as well as job-related titles such as chairperson, director, and supervisor *suggest* a general competence, and years of experience are often claimed to do the same. Neither the designations, the degrees, the titles, nor the years of experience, however, satisfy the common law requirement that occupational therapy personnel, as well as other health professionals, be expressly qualified for the separate individual duties that their specific job description includes. An occupational therapy manager or supervisor should use additional evaluative measures such as entry-level tests, references, probationary employment, observations, and conferences to determine an individual's competence. Matching an individual's competence to a particular job's demands and duties requires that the supervisor have a good understanding of the job specifications and the duties involved. A supervisor may be liable for negligent supervision if he or she knows or should have known that an employee was not qualified (4).

Some important generalizations can be made here:

1. People who are designated by their professional credentials as generally qualified will vary considerably in both depth and breadth of competence.
2. Those found to be fully qualified to work in one aspect of a program may not be qualified to rotate to another assignment or even to cover for a vacationing employee.
3. Some personnel may be highly qualified by virtue of prior or additional education to accept special assignments such as research, teaching, supervision, coordination, fabrication of adaptive equipment or devices, and so on.

To allow occupational therapy personnel to perform functions for which they are not qualified is not only unethical, but it exposes them, their supervisor, and their employer to liability (4).

Recommendations. Statements of one's own competence and/or experience that are not in accord with the facts are termed fraudulent, and a contract for employment arising from them will not be enforced (3). Further, fraudulent statements may form the basis for sanctions applied by the AOTA. If a fraud causes legal injury, it is actionable in the courts. Moreover, those who recommend others for jobs must do so in accord with the facts and without any personal ulterior motives.

Responsibility for competence. Responsibility for the competence of health care personnel has become shared in some ways. The employer is required by law to show "due care in selection" (5, pp 56–59) of professional staff. As mentioned, a supervisor must assign people to duties within their known competence. The professional association, at both the national and the state levels, offers conferences, workshops, research support, publications, and consultation to assist occupational therapy personnel in maintaining their competence. Colleges and universities offer basic and advanced educational programs that meet established standards. Such opportunities and assistance are evidence that the health care provider system shares a concern for the competence of personnel. In the final analysis, however, *an individual is responsible for his or her own competence*. Fulfilling this responsibility requires continued study throughout one's professional career. Graduation from an approved or accredited program is only a good start on the road to full competence.

III. [PRINCIPLES] RELATED TO RECORDS, REPORTS, GRADES AND RECOMMENDATIONS

The occupational therapist shall conform to local, state and federal laws and regulations, and regulations applicable to records and reports. The occupational therapist abides by the employing institution's rules. Objective data shall govern subjective data in evaluations, grades, recommendations, records and reports.

Guidelines: *Occupational therapists realize that reports are a required function of any position. Occupational therapists accurately record information and report information as required by AOTA standards, facility standards and state and national laws.*

Occupational therapists fulfilling a teaching role utilize objective data in determining student grades.

All data recorded in permanent files or records should be supported by the occupational therapist's observations or by objective measures of data collection.

Students' records can only be divulged as authorized by law or the students' consent for release of information.

Commentary

Uses of records. Records are absolutely integral in the use of occupational therapy personnel and things to treat patients/clients. Records are important as evidence of what has been done. The principle is that whatever duties the law requires to be done should be recorded, and the record should be executed promptly after the event it documents. Courts do not give much credence to the recollection of professional personnel because they see so many patients/clients. Conversely, the courts do give weight to the recollection of a patient/client as a plaintiff for whom medical care and any particular events that occurred were unique experiences the details of which stand out clearly (4).

Records should be written regularly and promptly in the course of providing services. Such records have been critical in the determination of a dispute. Those written only when an untoward medical event (as defined earlier) occurs may be considered self-serving and therefore invalid (4).

Management in health care today recognizes that records have a variety of uses:

1. Documenting a patient's/client's state of health before and after treatment
2. Offering evidence that services were given
3. Providing data for use in evaluation of both individual and group patient/client response to care and treatment
4. Justifying billed charges
5. Evaluating and supervising personnel
6. Giving evidence of maintenance of standards
7. Substantiating contributory negligence, if any
8. Supporting administrative program changes and requests.

One record might be employed for all these purposes and more. Above all, records should help give quality care to patients/clients.

Both ethical principles and the law allow and encourage that records be used for all the listed purposes. Therefore it is essential that they be written correctly. Guidance in the proper execution of records is beyond the scope of this chapter; teaching and supervision should provide it.

Responsibility for writing a record. There is an ethical and legal aspect to who writes a record. Those who perform a service for a patient/client have a right and often an obligation to write a record. No administrative process should prevent them from doing so, because a record they have written may serve as their defense if it should be needed. Students should write attendance records, progress notes, records of safety checks on equipment, supply records, incident reports, and so forth, and should be taught by staff how to do so. Obviously, professional staff have a legitimate professional concern with the quality of the record that appears on a patient's/client's chart or in some other place where it is read by other personnel.

Where fieldwork students' records are made and kept is an administrative decision determined at the departmental level. It should be remembered, however, that anyone who signs a note, a report, or other documentation is not merely approving its inclusion, but is attesting to the truth of all of the contents. Those who sign notes or records that others have written, or even countersign them, are thus accountable for the contents.

A basic principle is that one writes about things, events, treatments, incidents, teaching, supervision, and so on that are (a) within one's own professional purview and (b) performed by oneself. One does not write about things done by other services or things that are hearsay. This is not to imply that supervisors cannot write records and reports; they should do so, because the work of their supervisees is within their purview.

Storage of records. Patients/clients have a legal right to have no one except the responsible family member and the personnel who care for them know that they are patients/clients in a given facility or what their problems are. This means that patient/client records should not be taken outside so that notes can be written at home. It also means that records should be kept in a place where their confidentiality can be ensured. It means further than one should not identify any patient/client in casual conversation.

Discussing these prohibitions may dampen the enthusiasm that students and new staff find in their work. Teaching and supervision should offer guidance regarding subjects that may be shared with family and friends oustide the organization. Appropriate topics to share with outsiders include the types of services offered, the kinds of patients/clients seen, the research and the teaching being done, the physical facilities and equipment used, even the resources needed by the program.

(Commentary on grades appears under the Principles Related to Education; commentary on recommendations is offered under the Principles Related to Competence.)

IV. [PRINCIPLES] RELATED TO INTRA-PROFESSIONAL COLLEAGUES

The occupational therapist shall function with discretion and integrity in relations with other members of the profession and shall be concerned with the quality of their services. Upon becoming aware of objective evidence of a breach of ethics or substandard service, the occupational therapist shall take action according to established procedure.

Guidelines: *Information gained or data gathered on a client shall only be divulged as expedient to other professional colleagues, students, referring practitioner, and employer. This includes data used in the course of in-service programs, professional meetings, prepared papers for presentation or publication, and educational materials. Undue invasion of privacy should be of utmost con-*

cern. Any reference to quality or service rendered by, or the integrity of a professional colleague will be expressed with due care to protect the reputation of that person.

It is the obligation of occupational therapists with first-hand knowledge of a breach of the ethical principles of this Association, by a colleague or student, to attempt to rectify the situation. If informal attempts fail, such activities or incidents against the ethical principles of this Association, should immediately be brought to the attention of the appropriate local, regional or national Association committee/commission on ethical standards. Designated procedures should be followed and at all times the confidentiality of the information must be respected to protect the alleged party.

Practices by an employer which are in conflict with the ethical principles of this Association, should also be brought to the immediate attention of the appropriate body(ies).

Information gained in peer review procedures should be held within the realm of confidentiality and be dealt with according to established procedures.

Publication credit for material developed by colleagues must be given. Also, credit for materials used in the classroom, manuals, in-service training, and oral or written reports, for example, should acknowledge the name of the individual or group who developed the material.

Commentary

Although the guidelines for these principles are fairly complete, their implementation is often difficult. It usually seems easier to do one's own job and let others do theirs, and not interfere. This feeling is widespread and understandable, yet the question of relationships with one's colleagues bears deeper thinking. The ethics here are quite clear, but the law is cloudy. Ethically, occupational therapy personnel are members of a profession and a professional association, the AOTA. Degrees, diplomas, certificates, and licenses give individuals who hold them permission to function in occupational therapy provided standards are maintained. A commitment is thus created to uphold the profession. To this end occupational therapy personnel teach, consult, supervise, collaborate with, and otherwise assist one another. However, they must also be concerned with substandard or unethical performance as described in the guidelines—for example, falling below standards of care, participating in unethical relationships, spreading libelous information that could damage someone's reputation, even injuring a person.

There are other questionable practices that may diminish colleagues, without the offender's so intending. Adding one's name to another's paper even though one has not written any of it serves largely to decrease the visibility of the originating author. If by adding his or her name, a more experienced person intends to support the writer, this can be done more ethically and effectively by a signed review of the paper.

Another undesirable practice involves an outsider's approaching administrators or other personnel in an organization without first contacting his or her professional colleagues there. Occupational therapy personnel in the organization contacted expect to collaborate with their fellow professionals in all occupational-therapy-related contacts and arrangements. Separate and independent contacts by an outsider may seriously compromise the position of in-house occupational therapy personnel.

Developments since the revision of the Principles in 1979 somewhat alter the procedures to be followed if informal attempts to rectify an instance of unethical conduct fail. In states with licensure the violation should be reported to the licensure board first, then to the chairperson of the AOTA's Standards and Ethics Commission. In states without licensure the matter should be referred to the ethics committee of the state occupational therapy association and, if necessary, to the chairperson of the AOTA's Standards and Ethics Commission.[2]

V. [PRINCIPLES] RELATED TO OTHER PERSONNEL

The occupational therapist shall function with discretion and integrity in relations with personnel and cooperate with them as may be appropriate. Similarly, the occupational therapist expects others to demonstrate a high level of competence. Upon becoming aware of objective evidence of a breach of ethics or substandard service, the occupational therapist shall take action according to established procedure.

Guidelines: *Occupational therapists understand the scope of education and practice of related professions, and make full use of all the professional, technical and administrative resources that best serve the interests of consumers.*

Occupational therapists do not delegate to other personnel those client related services where the clinical skills and expertise of an occupational therapist is required. Other personnel or students may support treatment or educational goals, but must have demonstrated competency in each aspect of service to the occupational therapist before the responsibility can be delegated.

Occupational therapists who employ or supervise other professionals or technicians, or professionals or technicians in training, accept the obligation to facilitate their further development by providing suitable working conditions, consultation and experience opportunities.

Occupational therapists protect the privacy of all persons with whom professional collaboration occurs. If, however, an occupational therapist has first-hand knowledge of a colleague's performance which is in conflict with ethical standards, the therapist shall attempt to rectify the situation. Failing an informal solution, the occupational therapist shall utilize procedures established within the facility or agency, or to call the behavior to the attention of management, or utilize procedures established by the profession to handle such situations. Under no circumstances should the occupational therapist remain silent when a client, student or facility's status is in jeopardy.

Commentary

Limitations. Cooperation with other disciplines should not be so construed that duties and responsibilities are mingled and shared. People should not perform services that are not in the accepted scope of their

---

[2]Enforcement Procedures are available from the Standards and Ethics Commission. Requests should be addressed to AOTA, 1383 Piccard Drive, Rockville, MD 20850. Complaints should be addressed to the chairperson of the Standards and Ethics Commission, 1383 Piccard Drive, Rockville, MD 20850.

own profession and for which they are not fully trained, unless the following conditions are met (6):

1. An adequate and approved education program covering the services has been given.
2. A "white paper" or a document has been prepared that outlines the conditions under which the services will be performed and that has been approved by the administrator, the medical director, and the legal counsel of the organization.
3. Proper supervision of those performing the services will be provided.

Teaching others. Occupational therapy personnel's teaching of professionals in other disciplines is appropriately directed toward the understanding and the use of occupational therapy, and such follow-up activities as can be properly carried out by others. It is widely accepted that education for occupational therapy, as well as for other health disciplines, occurs in a long, thorough approved or accredited program. Teaching or learning to practice one or more of the activities or techniques of another profession does not qualify the individual to function in place of the professional whose techniques he or she has been shown. A person who performs the services of other professions may be found incompetent, and the person, his or her supervisor, and the employing organization may be found liable.

New activities. The principle regarding new learnings, if carried to the extreme, could serve to prevent change and the development of new services and programs. No one can function indefinitely using only the knowledge and the skill learned in basic professional education. Continuing education and postgraduate study are some answers. Also, the courts have allowed professional personnel to perform new functions under the conditions just enumerated under Limitations.

Responsibility for others. One problem in relation to other health care professionals has caused occupational therapy personnel some discomfort. The guidelines emphasize that occupational therapy personnel have a responsibility for taking some form of action when they have personal knowledge of unethical conduct or substandard performance by a person in another profession. There will be times when the nurse will be a good resource for occupational therapy personnel in this regard, because the nursing profession and the courts make the nurse responsible for seeing that the patient/client actually receives care and treatment as ordered. Occupational therapy personnel are well advised to cultivate and educate their nursing colleagues in advance of calling on them as a resource.

A word of caution may also be appropriate. It is often easy to libel a colleague without so intending. One need only say to a patient/client, "I wonder why the doctor ordered that treatment for you" or "Why did the physical therapist give you that?" to cast doubt about those providers' qualifications and the quality of care received from them.

When unethical conduct or substandard performance is suspected, occupational therapy personnel should first document what they have personally observed. Often, careful inquiry supports the ethicality or the adequacy of what initially appeared to be unethical or substandard practice. If it does not, further action should be taken. After a conference with one's supervisor, the problem should be reported—in states with licensure, to the licensure board of the profession in question, and in states without licensure, to the state ethics committee of that profession (or to the state association if there is no ethics committee per se). The courts have found those who do nothing about the obviously unethical or substandard practice of another professional guilty themselves of substandard practice.

VI. [PRINCIPLES] RELATED TO EMPLOYERS AND PAYERS

The occupational therapist shall render service with discretion and integrity and shall protect the property and property rights of the employers and payers.

Guidelines: *Occupational therapists function within the parameter of the job description or the goals established mutually between the employer or agency, and the occupational therapist. Occupational therapists use the utmost integrity in all dealings with the facility, university/college or contracting agency. Established procedures are followed regarding purchasing and bids.*

Occupational therapists recommend appropriate fees for services and gain necessary acceptance for fees from the facility, agency and payers. Fees must be based upon cost analysis or a factor that can be justified upon request.

Occupational therapists shall not use the property, such as supplies and equipment, of the employer for their own personal use and aggrandizement.

Commentary

There are both legal and ethical relationships between employers and employees. An employer's duties to employees are stated in labor laws, wage and hour laws, fair employment practices legislation, antidiscrimination laws, and other laws and regulations. All these are beyond the scope of this commentary. Occupational therapy managers, as agents of an employer or as employers themselves, are well advised to become informed about the many provisions involved.

Common law. It is more difficult to learn about the many applications of case law or common law. Some are discussed here.

The guidelines for Principles Related to Employers and Payers state that occupational therapy personnel function within their individual job descriptions. These should include what the duties of a job are, where they are to be performed, and what supervision is to be given and received. When duties change, the job description should be changed accordingly. An employer has vicarious liability for the work of all employees and thus has the right to know, as does the insurance carrier, what the duties are and the general location in which they are performed, such as in the facility, in a patient's/client's home, or in the community. Insurance carriers have declined to pay for untoward medical events (as defined earlier) that have occurred during employee activities that were unknown to the employer or outside the usual place of employment.

Use of one's own car. From time to time most occupational therapy personnel use their lunch hour to rush out for some needed supplies or to take an outpatient home when his or her ride fails. There may be serious consequences if an accident or untoward medical event (as defined earlier) occurs while the occupational therapist or occupational therapy assistant is using his or her own car for what is really the business of the employer. The employee is, of course, personally liable, and his or her insurance will be levied on first, up to the limits of coverage. If he or she is legally determined to be doing the employer's work at the time of the accident or the event, the employer may also be liable under the doctrine of vicarious liability and may be required to pay the balance of a judgment in excess of the limits of the employee's policy. On the other hand, if the employee is legally determined to be on a personal errand, the employer is not liable. Any occupational therapist or occupational therapy assistant using his or her own car for any purpose that could be termed the employer's business should advise the employer to this effect and provide in writing (a) the name of his or her insurance carrier, (b) the amount of coverage carried, and (c) the effective dates and the limits of the policy. The employer can then either prevent the activity, provide a car belonging to the organization, or carry insurance for nonowned automobiles. Employees should check their personal automobile insurance coverage to be sure that it covers them when using the care for the employer's business.

The employer's property. An employer, either an individual, a partnership, or a corporation, has two valuable assets that employees are legally obligated to protect: physical property and reputation. Regarding the first asset, with administration approval it is acceptable for employees to use the employer's physical facilities for both professional and educational activities, because presumably these indirectly benefit the organization and its patients/clients. Two widespread abuses, however, are very costly—the use of the telephone for personal purposes and the misuse of time. Roughly 75 percent of the cost of health care is for employee time, all of which belongs to the employer, just as the facilities and the equipment do. Lateness to work, long coffee breaks, and visiting with fellow employees can use up a significant and costly amount of time.

Regarding the second asset, employers, like patients/clients and employees, have a right to their good reputation. Loose and derogatory talk benefits no one. A little thought and planning help define the topics that should be kept in house and those that can be shared with outsiders.

VII. [PRINCIPLES] RELATED TO EDUCATION

The occupational therapist implements a commitment to the education of society and the consumer of health services as well as to the education of health personnel in matters of health which are within the purview of occupational therapy.

Guidelines: *Occupational therapists do not only provide direct service to alleviate specific problems with clients, programs or a community, but in addition, include education of all phases of services which can be provided to the public. This should include education of situations and conditions for which the competency of occupational therapists is recognized to assist in alleviating barriers limiting a person's ability to function socially, emotionally, cognitively or physically.*

The public includes not only individuals concerned with the well-being of a member of their family, but also federal, state and local governmental agencies, educational systems and social agencies dealing with the health and well-being of the public.

Commentary

Standards for student selection. Standards and objective procedures for the selection of students are essential to safeguard the interest of each component of the educational process: the student, the college or university, the faculty, the clinical center (including the supervisor), and the patient/client. Such standards and procedures should not discriminate on the basis of race, creed, color, national origin, age, or state of health, *except* that they should relate to criteria for effective and safe professional function. Deficits that are legal and valid bases for exclusion usually include those that present a probable hazard to the individual or his or her patients/clients.

This standard is somewhat in conflict with a student's legal right to an education. Some applicants have tried to interpret the law to mean that they are entitled to *any* education of their choice. It is not a favor to applicants to admit them if it is objectively determined that they are definitely not suited to a career in occupational therapy.

In other words, it cannot be considered ethical to admit, retain, or graduate students who cannot ultimately be recommended for a job as an occupational therapist or an occupational therapy assistant, as appropriate. Employers have a legal duty to show "due care in selection" (5, pp 56–59) of those who will treat patients/clients. It may be fraud and negligence knowingly to recommend to an employer someone who cannot meet the test of "due care."

Although some graduates will not work at all, it should be remembered that the purpose of education in occupational therapy is to prepare graduates to work in the profession. They have a right to a realistic expectation of a job, provided they have completed a program successfully and been certified.

The catalog and its component courses. An educational program in occupational therapy and its component courses are developed in accordance with established "Essentials" (7, 8). A university or college catalog and other *official* bulletins and publications have been interpreted by the courts as a contract with students. The implication is that courses as given must actually include the content listed and be adequate to qualify students as intended, enabling them to find employment in the career selected. Faculty should sign and date their teaching outlines, notes, or lectures and record student attendance, thus providing evidence of material actually taught and to whom. Students bear the final responsibility for their own active participation in the program and their own learning.

Grades and recognitions. These should be based on the measurable attainment of established objectives and relevant learning experiences and should not be influenced by special favors or exhortations.

Counseling of students. Counseling and personal contacts between faculty (either academic or clinical) and students should be designed to further the educational objectives of the program. Such contacts should be guided by the educational needs of the students and the reasonable time limitations of the faculty. Moreover, they should be such as can be offered to any and all students in the program. Students have a right to their privacy. Faculty and supervisors are essentially academic advisers, rather than trained counselors. They should avoid giving personal counseling or therapy to students even if they happen to be qualified to do so. It is quite appropriate, however, to refer students to a counseling service if they need it.

Education as a shared commitment. Faculty and students share a commitment to the quality of the educational program in which they participate. They should protect the reputation and safeguard the privacy of one another, and work together for the success of the enterprise. A student should understand, for example, that casual negative remarks about an instructor's ability or the program's quality may damage the reputation of the instructor or the department without the student's intending them to do so or knowing that they have. Students' objective and thoughtfully prepared recommendations for their own education or for the program itself often contribute significantly to education in occupational therapy.

Education of other personnel. A well-designed rationale should guide occupational therapy personnel's teaching of or about occupational therapy to others. The term *teaching* is used here in the broadest sense to refer not only to courses, but to workshops, exhibits, conferences, observation periods, preparation of educational materials, and so on. The rationale and the preparation for what is taught in such contexts merit more attention than it has often received, because dangers are involved.

The objectives of teaching others may be to have them learn (a) what occupational therapy can do for them and their patients/clients, (b) how they can help occupational therapy personnel give more service to their patients/clients, (c) how occupational therapy can shorten a hospital stay or decrease the time needed to return to work, and (d) why occupational therapy merits a budget expenditure. One needs first to determine what *others* need to know about occupational therapy in order to do *their* job. Different personnel need different information. Considerable harm can be done if the content of teaching is not matched to the job-related needs of the audience. Moreover, one does not teach other professionals in a few easy demonstrations to function *as* occupational therapy personnel. Similarly an occupational therapist or an occupational therapy assistant cannot adequately do the job of other professionals just by being shown a few of their procedures. Professional standards are maintained only when services are provided by those who are fully trained and qualified to perform them.

Education of the public. It is in occupational therapy's interest to be known and understood by the public. The public includes not only families of patients/clients and agency personnel, as described in the guidelines, but also the insurance industry, legislators, school and college counselors, parent associations, service clubs, Golden Age groups, and organizations concerned with the many different disabilities. Each group, however, needs a message appropriate to what its interests are and what it should know (Chapter 16 discusses targeting communications to selected audiences).

VIII. [PRINCIPLES] RELATED TO EVALUATION AND RESEARCH

Occupational therapists shall accept responsibility for evaluating, developing and refining service and the body of knowledge and skills which underlie the education and practice of occupational therapy and at all times protects the rights of subjects, clients, institutions and collaborators. The work of others shall be acknowledged.

Guidelines: *Clients' families have the right to have, and occupational therapists have the responsibility to provide explanations of the nature, the purposes, and results of the occupational therapy services unless, as in some employment or treatment settings, there is an explicit exception to this right agreed upon in advance.*

In reporting test results, occupational therapists indicate any reservations regarding validity or reliability resulting from testing circumstances or inappropriateness of the test norms for the person tested.

In performing research and reporting research results, occupational therapists must use accepted scientific methodology.

Commentary

In occupational therapy one finds the total range of efforts that in their most disciplined and advanced form are termed research. The profession recognizes the need to substantiate the theoretical base that undergirds practice and has prepared manuals, workshops, courses, and consultation services to assist practitioners. All who can should profit from these materials and activities and undertake some research in their area of interest. However, inquiry, analysis, evaluation, and organized data collection should characterize *all* occupational therapy. Programs of quality assurance are excellent evidence of attention to standards and ethical practice. Moreover, such programs often form the substance of papers and further studies.

Occupational therapy personnel will find it helpful to be knowledgeable about research being done in their own organization and in the profession at large. This may help them identify sources of collaboration and support, and suggest projects in which they might participate.

Any research that involves experimentation with humans should be conducted according to accepted guidelines for the protection of human subjects. Many organizations have developed such guidelines or have adopted existing guidelines—for example, those of the American Psychological Association (9). By law, many organizations also have an Institutional Review Board that must review proposals for research that their employees propose to conduct with human subjects. Most research in which occupational therapy personnel engage uses humans, and so these conditions apply. Program evaluation normally does not involve direct experimentation with humans but must meet these conditions when it does (e.g., when a survey of former patients/clients is proposed). In informing themselves about research, occupational therapy personnel should search the literature on the protection of human subjects and read some of the resources listed at the end of this chapter.

IX. [PRINCIPLES] RELATED TO THE PROFESSION

The occupational therapist shall be responsible for gaining information and understanding of the principles, policies and standards of the profession. The occupational therapist functions as a representative of the profession.

Guidelines: *Occupational therapists should provide accurate information to the public about the profession and the services that can be provided. Occupational therapists should remain informed about changes in the profession and represent the profession accurately to the consumer.*

Occupational therapists should conduct themselves in a manner befitting professionals. The profession is judged in part by the conduct of its members as they carry out their functions.

Occupational therapists should show support and loyalty to the Association by cooperating with the Representatives in collecting information regarding proposed Association policy, replying to official requests for information and supporting the policies of the Association. It is the member's duty if he disagrees with an Association policy to work through existing channels to effect change.

Occupational therapists who engage in work or volunteer activities in addition to professional occupational therapy responsibilities, shall not violate the ethical principles of the Association in such activities.

Commentary

The organized occupational therapy profession has made possible the education, jobs, recognition, salaries, and status enjoyed by all occupational therapy personnel today. The AOTA and its component groups support the practice of occupational therapy by fostering research, establishing and maintaining standards, working for better legislation, and more. The AOTA has the legal duty to inform its members of the actions it takes and the standards it establishes. This information must be contained in an official publication, which may be the *American Journal of Occupational Therapy* or *Occupational Therapy News*. Members have a legal duty to inform themselves of materials so published.

Sometimes occupational therapy personnel who retire or leave the field think that they are no longer occupational therapy personnel. Once educated and certified as occupational therapists or occupational therapy assistants, however, they are so designated in the thinking of the public. This is not to say that such people are qualified to practice (commentary on this subject appears under the Principles Related to Competence). It does suggest that they represent their profession. If a person left the field and were no longer identified with it by the public, the ethical standards would not apply unless they were in fact still doing some type of occupational therapy.

X. [PRINCIPLES] RELATED TO ADVERTISING

Advertising by therapists under their professional title shall be in accordance with propriety and precedent in health professions.

Guidelines: *Occupational therapists may provide information to the public about available services through procedures established by the employing facility or contracting agency. If an occupational therapist provides an independent service, it is appropriate to advertise those services.*

The occupational therapist shall not use, or participate in the use of, any form of communication containing a false, fraudulent, misleading, deceptive, self-laudatory or unfair statement or claim. Testimonials or statements which promise a favorable result shall be avoided.

Commentary

If advertising is considered to be providing information rather than promoting oneself or one's organization, acceptable approaches will be much clearer. It is appropriate to include any or all of the following in advertising: the names and the designated qualifications of personnel, the services available, their location, and the hours they are offered. It is not appropriate to include any statement promising results or suggesting that the services or the personnel of the advertising organization are better than those of another.

XI. [PRINCIPLES] RELATED TO LAW AND REGULATIONS

The occupational therapist shall seek to acquire information about applicable local, state, federal and institutional rules and shall function accordingly thereto.

Guidelines: *Occupational therapists are obligated to function professionally as a practitioner within the limits of all laws related to the delivery of health services, and applicable to the practice of occupational therapy. Occupational therapists will not engage in any cruel, inhumane or degrading practices in the treatment of clients or in the education of students, or in supervision of others or in peer relationships with other individuals.*

It is the responsibility of occupational therapists to make known to their employers, employees and colleagues, those laws applicable to the practice of occupational therapy and education of occupational therapists.

Commentary

The law is like the sea of some ways. There are many named bodies of water, which are spoken of as the Pacific Ocean or the Black Sea or whatever. It is equally correct to speak of "the sea" generically and to say, "I love the dark sea in winter." Law today is of several types and is derived from a number of sources. Constitutional law and statutory law consist of laws enacted by Congress and by the legislatures of each state. Laws written by counties and cities are called ordinances. Regulations are prepared to implement all these types of laws and are enforced by the authority provided in the laws they implement. Thus regulations are included in what is known as the law.

A last type of law is known as common law or case law. It consists of decisions handed down by the courts throughout the country. (Much of this law has its origins in British common law.) A subspecialty of common law is tort law. A tort is "a legal wrong committed upon the person or property independent of contract" (2, p 1335). Tort law concerns alleged injuries between individuals for which the courts may provide a remedy called damages, usually money, as compensation. The injuries may include personal injuries (assault and battery) of all sorts, damage to an individual's reputation (libel and slander), invasion of privacy, interference with the right to earn a living, and abrogation of the right to enjoy (own) property (a fuller discussion of these rights and the possible abrogation of them by occupational therapy personnel appears under the Principles Related to the Recipient of Service).

Occupational therapy personnel should have a good knowledge of statutory law and regulations covering employment practices and common law pertaining to relationships and the giving of health care services. The resources listed at the end of the chapter will be useful in this regard.

XII. [PRINCIPLES] RELATED TO MISCONDUCT

The occupational therapist shall not appear to act with impropriety nor engage in illegal conduct involving moral turpitude and will not circumvent the principles of occupational therapy ethics through actions of another.

Guidelines: *As employees, occupational therapists refuse to participate in practices inconsistent with legal, moral and ethical standards regarding the treatment of employees or the public. For example, occupational therapists will not condone practices that are inhumane, or that result in illegal or otherwise unjustifiable discrimination on the basis of race, age, sex, religion, handicap or national origin in hiring, promotion or training.*

In providing occupational therapy services, occupational therapists avoid any action that will violate or diminish the legal and civil rights of clients or of others who may be affected.

As practitioners and educators, occupational therapists keep abreast of relevant federal, state, local and agency regulations and American Occupational Therapy Association Standards of Practice and education essentials concerning the conduct of their practice. They are concerned with developing such legal and quasi-legal regulations that support the interests of the public, students and the profession.

Commentary

For occupational therapy personnel to be found guilty of illegal practices, there must have been an actual breaking of some law or pertinent regulation. For occupational therapy personnel to be found liable by the courts for a tort or personal injury, the following conditions must usually be met:

1. A professional relationship must have been created in which the defendant owed a duty to the plaintiff.
2. There must have been a breach or a dereliction of duty of the defendant. In other words, the defendant must have fallen below the legally required standard of care.
3. There must have been actual damage to the plaintiff.
4. The plaintiff's damage or injury must have been caused directly by the defendant's substandard care of him or her.

For occupational therapy personnel to be found guilty of unethical conduct, there must be objective evidence of a serious breach of ethical standards or actual damage to another through the commission of an unethical act. The guidelines and the commentary under Principles Related to Intra-Professional Colleagues explain procedures for dealing with unethical practices.

XIII. [PRINCIPLES] RELATED TO BIOETHICAL ISSUES AND PROBLEMS OF SOCIETY

The occupational therapist seeks information about the major health problems and issues to learn their implications for occupational therapy and for one's own services.

Guidelines: *The principle is a philosophical statement that encourages occupational therapists to be global in their views of health in relationship to society.*

Commentary

Overview of the issues and problems. Society today has an enormous interest in and concern with bioethical issues. The concern is fostered by the media. Events such as human, mechanical, and animal heart transplants have been publicized. Issues about birth have been widely aired, including surrogate mothering, test-tube fertilization, abortion, the right to life, and birth control. At the other end of life, people are thinking about the right to die, suicide, euthanasia, definitions of death, do-not-resuscitate orders, "pulling the plug," living wills, organ banks, and more. Of equal concern are the rights of individuals to decide for themselves, and perhaps for their families, what they should eat, what medications they should take, and whether or not they should smoke, drink, or use drugs and other harmful substances. The rights of individuals in this area are balanced against the obligation or the right of the state to make decisions for both individuals and society. People's involvement with some of these issues is often emotionally charged because of poignant events and situations very close to them. Decisions become difficult and harm may be done.

The role of occupational therapy. Occupational therapy personnel should maintain an active interest in these kinds of issues and have an informed understanding of the implications for patients/clients who are intimately involved with the issues. Occupational therapy personnel can then help patients/clients in their decision making and support the best quality of life possible under the circumstances.

Problems may result from an uninformed eagerness to deal with bioethical issues. Such problems are more often caused by the public than by health professionals, but caution pays. Activities such as witch-hunting, public exposure, and trying cases in the press usually do more harm than good.

Triage. A few bioethical issues actively concern occupational therapy personnel. Resources such as staff, space, equipment, and time may not be adequate to treat all who need service. What is the most ethical solution? Do a little for each one? Make some wait? Triage, or selecting those who need care most and can profit from it, is practiced in the emergency room and should be practiced in occupational therapy if needed.

Legitimate criteria for deciding who is treated will differ in each setting, so none are listed here. Occupational therapists are well advised to seek help, gather data, formulate objective criteria, and develop plans for implementing them.

Dealing with the media. Occupational therapy personnel have an obligation not only to protect their employer's reputation and ensure the privacy of their patients/clients, but also to create public understanding of occupational therapy. Better and more accurate education of the public will be achieved if it is planned. Planning includes the following:

1. Preparing an information sheet for the press in advance
2. Getting releases for photographs ahead of time
3. Analyzing beforehand what message would do the most for occupational therapy with the intended audience
4. Collaborating with professional public relations personnel, including those of related organizations with which the public information program may be coordinated
5. Preparing a list of needs that the community can help meet and considering how the community's doing so will help it.

Information prepared for release should be in accord with the policies of one's organization. Public relations may not initially appear to relate to ethics, but indeed they do. Information that is full of errors or poorly chosen can be very damaging to patients/clients, to staff, and to an organization and its programs.

CONCLUSION

The formulation of ethical standards and enlightened legislation represents a sincere attempt to serve humanity better. As such, they are best used to educate, guide, and prevent; even to inspire a person to give his or her finest effort. Occupational therapy's ethical standards should be widely taught, well understood, and frequently used. Although problems may occasionally arise and call for corrective action, may the primary purpose of the standards be to guide occupational therapy personnel everywhere in giving their best.

SUMMARY OF COMMENTARY

Ethics set a standard of behavior for individuals and groups, including professions. Most ethical standards are supported by law in some form. Therefore, ethics should not be considered separately from law. The ethical standards of a profession apply to all its members. In ethics concern is with outcomes, not intentions.

In the selection of patients/clients, triage—serving those who can profit most—should be practiced, if necessary. Patients/clients have the right to freedom from bodily harm, which means that they must consent to treatment. They also have the right to privacy, which means keeping confidential their presence in a facility and their diagnosis and treatment. It also means that their consent should be sought if they are to be used in teaching or be photographed.

Occupational therapy personnel have a right to be paid for their services. In regard to quality of treatment, however, the ethical principles make no distinction as to whether or not personnel are paid.

Supervisors and consultants have different relationships to recipients of service. The law expects supervisors to match *people* with *duties* based on objective assessments of both, and to evaluate the success of the assignments they make. If those obligations have been met, a supervisor cannot be held liable for a supervisee's incompetence. A consultant should document his or her teaching and recommendations and the names of the people to whom they were given.

Occupational therapy personnel must be expressly qualified for the duties included in their job description. A supervisor may be liable for negligent supervision if he or she knows or should have known that a supervisee was not qualified.

Statements of one's own competence or experience that are not in accord with the facts are actionable if they cause legal injury. Responsibility for competence is shared in some ways, but the individual bears the ultimate responsibility to be competent in his or her job.

Records are important evidence of what has been done. They should be written regularly and promptly. They have many legitimate uses, the primary one being documenting the state of health of a patient/client before and after treatment. Those who perform a service have a right and often an obligation to write a record of it. A basic principle is that one writes about what is within one's own purview and performed by oneself. Records should be confidential. Patients/clients should not be identified in casual conversation.

Occupational therapy personnel must be concerned with substandard or unethical performance, avoiding it themselves and acting to rectify it when they witness it in fellow professionals. When they suspect unethical conduct by other health care professionals, they should also take corrective action. If they do not, they may be guilty themselves of substandard practice.

Teaching of occupational therapy to others is appropriately directed toward their understanding and using occupational therapy and carrying out follow-up activities. People should not perform services that are not in the accepted scope of their profession. New functions can be performed with appropriate continuing education or postgraduate study, or under certain conditions laid down by the courts.

Employers have vicarious liability for the work of their employees. Thus caution must be taken in such matters as using one's personal car for the employer's business. Employees, for their part, are obligated to protect their employer's physical property and reputation.

Standards and procedures for selecting occupational therapy students must be nondiscriminatory. However, students may be denied admission because of deficits that present a probable hazard to them or their patients/clients. The official publications of a college or university are considered contracts with students, and thus courses as given must include the content listed in these publications and qualify students to find employment in their chosen career. Counseling and personal contacts between students and faculty should be designed to further the educational objectives of a program.

A well-designed rationale should guide occupational therapists' teaching of or about occupational therapy to others. Considerable harm can be done if the content is not matched to the audience's job-related needs. The public too needs messages appropriate to its interests.

All occupational therapy personnel who can should profit from continuing education materials and activities that encourage research to build the profession's theoretical base. Inquiry, analysis, evaluation, and organized data collection should characterize all occupational therapy, however.

The AOTA has the legal duty to inform its members of its actions and its standards. AOTA members are legally obligated to inform themselves of these actions and standards.

Appropriate advertising involves providing the following information: the names and the designations of personnel, the services available, their location, and the hours of operation.

Occupational therapy personnel should have a good knowledge of statutory law and regulations covering employment practices and common law pertaining to relationships and the giving of health care services. For occupational therapy personnel to be guilty of illegal or unethical conduct, or to be found liable for a tort, certain conditions must obtain.

Occupational therapy personnel should maintain an active interest in bioethical and social issues such as triage, and be informed about the implications of these issues for patients/clients.

Occupational therapy personnel have an obligation to create public understanding of their profession. Better and more accurate education of the public will be achieved if it is planned.

References

1. Principles of occupational therapy ethics. *Am J Occup Ther* 38:799–802, 1984
2. Black HC: *Black's Law Dictionary*, 5th edition. St. Paul, MN: West Publishing Co, 1979
3. Creighton H: *Law Every Nurse Should Know*. Philadelphia: WB Saunders Co, 1970
4. Welles C: Liability considerations in the occupational therapy practice environment. *Occup Ther Health Care* 1(4):35–45, 1984
5. Hayt E, Hayt LR: *Law of Hospital and Nurse*. New York: Hospital Textbook Co, 1958
6. Magit v Board of Medical Examiners of the State of California, 75C2d74 (1961)
7. American Occupational Therapy Association. Essentials of an approved program for occupational therapy assistants. In *Reference Manual of the Official Documents of the American Occupational Therapy Association*. Rockville, MD: American Occupational Therapy Association, 1983
8. American Occupational Therapy Association. Essentials of an accredited program for occupational therapists. In *Reference Manual of the Official Documents of the American Occupational Therapy Association*. Rockville, MD: American Occupational Therapy Association, 1983
9. American Psychological Association: *Ethical Principles in the Conduct of Research with Human Participants*. Washington, DC: American Psychological Association, 1982

Additional Resources

Abrams N, Buckner M, Editors: *Medical Ethics*. Boston: MIT Press, 1983

Annas G: *The Rights of Hospital Patients*. New York: Avon Books, 1975

Fiesta J: *The Law and Liability, A Guide for Nurses*. New York: John Wiley & Sons Inc, 1983

The Hastings Center Report. Hastings-on-Hudson, NY: Institute of Society and Ethics and Life Sciences. Published six times a year

Law, Medicine and Health Care. Boston: American Society of Law and Medicine. Published six times a year. (Address: 765 Commonwealth Avenue, Sixteenth Floor, Boston, MA 02215)

MPR The Malpractice Reporter. New York: Public Reporting Services. Published eight times a year

Posgar G: *Legal Aspects of Health Care Administration*. Rockville, MD: Aspen Systems Corp, 1979

Tancredi LR, Editor: *Ethics in Health Care*. Washington, DC. National Academy of Sciences, 1974

Welles C: The implications of liability: Guidelines for professional practice. *Am J Occup Ther* 23:18–26, 1969

Welles C: Specialization: Legal and administrative implications. *Am J Occup Ther* 33:118–119, 1979

Appendix A: Conducting Productive Meetings

Madelaine S. Gray, MPA, OTR, FAOTA

The standard complaint is heard everywhere: Oh no, not another meeting! There is much negativism about meetings. People do not look forward to them. On the other hand, they are often essential for communication, deliberation, decision making, and planning. Managers who set a precedent for productive meetings that make good use of people's time, energy, and effort get more cooperation from staff and others who participate. Following are some important points to consider in planning and conducting meetings.

BEING SURE THAT MEETINGS HAVE A PURPOSE

Meetings should have a purpose, and it should be clear to participants. For example, a meeting can be helpful when a manager is faced with a complex issue on which the advice of colleagues or staff is needed. A meeting can also be helpful when a manager senses resistance to a task or recognizes great differences of opinion on an issue. In such circumstances meetings can serve to explore possible actions, uncover critical information, create new ideas, thrash out differences, seek consensus, develop commitment, generate team spirit, and so on. If they are handled skillfully, they can be productive and satisfying. At the least they can provide an opportunity for a manager to clarify issues, clear the air, and indicate before the group the official policy or position.

Good meetings are challenging, stimulating, and enlightening to participants. They involve thinking, problem solving, and interaction, and they produce results. Participants become a part of the activity.

On the other hand, meetings are often not that way. Sometimes they involve routine tasks that have little ambiguity or challenge, that could readily be handled by a single person. For instance, developing standard operating procedures is a fairly straightforward task. Instead of calling a meeting to accomplish it, a manager might ask a staff member to draft some procedures and send them out for review. When the comments come in, a meeting might then be appropriate.

Madelaine S. Gray was a clinician and an educator for eight years and has been a manager for thirteen. She is AOTA's Associate Executive Director, Department of Professional Services. Her graduate degree is in management.

AGENDAS

Preparation for a meeting should include the development of a written agenda. Some of the issues to think about are: What needs to be discussed? Who will be responsible for an agenda item? What background materials are needed? Are there some items of information that the people attending the meeting should bring? How will the agenda item be handled—by a presentation or through a problem-solving process? How much time will be devoted to it? Timing is very important sometimes in how a decision is made. What are the desired outcomes?

In developing an agenda, an effective strategy is to involve staff or others who will attend the meeting so that the manager can learn directly what is on their minds and what they think needs to be discussed. Their input can be sought by telephone or memo. If it is not possible to get input in advance, the manager might ask at the end of the meeting, "Are there any topics you'd like me to put on the agenda for the next meeting?"

When a meeting is called, an agenda should be circulated in advance so that people know what to expect. Even so, a manager should be open to discussion of issues not on the written agenda, provided the issues being raised do not overwhelm the official purpose of the meeting.

SCHEDULING A MEETING

A manager with a large staff may schedule regular meetings in order to set aside a standard time to discuss problems and exchange information. On occasion, a special meeting might be called—for example, when legislation affecting occupational therapy has just been passed and immediate discussion is essential. With a small staff, meetings might be scheduled irregularly, as topics come up that need to be discussed. If meetings are not regularly scheduled, a good way to give sufficient notice is to set the date for the next meeting at the end of a current meeting. For special meetings, as much advance notice should be given as is possible.

ATTENDANCE AT MEETINGS

Who should attend a meeting is usually well set. Either an established group or a task-oriented group is convened to deal with a particular problem or issue. The manager might at times, however, want to have a consultant or a guest speaker. Also, it is important to invite all the people who will be affected by the work of a group. If the people who will have to carry out the decisions of a group are left out, they may not fully understand the task and the reasons behind it, and therefore they may not be committed to the decisions. For instance, an occupational therapy consultant who is developing guidelines for school systems would want to involve several key people in those systems and any people who serve linkage functions to explain the guidelines to school systems.

THE ROLE OF THE MANAGER IN CONDUCTING A MEETING

A manager usually chairs meetings and tries to

- Facilitate discussion
- Ensure that everyone is heard
- Ensure that ideas are understood
- Seek compromise when necessary
- Summarize at appropriate points
- Call for decisions
- Move the agenda along
- See that a record of the meeting is kept.

With all those (and more) chores as chair, a manager often has little opportunity to participate in discussions. Some managers chairing meetings strive to be neutral, thinking of themselves more as a facilitator of discussion than as a part of the group. For occupational therapy managers who want to participate in meetings and still maintain final control, the approach described in Doyle and Straus's *How to Make Meetings Work* (1) may be appropriate. The authors propose the interaction method, in which the manager appoints a skilled person to facilitate the meeting as a neutral player. That allows the manager to participate freely in discussion. A manager who is chairing a meeting cannot always participate as effectively as he or she might want. Also, how much does a manager want to dominate, functioning not only as the head of the occupational therapy organization but also leading all the meetings?

A manager who decides to try the Doyle and Straus method should explain it to the group ahead of time. The manager is, in a sense, delegating authority, even though the facilitator does not contribute content ideas to the meeting. The facilitator deals only with process ideas, keeps the group focused on the task, and suggests methods for protecting group members from attacks on their ideas. The facilitator looks for ways to encourage nonjudgmental behavior and calls attention to judgmental behavior if it interferes with group participation. He or she helps the group find win-win solutions, searches for ways to compromise, if necessary, and coordinates pre- and postmeeting logistics.

Another option is for the manager to move in and out of chairing a meeting. He or she could say, "I'm going to chair this portion of the meeting, but for the next portion, when we're going to be talking about such-and-such an issue, I've asked so-and-so to be a facilitator."

CONSIDERING THE PHYSICAL ENVIRONMENT OF THE MEETING ROOM

The physical environment of the meeting room can be very important. For example, a round table, versus the authoritarian rectangular table with the manager at the head, can make a difference in terms of interaction and participation. The comfort level of the room is another consideration: Is the room too hot or too cold? Is it stuffy? Is it smoke filled? Figure 1 is a checklist of important variables in relation to the physical environment.

FIGURE A–1
Checklist for Physical Arrangements

	Yes	No
Is the meeting room appropriate—not too small, not too big?	____	____
Is the lighting adequate?	____	____
Can the lights be worked conveniently, if need be, by the conference leader?	____	____
Is a lectern available?	____	____
Is the seating arrangement appropriate for the meeting?	____	____
Are the chairs comfortable?	____	____
Will conferees have tables or some other hard surface on which to write?	____	____
Can the seating be arranged so that conferees can enter and exit from the rear of the room?	____	____
Is the arrangement such that conferees will not be distracted by outside activities?	____	____
If the meeting is being held outside company facilities, has someone checked to make certain that no distracting activities will be taking place in adjacent rooms?	____	____
Is water available?	____	____
Have arrangements been made for coffee breaks that will not disturb the meeting?	____	____
Are ashtrays available? Is the ventilation adequate to permit smoking?	____	____
Are name plates, pencils, and writing paper available?	____	____
Are all props in order? Are sufficient and convenient outlets available for planned visual aids?	____	____
Is the room absolutely clean?	____	____

WRITING MINUTES

Minutes are important records of meetings and can be useful in keeping track of decisions, issues, assignments, and policies. Guidelines for writing minutes are available from The American Occupational Therapy Association, Department of Professional Services.

EVALUATING THE MEETING

Figure 2 is a checklist that managers can use to analyze a meeting that did not go well, or just to review a meeting. The checklist helps a manager think through what happened in a meeting in terms of the content, or the process that was used.

FIGURE A–2
Checklist for Evaluating Meetings

The Meeting Itself

1. Were the right persons present?
2. Were the physical facilities adequate?
3. Were most of the proposed points in the discussion guide covered?
4. Was participation in the discussion generally good?
5. Was any individual unfairly squelched?
6. Were there any breaches of the rules as regards rank?
7. If the result was that something had to be done, were the *what, who,* and *when* explicitly covered?
8. Was an adequate summary statement made?
9. Does a good set of notes exist to use in drawing up the minutes?

The Follow-Up

10. What do the minutes say about who is to do what and when?
11. Have the minutes been distributed to all concerned—nonparticipants as well as participants—and promptly?
12. How is the apparent reconciliation, solution, or decision obtained in the meeting actually working out?
13. What will be done about tabled matters?
14. Is a tactful follow-up with certain individuals called for as a result of a highly controversial meeting?
15. Is individual discussion of minutes called for?
16. Should memos be sent to certain individuals?
17. Is an explanation necessary to anyone because of management action contrary to a conference recommendation?

Reference

1. Doyle M, Straus D: *How to Make Meetings Work: The New Interaction Method.* New York: Playboy Paperbacks, 1976

Additional Resources

How committees work. *Principles of Association Management.* Washington, DC: American Society of Association Executives, 1975

How to run worthwhile meetings. *Executive Skills* 2(79-6):1–10, 1979

Jay A: How to run a meeting. *Harvard Business Review,* March–April 1976

Schneier CE, Beatty RW, Goktepe JR: How to manage a committee. *Association Management's Leadership,* December 1984

Appendix B: Occupational Therapy Personnel Classifications*

CLASSIFICATION: Staff occupational therapist, registered (OTR) entry level

PRIMARY FUNCTION

To provide occupational therapy services to patients/clients, including assessment, treatment program planning and implementation, related documentation, and communication.

QUALIFICATIONS

1. *Education:* Graduate of an accredited occupational therapy program or completion of the AOTA career mobility program, or graduate of a World Federation of Occupational Therapy WFOT-approved occupational therapy program; successful completion of a minimum of six months, Level II Fieldwork experience; successful completion of AOTA Certification Examination for Occupational Therapist, Registered.
2. *Certification and Licensure:* Current AOTA certification; licensed as an occupational therapist where required by state law.
3. *Experience:* Less than one year as an OTR.
4. *Skills:* Professional competency as a general practitioner of occupational therapy, as defined by AOTA through successful completion of AOTA certification or state licensure process.

EXAMPLES OF CRITICAL PERFORMANCE AREAS

- Responds to requests for service and initiates referrals where appropriate.
- Screens individuals to determine need for intervention.
- Evaluates patients/clients to obtain and interpret data necessary for treatment planning and implementation.
- Interprets evaluation findings to patients/clients, family, significant others, and care team.
- Develops treatment plans, including goals and methods to achieve identified goals.
- Coordinates treatment plan with patients/clients, family, significant others, and care team.

*Material taken from "Guide to Classifications of Occupational Therapy Personnel," an official document approved by the AOTA Representative Assembly in April 1985 that will be published in the December 1985 issue of *The American Journal of Occupational Therapy.*

CLASSIFICATION: Staff certified occupational therapy assistant (COTA) entry level

PRIMARY FUNCTION

To implement occupational therapy services for patients and clients under the supervision of an occupational therapist (OTR). These services include structured assessments, treatment, and documentation.

QUALIFICATIONS

1. *Education:* Graduate of an AOTA-approved occupational therapy assistant education program; successful completion of a minimum of two months supervised Level II Fieldwork experience; successful completion of the certification process for Occupational Therapy Assistant.

2. *Certification and Licensure:* Current AOTA certification; licensed as an Occupational Therapy Assistant where required by state law.

3. *Experience:* Less than one year of practice experience as a COTA.

4. *Skills:* Competent in the delivery of occupational therapy treatment, under the direction of an OTR as delineated in the AOTA Entry-Role Delineation for OTRs and COTAs.

EXAMPLES OF CRITICAL PERFORMANCE AREAS

● Indicates basic critical performance areas.

● Indicates performance areas at higher levels.

● Responds to requests for service by relaying information and referral to an OTR.

● Determines patient's/client's need for services in collaboration with an OTR.

● Contributes to the assessment process under supervision of an OTR.

● Assists OTR in developing treatment plans and techniques to implement plans.

● Monitors patient's/client's response to treatment and modifies treatment during sessions as indicated in collaboration with an OTR.

● Reports observations of patient's/client's performance and responses to services to the OTR.

● Implements treatment directly or supervises treatment by a certified occupational therapy assistant.

● Monitors patient's/client's response to intervention and modifies treatment as indicated to attain goals.

● Develops appropriate home or community programming to maintain and enhance the performance of the patients/clients in their own environments.

● Terminates services when maximum benefit has been achieved.

● Documents results of patient's/client's assessment, treatment, follow-up, and termination of services.

● Reviews the quality and appropriateness of the total services delivered and of individual occupational therapy programs for effectiveness and efficiency, using predetermined criteria.

● Maintains service-related records.

● Follows billing and reimbursement procedures.

- Provides inservice education to members of the patient's/client's care team and education to the community.
- Complies with established agency standards and evaluates compliance.
- Identifies own continuing education and consultation needs.
- Supervises COTAs, occupational therapy aides, and volunteers.
- Supervises occupational therapy and occupational therapy assistant Level I Fieldwork students.

SUPERVISORY SUPPORT NEEDED

1. *Clinical:* Close supervision (i.e., daily direct contact on-site) by an intermediate or advanced level OTR is preferred. If not provided, general supervision (i.e., less than daily) or consultation, or both, by an intermediate or advanced level therapist is recommended. Frequency and manner of contact is determined by the supervising OTR, with on-site contact occurring at least monthly. Therapists may require consultation by an advanced level OTR in special areas in which they have minimal experience.
2. *Management/Administrative:* Administrative supervision is recommended for implementation of policies, quality assurance, and materiel management. In addition, supervision or consultation, or both, by an OTR with administrative experience is recommended in the development of service operations, policies, and procedures related to billing, reimbursement, and adherence to state and federal regulatory requirements.

- Recommends termination of patient/client services to the supervisor.
- Documents and maintains service-related records, as directed by supervising OTR.
- Assists in providing inservice education.
- Complies with established agency and service standards.
- Identifies own continuing education needs in consultation with OTR.

SUPERVISORY SUPPORT NEEDED

1. *Clinical:* Close supervision (i.e., daily direct contact on-site) is required from an OTR or intermediate or advanced level COTA.
2. *Management/Administrative:* General supervision by an experienced OTR or an experienced COTA is required for implementation of policies and procedures related to delivery of occupational therapy services.

Appendix C: Significant Employment Legislation

John W. Schell, PhD

Legislation	Major Features
Civil Rights Act of 1964, Titles VI & VII (as amended in 1972)	*Title VI* 1. Prohibits employment discrimination in all programs receiving federal funds. *Title VII* 1. Prohibits discrimination in employment based on race, sex, religion, color, or national origin. 2. Provides criteria for bona fide occupational qualification (BFOQs) that allow for legal discrimination based on the concept of "disruption of normal operation." 3. Requires compliance by most public and private organizations including employment agencies and labor unions. 4. Is enforced by the Equal Employment Opportunity Commission (EEOC) through the following activities: a. Investigation of discrimination complaints b. Conciliation of discrimination charges c. Litigation in federal courts.

Legislation	Major Features
Executive Order 11246 (as amended by E.O. 11375)	1. Prohibits employment discrimination (same as Title VII). 2. Mandates federal contractors with 50+ employees to develop Affirmative Action Plans.
Age Discrimination in Employment Act of 1967	1. Prohibits employment discrimination among workers aged 40 to 70 years old. 2. Requires compliance by employers with 25+ employees.
Equal Pay Act of 1963 (as amended in 1972), an amendment to the Fair Labor Standards Act	1. Requires employers to pay males and females equally, based on the concept of "equal work." 2. Bases "equal work" on analysis of a specific job. 3. Allows pay differentials for reasons of productivity, merit, and seniority. 4. Is enforced by EEOC.
Vietnam-Era Veterans Readjustment Act of 1974	1. Requires firms holding federal contracts to take affirmative action in employment and advancement of Vietnam-era veterans (and disabled veterans).
Rehabilitation Act of 1973, Section 504	1. Requires nondiscriminatory hiring by employers receiving federal assistance. 2. Broadly defines term *handicapped* to include the following: a. Physical or mental impairment . . . limiting one or more of such person's major life activities. b. A record of such impairment.

Legislation	Major Features
	c. Is regarded as having such an impairment. 3. Extends protection to only those capable of performing a particular job with "reasonable accommodation."
Fair Labor Standards Act	1. Establishes minimum wages, maximum hours, and overtime requirements. 2. Exempts most "professional employees" from minimum wages, maximum hours, and rates of overtime.
Uniform Guidelines on Employee Selection Procedures	1. Set forth uniform federal guidelines, jointly published by the U. S. Civil Service Commission, EEOC, the Justice Department, and the Department of Labor. 2. Purpose: The guidelines establish the technical methods for development of legal employment testing and selection procedures. 3. Adverse Impact: If employer policies or practices create an adverse impact on employment opportunities based on race, sex, or ethnic group, employers must statistically validate their selection devices. Such devices include educational and employment experience levels, interview results, and test scores. 4. The Four-Fifths Rule: The selection rates for minority applicants (minorities can

Legislation	Major Features
	be any group when compared with the majority of applicants) must be 80 percent of the selection rates for nonminorities. 5. The "Bottom Line" Concept: Employers are not required to validate all parts of their selection procedures if the overall process is predictive of future job performance.

Appendix D: Applicant Interview Analysis*

Name of Applicant: ____________________ **Date of Interview:** ____________________

Candidate For: ____________________ **Interviewer:** ____________________

PLEASE REPORT YOUR INTERVIEW IMPRESSIONS BY CHECKING THE ONE MOST APPROPRIATE BOX IN EACH AREA

1. APPEARANCE
- ☐ Untidy
- ☐ Somewhat careless about personal appearance.
- ☐ Satisfactory personal appearance.
- ☐ Better than average appearance

2. PERSONALITY
- ☐ Appears very distant and aloof.
- ☐ Approachable; fairly friendly.
- ☐ Warm; friendly; sociable.
- ☐ Very sociable and outgoing.

3. POISE-STABILITY
- ☐ Ill at ease; is "jumpy" and appears nervous.
- ☐ Somewhat tense; is easily irritated.
- ☐ About as poised as the average person.
- ☐ Sure of himself; well composed.

4. COMMUNICATION ABILITY
- ☐ Expresses himself poorly.
- ☐ Does less than average job at expressing himself.
- ☐ Average fluency and expression.
- ☐ Communicates well.

5. ALERTNESS
- ☐ Appears slow to "catch on."
- ☐ Appears rather slow; requires more than average explanation.
- ☐ Appears to grasp ideas with average ability.
- ☐ Appears quick to understand; perceives very well.

6. KNOWLEDGE OF FIELD
- ☐ Appears to have poor knowledge of field.
- ☐ Appears to have some knowledge of field.
- ☐ An average amount of knowledge is demonstrated.
- ☐ Appears to have excellent knowledge of field.

7. EXPERIENCE IN FIELD
- ☐ No relationship between applicant's background and job requirements.
- ☐ Fair relationship between applicant's background and job requirements.
- ☐ Average amount of meaningful background and experience.
- ☐ Excellent background considerable experience in field

8. DRIVE
- ☐ Appears to have poorly defined goals.
- ☐ Appears to set goals too low.
- ☐ Appears to have average goals.
- ☐ Appears to have high desire to acheive.

9. OVERALL
- ☐ Definitely unsatisfactory candidate.
- ☐ Substandard candidate.
- ☐ Average candidate
- ☐ Definitly above average candidate.
- ☐ Outstanding candidate.

NOTES:

THIS APPLICANT SHOULD BE CONSIDERED FURTHER ☐YES ☐NO IF NO, STATE REASON: ____________________

IF YES - REQUEST REFERENCE CHECK ☐YES ☐NO ____________________

IF NO, WOULD YOU RECOMMEND CONSIDERATION AT FUTURE DATE FOR THIS OR ANY OTHER POSITION?

☐YES ☐NO REMARKS: ____________________

ADDITIONAL COMMENTS: ____________________

SALARY QUOTE: ____________________

1/82 **Return Completed Form to Personnel Office**

**Reprinted with permission from Harmarville Rehabilitation Center, Inc., Pittsburgh, PA.*

Appendix E: Review of Performance

Name	______	**Date Hired**	______
Address	______	**Employee No.**	______
Department	______	**Social Security**	______

Date: 19 This is a ( ) 30–60 day ( ) 90–110 day ( ) 120–150 day ( ) annual ( ) special

Instructions to Reviewer:

1. In connection with each work trait considered, place a check mark at that point along the line which most nearly coincides with your opinion of the individual.
2. Consider only one trait or quality at a time. Don't let your judgment concerning one trait influence your judgment of other traits.
3. Consider the individual's entire work performance. Don't base your judgment on only one or two occurrences.

1. Quality of work. Consider how work measures up to department's standard: accuracy, neatness, thoroughness, technical excellence, etc. (Disregard volume of work.)

Highest quality work always	Good, almost always accurate	Fair, occasional errors	Careless, frequent errors	Unsatisfactory. Work slipshod, errors very frequent

2. Quantity of work. Consider only volume of work produced and how it compares to your department's standard. Consult available production records.

Unusually fast worker	High rate of production	Works at steady average speed	Low production	Excessively slow worker

3. Cooperativeness. Consider his or her attitude toward his or her job and toward co-workers, and how they react toward him or her. Is he or she a good team worker?

Always gives and gets exceptionally fine cooperation	High degree of cooperation	Satisfactory	Sometimes "difficult." Tends to be balky and to irritate others.	Frequently unpleasant and uncooperative.

In one sentence, describe why you gave the employee this rating ______

______

4. Dependability. Consider general application to work. Can you always count on this person to be punctual, conscientious, industrious, accurate? Does he or she require constant supervision or direction?

Dependable in highest degree.	Superior, occasional supervision needed.	Conscientious but needs regular supervision.	Can't be sure of him or her. Needs considerable supervision.	Undependable, needs constant direction and watching.

5. Adaptability. Consider his or her ability to meet changing conditions, to pitch in on emergency jobs, to respond to new procedures.

Most adaptable and flexible.	Usually responds well to changing needs, jobs, procedures.	Moderately adaptable.	Rather slow and reluctant to accept or adapt to changes.	Inflexible, resists change.

6. Judgment, Common Sense, Initiative. Consider his or her ability to proceed with his or her job without being told every detail, to make suggestions, to solve problems, to be generally resourceful.

Sound judgment and high degree of resourcefulness at all times.	Well above average.	Judgment reasonably sound. Fairly resourceful.	Thoughtless. Frequently fails to "use his or her head."	Judgment can't be relied on. Shows no initiative.

Compared to other employees in similar jobs, this employee ranks

Marginal	Below Average	Average	Above Average	Excellent

Is employee promotable? ______________ If so, to what jobs? ______________

If unable to define jobs, what skills does he or she possess over requirements of present job? ______________

What further training does employee need in present position or to enhance his or her chances for promotional opportunities?

General remarks and recommendations ______________

Reviewed with Employee on ______________ ______________

(Date) Signature of Reviewer

Comments by Employee ______________

____

Employee Signature

Appendix F: Article 3101.9—Medicare Coverage for Occupational Therapy Services*

3101.9 *Occupational Therapy Furnished by the Hospital or by Others under Arrangements with the Hospital and under its Supervision.*

A. *General.* Occupational therapy is medically prescribed treatment concerned with improving or restoring functions which have been impaired by illness or injury or, where function has been permanently lost or reduced by illness or injury, to improve the individual's ability to perform those tasks required for independent functioning. Such therapy may involve:

1. the evaluation, and reevaluation as required, of a patient's level of function by administering diagnostic and prognostic tests;

2. the selection and teaching of task-oriented therapeutic activities designed to restore physical function, e.g., use of wood-working activities on an inclined table to restore shoulder, elbow and wrist range of motion lost as a result of burns;

3. the planning, implementing, and supervising of individualized therapeutic activity programs as part of an overall "active treatment" program for a patient with a diagnosed psychiatric illness, e.g., the use of sewing activities which require following a pattern to reduce confusion and restore reality orientation in a schizophrenic patient;

4. the planning and implementing of therapeutic tasks and activities to restore sensory-integrative function, e.g., providing motor and tactile activities to increase sensory input and improve response for a stroke patient with functional loss resulting in a distorted body image;

5. the teaching of compensatory technique to improve the level of independence in the activities of daily living, e.g., teaching a patient who has lost the use of an arm how to pare potatoes and chop vegetables with one hand, teaching an upper extremity amputee how to functionally utilize a prosthesis, or teaching a stroke patient new techniques to enable him to perform feeding, dressing, and other activities as independently as possible;

6. the designing, fabricating, and fitting of orthotic and self-help devices, e.g., making a hand splint for a patient with rheumatoid arthritis to maintain the hand in a functional position or constructing a device

*Reprinted from *Occupational Therapy Medicare Handbook.* Rockville, MD: American Occupational Therapy Association, Government and Legal Affairs Division, 1982, pp. B-1–B-5.

which would enable an individual to hold a utensil and feed himself independently; and

7. vocational and prevocational assessment and training.

Only a qualified occupational therapist has the knowledge, training, and experience required to evaluate and, as necessary, reevaluate a patient's level of function, determine whether an occupational therapy program could reasonably be expected to improve, restore, or compensate for lost function and, where appropriate, recommend to the physician a plan of treatment. However, while the skills of a qualified occupational therapist are required to evaluate the patient's level of function and develop a plan of treatment, the implementation of the plan may also be carried out by a qualified occupational therapy assistant functioning under the general supervision of the qualified occupational therapist. ("General supervision" requires initial direction and periodic inspection of the actual activity; however, the supervisor need not always be physically present or on the premises when the assistant is performing services.)

B. *Coverage Criteria.* To constitute covered occupational therapy for Medicare purposes the services furnished to a beneficiary must be (1) prescribed by a physician, (2) performed by a qualified occupational therapist or a qualified occupational therapy assistant under the general supervision of a qualified occupational therapist, and (3) reasonable and necessary for the treatment of the individual's illness or injury.

Occupational therapy designed to improve function is considered reasonable and necessary for the treatment of the individual's illness or injury only where an expectation exists that the therapy will result in a significant *practical* improvement in the individual's level of functioning within a reasonable period of time. Where an individual's improvement potential is insignificant in relation to the extent and duration of occupational therapy services required to achieve improvement, such services would not be considered reasonable and necessary and would thus be excluded from coverage by 1862(a)(1). Where a valid expectation of improvement exists at the time the occupational therapy program is instituted, the services would be covered even though the expectation may not be realized. However, in such situations the services would be covered only up to the time at which it would have been reasonable to conclude that the patient is not going to improve. Once a patient has reached the point where no further significant practical improvement can be expected, the skills of an occupational therapist or occupational therapy assistant will not be required in the carrying out of any activity and/or exercise program required to *maintain function* at the level to which it has been restored. Consequently, while the services of an occupational therapist in *designing* a maintenance program and making infrequent but periodic evaluation of its effectiveness would be covered, the services of an occupational therapist or occupational therapy assistant in *carrying out* the program are not considered reasonable and necessary for the treatment of illness or injury and such services are excluded from coverage under section 1862(a)(1).

Generally speaking, occupational therapy is not required to effect improvement or restoration of function where a patient suffers a temporary loss or reduction of function (e.g., temporary weakness which may follow prolonged bedrest following major abdominal surgery) which could reasonably be expected to spontaneously improve as the patient gradually resumes normal activities. Accordingly, occupational therapy furnished in such situations would not be considered reasonable and necessary for the treatment of the individual's illness or injury and the services would be excluded from coverage by 1862(a)(1).

Occupational therapy may also be required for a patient with a specific diagnosed psychiatric illness. Where such services are required they would be covered, assuming the coverage criteria set forth above are met. However, it should be noted that where an individual's motivational needs are not related to a specific diagnosed psychiatric illness, the meeting of such needs does not usually require an individualized therapeutic program. Rather, such needs can be met through general activity programs or the efforts of other professional personnel involved in the care of the patient, patient motivation being an appropriate and inherent function of all health disciplines which is interwoven with other functions performed by such personnel for the patient. Accordingly, since the special skills of an occupational therapist or occupational therapy assistant are not required, an occupational therapy program for such individuals would not be considered reasonable and necessary for the treatment of an illness or injury, and services furnished under such a program would be excluded from coverage by 1862(a)(1). See D for discussion regarding coverage of patient activity programs.

As indicated, occupational therapy includes vocational and prevocational assessment and training. When services provided by an occupational therapist and/or assistant are related *solely* to specific employment opportunities, work skills or work settings, they are not reasonable or necessary for the *diagnosis or treatment* of an illness or injury and are excluded from coverage under the program by 1862(a)(1). However, care should be exercised in applying this exclusion, because the assessment of level of function and the teaching of compensatory techniques to improve the level of function, especially in activities of daily living, are services which occupational therapists provide for both vocational and nonvocational purposes. For example, an assessment of sitting and standing tolerance might be nonvocational for a mother of young children or a retired individual living alone, but would be a vocational test for a sales clerk. Training an amputee in the use of a prosthesis for telephoning is necessary for every-day activities as well as for employment purposes. Major changes in life style may be mandatory for an individual with a substantial disability; the techniques of adjustment cannot be considered exclusively vocational or nonvocational.

C. *Supplies.* Occupational therapy frequently necessitates the use of various supplies, e.g., looms, ceramic tiles, leather, etc. The cost of such supplies may be included in the occupational therapy cost center. However, to prevent possible abuse in this area these costs should be carefully reviewed by the intermediary to ensure that they are reasonable.

D. *Patient Activity Programs.* In the inpatient setting, organized patient activity programs are utilized to provide diversion and general motivation to inpatients. Although occupational therapists and occupational therapy assistants may be involved in directing and supervising such programs, these activity programs are part of a generalized effort directed to the health and welfare of all patients and such programs *do not* constitute occupational therapy and no ancillary charges may be recognized for such services. However, since these programs do constitute an integral part of good inpatient care they would be considered covered services related to the routine care of patients, providing: (1) the program is one ordinarily furnished by the provider to its inpatients, and (2) it is of a type in which Medicare patients requiring a covered level of inpatient care may reasonably be expected to participate. For example, patients requiring the level of inpatient care covered under the program might engage in games such as checkers or chess, handicrafts such as sewing or weaving, and they might attend movies, etc. But, it would not be expected that such patients would be able to go on field trips, engage in strenuous athletics, or participate in other activities which are inappropriate for patients requiring the level of care covered under the program. (The capacities of physically healthy psychiatric patients would vary from those of patients whose ailments are physical.)

*Appendix G: What to Do if Medicare Denies Payment**

Run through the following checklist:

1. *Is your patient Medicare eligible?*
2. *Is your facility Medicare certified?*
3. *Are you providing services covered under the law?*
4. *Do you have a physician prescription?*

According to the Health Care Financing Administration (HCFA) (the federal agency that administers the Medicare program), the following constitutes an appropriate prescription for Medicare purposes:

a. The physician orders occupational therapy, occupational therapy evaluation, or occupational therapy for a specific problem.
b. The occupational therapist evaluates the patient and submits a report containing the results of the evaluation and the occupational therapy treatment plan for the patient. This report is placed in the patient's medical record.
c. The physician indicates in the patient's medical record, in some manner, that the treatment plan has been approved and treatment may proceed.

5. *Is a qualified occupational therapist or certified occupational therapy assistant (COTA) providing the services?*

If a COTA provides services, it must be under the general supervision of an occupational therapist (see p. B-3, line 7, of Medicare guidelines for definition of general supervision).

6. *Are the occupational therapy services reasonable and necessary for the treatment of the individual's illness or injury?*

Occupational therapy designed to improve function is considered *reasonable and necessary* for the treatment of the individual's illness or injury only where an expectation exists that the therapy will result in a significant *practical* improvement in the individual's level of functioning *within a reasonable period of time.*

In order to comply with the above definition, the occupational therapy notes must contain information indicating that treatment will improve the patient's function and a prognosis indicating when goals outlined will be achieved, e.g., (a) patient is a good rehabilitation candidate, and (b) daily occupational therapy treatment should result in the patient's independence in grooming and dressing within two weeks.

7. *Have you properly documented treatment in the medical record?*

Notes must indicate the need for continued treatment as well as the

*Reprinted from *Occupational Therapy Medicare Handbook.* Rockville, MD: American Occupational Therapy Association, Government and Legal Affairs Division, 1982, pp D-1–D-4.

need for *skilled* occupational therapy treatment. For example, documenting that activities of daily living (ADL) was done with a patient is insufficient. Documentation needs to indicate that the occupational therapist is teaching a patient compensatory techniques to improve the patient's level of independence.

Words such as *teach, plan, design* are acceptable words to use. Remember, Medicare does not pay for maintenance treatment. However, the services of an occupational therapist in *designing* a maintenance program and making infrequent but periodic evaluation of its effectiveness would be covered. The services of an occupational therapist or occupational therapy assistant in *carrying out* the maintenance program are not considered reasonable and necessary for the treatment of illness or injury, and such services are excluded from coverage.

8. *Does your treatment provided in occupational therapy sound like physical therapy?*

If your therapy documentation is very similar to the physical therapy documentation, the occupational therapy treatment may be denied because of duplication of services. Also if any traditional physical therapy modalities are documented in occupational therapy notes (e.g., hydrocollator, whirlpool or ultrasound), Medicare may not pay because these modalities are specifically mentioned in the physical therapy Medicare guidelines as physical therapy treatment.

9. *Have you overtreated the patient?*

Medicare will not always continue paying for treatment until the patient is totally recovered and/or independent. An example is their thoughts on reimbursement for ADL treatment:

> The Health Care Financing Administration interprets reimbursable ADL activities to be those which enable the patient to achieve a level of *semi-independence.* Clear examples of these types of activities are eating, dressing, and personal hygiene. Activities designed to reach a level of *total independence* are not considered reimbursable. A narrow distinction frequently separates the two types of activities. Borderline cases will require an individual assessment of all the factors involved in the situation.

If you have followed all the coverage criteria and your documentation is in order and payment continues to be denied, you need to contact your local Medicare intermediary and request its reasons for denying coverage. If the reasons have no relationship to fact, that is, to the Medicare law, regulations, or occupational therapy guidelines—for example, "We only pay for occupational therapy when the diagnosis involves the upper extremities," "We can only authorize ten occupational therapy visits with stroke patients," or "We only cover the materials for splints, not the therapist's time to fabricate splints"—then it is suggested that you bring the Occupational Therapy Medicare Guidelines and proof of your compliance to your Medicare intermediary.

If the intermediary fails to acknowledge your compliance with the law and the Medicare guidelines, contact the Government and Legal Affairs Division of the AOTA, 1383 Piccard Drive, Rockville, MD 20850, (301) 948-9626.

Appendix H: Procedural Safeguards Fact Sheet*

What guarantee of procedural safeguards including due process is there for handicapped children?

Public Law 94-142 requires any state, intermediate, or local education agency that wants to be eligible to receive federal funds for the education of handicapped children must provide procedures to assure that handicapped children and their parents or guardians are guaranteed procedural safeguards with respect to identification, evaluation, and educational placement or the provision of a free appropriate public education.

What are the procedural safeguards guaranteed to parents or guardians by Public Law 94-142?

Public Law 94-142 offers the following guarantees to parents and guardians:

- Written notification before evaluation. In addition, the right to an interpreter/translator if the family's native language is not English (unless it is clearly not feasible to do so).
- Written notification when initiating or refusing to initiate a change in educational placement.
- Opportunity to present complaints regarding the identification, evaluation, placement, or the provision of a free appropriate education.
- Opportunity to obtain an independent educational evaluation of the child.
- Access to all relevant records.
- Opportunity for an impartial due process hearing including the right to: (a) receive timely and specific notice of the hearing; (b) be accompanied and advised by counsel and/or individuals with special knowledge or training in the problems of handicapped children; (c) confront, cross examine, and compel the attendance of witnesses; and (d) present evidence, such as the written or electronic verbatim record of the hearing and written findings of fact and decisions.
- The right to appeal the findings and decision of the hearing.

Under what conditions can a surrogate parent be appointed for a child?

According to the law, assignment of a surrogate parent for children occurs when the child's parent or guardian is not known, the child's parents are unavailable, or the child is a ward of the state.

*Source: The ERIC Clearinghouse for Handicapped and Gifted Children, 1920 Association Drive, Reston, VA 22091.

What is the purpose of a surrogate parent?

The surrogate parent represents the child as a parent in all matters pertaining to the identification, evaluation, placement, and the provision of a free appropriate public education.

What situations could require the convening of an impartial due process hearing?

If a child is being considered for evaluation and permission is not granted by the parents, the education agency may request a hearing to present its reasons for wanting to conduct the evaluation.

If there is a disagreement about the recommended individual education program (including placement) or change in the program of a child, the parent or the local education agency may request a hearing.

If there is any complaint with respect to any matter relating to the identification, evaluation, or educational placement of a child or the provision of a free appropriate public education, such complaints may be reviewed at an impartial due process hearing.

What guarantee is there that the hearing will be impartial?

The law states that employees of local or state education agencies involved in the education or care of a specific child may not act as hearing officers for that case. The intent of this safeguard is to eliminate any bias that may be brought to the hearing by someone already involved in the matter.

What happens if one of the parties is not satisfied with the outcome of the local or intermediate education agency hearing?

An appeal may be made to the state education agency which shall conduct an impartial review of the hearing and render an independent decision. If the problem cannot be resolved to everyone's satisfaction by the review, either party has the right to bring civil action with respect to the complaint.

What happens to the child while proceedings are pending?

If the education agency and the parent agree on a temporary placement, the child will be placed. If an agreement cannot be reached then the child will remain in the same setting as before the action began.

If the case involves a child who is entering public school for the first time then the child shall be temporarily placed in a public school program, with the consent of the parent or guardian, until all proceedings have been completed.

Resources

A primer on due process—education decisions for handicapped children. Alan Abeson, Nancy Bolick, Jayne Hass. The Council for Exceptional Children, 1920 Association Drive, Reston, Virginia 22091 (Stock No. 104, $4.95).

A CEC training institute is available on due process. For additional information write CEC, Conventions Unit or call our toll free number (800) 336-3728. Virginia residents, please call collect (703) 620-3660.

*Appendix I: Standards of Practice for Occupational Therapy**

PREFACE

These standards will assist the AOTA members in the management of occupational therapy services and will serve as a minimum standard for occupational therapy practice that is applicable to all client populations and the programs in which clients are served.

These standards are for qualified occupational therapists (OTRs) that are currently certified or licensed where required by the state.

STANDARD I: SCREENING

1. Occupational therapists have the responsibility to identify clients who may present problems in occupational performance (work, self-care, and play/leisure) that would require an evaluation.
2. Occupational therapists screen independently or as members of a team.
3. Screening methods shall be appropriate to the client's age, education, cultural background, medical status, and functional ability.
4. Screening methods may include interview, observation, testing and record review.
5. Occupational therapists shall communicate the screening results and recommendations to all appropriate individuals.

STANDARD II: REFERRAL

1. A client is appropriately referred to occupational therapy for remediation, maintenance, or prevention when the client has, or appears to have, a dysfunction or potential for dysfunction in occupational performance (work, self-care, play/leisure) or the performance components (sensorimotor, cognitive, psychosocial).
2. Clients shall be referred to occupational therapy for evaluation, design construction of, or training in therapeutic adaptations that include, but are not limited to, the physical environment, orthotics, prosthetics, and assistive and adaptive equipment.
3. Occupational therapists respond to a request for service and enter a case at their own professional discretion and on their own cogni-

* Adopted April 1983 by the Representative Assembly, The American Occupational Therapy Association, Inc.

zance, and then assume full responsibility for the determination of the appropriate type, nature, and mode of service.

4. When physician referral is necessary to meet regulations (facility, state, federal, Joint Commission for Accreditation of Hospitals, licensure) or is required for third-party payment, the registered occupational therapist enters a case at the request of a physician; assumes full responsibility for the occupational therapy assessment; and, in consultation with the physician, establishes the appropriate type, nature, and mode of service.
5. Registered occupational therapists shall refer clients to other appropriate resources when, in the judgment of the occupational therapist, the knowledge and expertise of another professional is required.
6. Occupational therapists have the responsibility to teach appropriate persons how to make occupational therapy referrals.

STANDARD III: EVALUATION

1. Occupational therapists shall evaluate the client's performance according to the Uniform Occupational Therapy Checklist (AOTA-Adopted, 1981).
2. Initial occupational therapy evaluations shall consider the client's medical, vocational, educational, activity, social history, and personal/family goals.
3. The occupational therapy evaluation shall include assessment of the functional abilities and deficits as related to the client's needs in the following areas:
   a. Occupational Performance: work, self-care, and play/leisure.
   b. Performance Components: sensorimotor, cognitive, psychosocial.
   c. Therapeutic adaptations and prevention.
4. Initial occupational therapy evaluations shall be completed and results documented within the time frames established by facilities, government agencies, and accreditation programs.
5. All evaluation methods shall be appropriate to the client's age, education, cultural and ethnic background, medical status, and functional ability.
6. The evaluation methods may include observation, interview, record review, and the use of evaluation techniques or tools.
7. When standardized evaluation tools are used, the tests should have normative data for the client characteristics. If normative data are not available, the results should be expressed in a descriptive report.
8. Collected evaluation data shall be analyzed and summarized to indicate the client's current status.
9. Occupational therapists shall document evaluation results in the client's record and indicate the specific evaluation tools and methods used.
10. Occupational therapists shall communicate evaluation results to the appropriate persons in the facility and community.
11. If the results of the evaluation indicate areas that require intervention by other professionals, the occupational therapist should refer the client to the appropriate service or request consultation.

STANDARD IV: INDIVIDUAL PROGRAM PLANNING

1. Occupational therapists shall use the results of the evaluation to develop an individual occupational therapy program that is:
   a. Stated in measurable and reasonable terms appropriate to the client's needs and goals and expected prognosis.
   b. Consistent with current principles and concepts of occupational therapy theory and practice.
2. The planning process shall include:
   a. Identifying short- and long-term goals.
   b. Collaborating with client, family, other professionals, and community resources.
   c. Selecting the media, methods, environment, and personnel needed to accomplish goals.
   d. Determining the frequency and duration of occupational therapy services.
3. The initial program plan shall be prepared and documented within the time frames established by facilities; government agencies, and accreditation programs.

STANDARD V: INDIVIDUAL PROGRAM IMPLEMENTATION

1. Occupational therapists shall implement the program according to the program plan.
2. Occupational therapists shall formulate and implement program modifications consistent with changes in the client's occupational performance and performance components.
3. Occupational therapists shall periodically re-evaluate and document the client's occupational performance and performance components.
4. Occupational therapists shall document the occupational therapy services provided and the frequency of the services within time frames established by facilities, government agencies, and accreditation programs.

STANDARD VI: DISCONTINUATION OF SERVICES

1. Occupational therapists shall discontinue services when the client has achieved the goals or has achieved maximum benefit from occupational therapy.
2. Occupational therapists shall document the comparison of the initial and current state of functional abilities and deficits in occupational performance and performance components.
3. Occupational therapists shall prepare a discharge plan that is consistent with the occupational therapy, client, interdisciplinary team, family and goals, and the expected prognosis. Consideration should be given to appropriate community resources for referral and environmental factors or barriers that may need modification.
4. Occupational therapists shall allow sufficient time for the coordination of and the effective implementation of the discharge plan.
5. Occupational therapists shall document recommendations for follow-up or re-evaluation.

STANDARD VII: QUALITY ASSURANCE

1. The occupational therapist shall periodically and systematically review all aspects of individual occupational therapy programs for effectiveness and efficiency.
2. Occupational therapists shall periodically and systematically review the quality and appropriateness of total services delivered, using predetermined criteria that reflect professional consensus and recent development in research and theory.

STANDARD VIII: INDIRECT SERVICES

1. Occupational therapists shall provide supervision of other personnel as assigned in accordance with the AOTA *Guide for Supervision* (AOTA-Adopted, 1981).
2. Occupational therapists shall maintain records to meet facility, government agency, and accreditation program requirements.
3. Occupational therapists shall maintain a level of professional knowledge and skills to assure continued competency.
4. Occupational therapists shall facilitate research as it applies to the active practice of occupational therapy.
5. Occupational therapists shall provide administration and management services that ensure the use of AOTA standards.
6. Occupational therapists shall provide consultation services in order to develop or coordinate occupational therapy services, provide inservice education, adapt environments, and promote preventive health care in the home, client care facility, or community.

STANDARD IX: LEGAL/ETHICAL COMPONENTS

1. Occupational therapists shall maintain current AOTA certification or licensure where required by the state.
2. Occupational therapists shall practice and manage occupational therapy programs as defined by federal and state laws and regulations.
3. Occupational therapists shall be familiar with and abide by the ethical practices of the specific facility or system in which the service is provided.
4. Occupational therapists shall observe the ethical practices as defined by The American Occupational Therapy Association, Inc., *Principles of Ethics* (AOTA, Revised 1980).
5. Occupational therapists shall provide all aspects of direct and indirect services according to Standards and Policies of The American Occupational Therapy Association, Inc.

GLOSSARY*

Occupational Therapy Assessment—the process of determining the need for, nature of, and estimated time of treatment, determining the needed coordination with other persons involved, and documenting these activities.

* Uniform Terminology for Reporting Occupational Therapy Services, adopted March 1979 by The Representative Assembly, AOTA.

Evaluation—the process of obtaining and interpreting data necessary for treatment. This includes planning for and documenting the evaluation process and results. These data may be gathered through record review, specific observation, interview, and the administration of data collection procedures. Such procedures include, but are not limited to, the use of standardized tests, performance checklists, and activities and tasks designed to evaluate specific performance abilities.

Maintenance of Function—the process of preserving and supporting an individual's current abilities to engage in interpersonal relationships and to manipulate the nonhuman environment.

Occupational Performance—life tasks (self-care, work, play/leisure) that are all those activities that individuals must perform to meet their own needs and to be contributing members of the community.

Performance Components—the skill areas (sensorimotor, cognitive, psychosocial) a person develops to facilitate carrying out self-care, work and play/leisure.

Program Planning—the development of an individual client's treatment plan.

Screening—the review of the potential client's case to determine the need for evaluation and treatment.

Therapeutic Adaptations—the design and restructuring of the physical environment to assist self-care, work, and play/leisure performance. This includes selecting, obtaining, fitting, and fabricating equipment, and instructing the client, family, and staff in proper use and care of equipment. It also includes minor repair and modification for correct fit, position, or use. Categories of therapeutic adaptations consist of: orthotics, prosthetics, and assistive and adaptive equipment.

Index